Cognitive Behavior Therapy for Persistent Somatic Symptoms and Somatic Symptom Disorder

Cognitive Behavior Therapy for Persistent Somatic Symptoms and Somatic Symptom Disorder

Maria Kleinstäuber • Petra Thomas • Michael Witthöft
Wolfgang Hiller

Cognitive Behavior Therapy for Persistent Somatic Symptoms and Somatic Symptom Disorder

Springer

Maria Kleinstäuber
Department of Psychology
Emma Eccles Jones College of Education
and Human Services, Utah State University
Logan, UT, United States

Michael Witthöft
Forschungs- und Behandlungszentrum für
psychische Gesundheit (FBZ), Klinische
Psychologie und Psychotherapie
Ruhr-Universität Bochum
Bochum, Germany

Petra Thomas
Reha Rheinfelden
Rheinfelden, Switzerland

Wolfgang Hiller
Psychologisches Institut, Abteilung für
Klinische Psychologie und Psychotherapie
Johannes-Gutenberg-Universität Mainz
Mainz, Germany

ISBN 978-3-662-69725-2 ISBN 978-3-662-69726-9 (eBook)
https://doi.org/10.1007/978-3-662-69726-9

This book is a translation of the original German edition "Kognitive Verhaltenstherapie bei medizinisch unerklärten Körperbeschwerden und somatoformen Störungen," 2nd edition, by Maria Kleinstäuber et al., published by Springer-Verlag GmbH, DE in 2018. The translation was done with the help of an artificial intelligence machine translation tool. A subsequent human revision was done primarily in terms of content, so that the book will read stylistically differently from a conventional translation. Springer Nature works continuously to further the development of tools for the production of books and on the related technologies to support the authors.

Translation from the German language edition: "Kognitive Verhaltenstherapie bei medizinisch unerklärten Körperbeschwerden und somatoformen Störungen" by Maria Kleinstäuber et al., © Springer-Verlag GmbH Deutschland 2018. Published by Springer Berlin Heidelberg. All Rights Reserved.

This Springer imprint is published by the registered company Springer-Verlag GmbH, DE, part of Springer Nature.
The registered company address is: Heidelberger Platz 3, 14197 Berlin, Germany

For Annelies and Dr. Gerd Kleinstäuber
(M. K.)

Foreword

Somatic Symptom Disorders have been rather a "stepchild" in the field of psychotherapy research. If one considers the high number of therapy studies in the field of depression or anxiety disorders, it is surprising how little comparable research is available in the field of somatic symptom disorders. This is all the more alarming since somatic symptom disorders are at least as common as depression and anxiety disorders and, especially in Germany, many people with such disorders even receive inpatient treatment due to the large network of psychosomatic clinics. But also in the outpatient setting there is a high need for treatment in order to avoid that affected persons helplessly switch from one specialist to the next, from traditional medicine to alternative methods and back or to other promises of cure.

Against this background, it is particularly gratifying that a German treatment manual for a psychologically based, empirically validated intervention is finally being presented. While treatment guidelines have been increasingly developed in the past, a detailed treatment manual that describes steps of the therapeutic procedure offers working materials, and is all based on a good empirical foundation has been missing until recently. In addition, this book contains a great deal of background information that is necessary for a better understanding of the disease as well as for adequate treatment. The treatment guide provides the reader with numerous intervention options to motivate patients for a psychotherapeutic approach. Patients with somatic symptom disorders are provided with easily understood and readily accepted information and accompanying behavioral experiments that illustrate the complex interconnectedness of physical well-being and psychological processes. Thus the problem, which sometimes seemed unmanageable in the past, suddenly gets a solution: How do I win these patients for psychotherapy?

The group of authors is well qualified to create such a treatment manual: Their experience is not only based on years of practical work in this field, but under the same first authorship, a highly regarded meta-analysis on the treatment of somatic symptom disorders was also prepared and published. Thus, the present manual incorporates not only a great deal of practical experience, but also theoretical knowledge about many other treatment attempts in this field.

Against this background, the book is to be wished above all that it may receive the success to which it is entitled. For the practicing clinical psychologist, it represents a crucial aid in carrying out well-acceptable and successful treatment steps with this group of patients, who are often perceived as difficult. However, manualization also opens up new avenues for the psychotherapy researcher: Here is the treatment path by which others must be measured, and new and further therapeutic developments must also be measured against the manual of Kleinstäuber et al. This is the new standard of treatment for persons with somatic symptom disorders.

I therefore wish the book a wide circulation, also on behalf of the many patients who can benefit from it.

Winfried Rief
Marburg, Germany
September 2011

Preface

One must not tie the ship to a single anchor, nor life to a single hope. (Epictetus, Greek philosopher, 50–138 AD)

Epidemiological studies show that persistent somatic symptoms examined in German primary care practices cannot be explained medically in the vast majority of cases. Many years often pass before those affected receive adequate treatment, which also includes psychotherapeutic measures. During this time, many patients go through lengthy—sometimes unnecessary, sometimes even contraindicated—diagnostic procedures and treatments. In the process, they are in danger of tying their lives to a single hope—namely, the hope of finally addressing the cause and curing their ailments. Unfortunately, this hope is all too often disappointed and leads to frustration, despair and resignation.

International research shows that cognitive behavior therapy is very promising for this clinical group. It gives patients a new perspective on their symptoms. Instead of leaning back and passively hoping for a "cure-all", they are encouraged and guided to actively deal with their symptoms and related problems. The aim is to become active oneself and learn to achieve a higher level of well-being again despite the symptoms. The aim is to develop a new hope alongside the primary hope of a cure—for example, to maintain a good quality of life despite symptoms. Over the past two decades, cognitive behavior therapy has developed many fruitful approaches to understanding and treating persistent somatic symptoms. Scientific research confirms the effectiveness of these treatment approaches. However, despite these promising findings, no published therapy manual for cognitive behavior therapy of persistent somatic symptoms has yet been available in the German-speaking world. Therefore, with this book we combine the concern to make our experiences as well as the experiences of other working groups accessible to the practitioner.

In order to meet the goal of making this treatment program practical, we provide the reader with a variety of worksheets, practical exercises and associated instructional texts, as well as question examples for designing the therapy session. This is embedded in an overview of current epidemiological, etiological as well as diagnostic background information on persistent somatic symptoms. This book is therefore not exclusively a therapeutic aid for psychologists, but is also aimed at physicians in both outpatient and inpatient treatment settings who work with patients with multiple somatic symptoms.

As the Mongolian proverb "You can't tie a knot with one hand" aptly expresses, this book was not written alone, but is the product of a fruitful and enriching collaboration between the four authors. We would like to express our special thanks to Prof. Dr. Winfried Rief and Dr. Gaby Bleichhardt from the University of Marburg for their many-sided suggestions and expert support. In addition, we would like to thank in particular Dipl.-Psych. Carina Grama, Dipl.-Psych. Ann Christin Krämer, and Dr. Fabian Jasper, without whose cooperation the elaborate effectiveness evaluation of this treatment program would not have been feasible. We would like to express our special thanks to the patients who, due to their symptoms, visited our treatment focus "Somatic Symptom Disorders" of the Outpatient Clinic for Psychotherapy of the Johannes Gutenberg University Mainz, placed their trust in us and provided us with an enormous amount of support by filling out many questionnaires.

Although the topic of persistent somatic symptom is gaining more importance in the clinical context, the proportion of patients with these symptoms who do not receive adequate psychotherapeutic treatment remains enormously high. This is also due to the fact that too few clinical psychologists as well as physicians who work in the field of behavioral medicine and psychosomatics have sufficient knowledge about this disturbance pattern or about the treatment strategies for dealing with this particular group of disorders. We hope that with this manual we can provide our psychological as well as medical colleagues with a manual containing many practical tips and working materials as well as a therapeutic approach that is based on the current state of research. We would like to stimulate your interest in the treatment of a group of patients who have so far been severely neglected in psychotherapy, and to show you possibilities of how to carry out a therapy which is beneficial for the patient as well as for the therapist and physician who work with patients who are unfortunately still classified as "difficult to deal with".

Maria Kleinstäuber
Petra Thomas
Michael Witthöft
Wolfgang Hiller
Mainz, Germany
Spring 2017

Contents

Contributors

Wolfgang Hiller Psychologisches Institut, Abteilung für Klinische Psychologie und Psychotherapie, Johannes-Gutenberg-Universität Mainz, Mainz, Germany

Maria Kleinstäuber Department of Psychology, Emma Eccles Jones College of Education and Human Services, Utah State University, Logan, UT, United States

Petra Thomas Reha Rheinfelden, Rheinfelden, Switzerland

Michael Witthöft Forschungs- und Behandlungszentrum für psychische Gesundheit (FBZ), Klinische Psychologie und Psychotherapie, Ruhr-Universität Bochum, Bochum, Germany

Theory

Contents

Persistent Somatic Symptoms, Somatoform Disorders, and Somatic Symptom Disorders

Contents

M. Kleinstäuber et al., *Cognitive Behavior Therapy for Persistent Somatic Symptoms and Somatic Symptom Disorder*, https://doi.org/10.1007/978-3-662-69726-9_1

1.1 Phenomenology

Patients with persistent somatic symptoms have somatic symptoms which are associated with emotional distress and other psychological symptoms and which are more or less sufficiently explained by a medical cause. This introductory chapter provides a deeper insight into the appearance, diagnosis and epidemiology of persistent somatic symptoms. To start with, two case studies will give an impression of how heterogeneous the therapeutic starting position can be for patients with persistent somatic symptoms.

1.1.1 The Despair of Ms. O.

Ms. O. feels on the verge of a nervous breakdown. With high expectations she makes her first appointment with a psychotherapist today. This was recommended to her by her primary care physician. Up to now Ms. O. had no contact with psychiatry and psychotherapy.

When Ms. O. is asked to describe her symptoms during the first consultation, she blurts out: "First of all, I would like to emphasize that I do NOT have a psychological problem! I have had back pain for a long time, and the back has very little to do with the psyche. Well, and besides my back, there is my vegetative nervous system, which is totally crazy. I don't really like the fact that my family doctor has now referred me to you. I feel a bit pushed aside and not taken seriously. Of course all these physical symptoms get to the substance with time and also drain my mental strength, but believe me, if my body would function normally, then I would be the happiest person in this world. I don't know how you as a psychologist are going to help me in this matter now, but in times of need, as we all know, you grasp at any straw that appears in front of you."

Ms. O. is 43 years old, divorced, but in a relationship and mother of an 11-year-old daughter from a previous relationship. She is self-employed as a physiotherapist. Currently with a workload of 60%. She simply cannot manage more, although she is actually dependent on the money.

She complains of "hellish back pain" which first appeared 3 years ago. Since last summer, she has been permanently plagued, i.e. daily, by this pain, which also radiates to other parts of her body (neck, upper arms and hips). "You can't even imagine what it's like! I'm really at the end of my rope."

Ms. O. describes the following additional symptoms: "I sweat like crazy and don't know why. My hands and feet are often freezing cold. I also get exhausted very quickly. I often feel like lead after the slightest exertion. I also don't sleep well anymore. Again and again I wake up because of the pain and then I can't fall asleep anymore. Accordingly, I feel as if I am exhausted in the morning. No, this is really no life anymore. When I imagine that this is going to go on for the next 40 years, well, good night!"

When asked what she had done so far to have her symptoms clarified and treated, Ms. O. replied as follows: "Too much! I just don't understand it. No doctor can tell me what I have. This can't be true! In the last 3 years I must have been to at least 20 different so-called experts, but I have the feeling that everyone is overwhelmed with me and passes me on to the next specialist like a buck. As I said, no one takes me seriously and they just pass the buck. I've slowly lost faith in medicine. And, as for my family doctor, I'm disappointed in him beyond measure. You know, he made it pretty easy for himself. He passed me on to you and gave me some psych pill that's supposed to make the pain go away. So, what happened? I took this pill for 3 weeks as recommended, but then I stopped because of the strong side effects. You see, I wasn't myself anymore. I was like a zombie, wandering around. That can't be the point. No, no, I'd rather deal with the pain than be in a daze. Apart from swallowing pills for the rest of my life, that can't be the solution to my problem either."

When asked about psychosocial stress, Ms. O. reacts dismissively, almost indignantly. With her arms folded and her volume turned up, she takes the floor: "Now please don't try to analyze me! My childhood was happy and I have nothing to work up. I am not traumatized or otherwise disturbed. I have a wonderful child and a partner who is there for me.—Believe me, I have my life under control, apart from the usual problems that everyone carries around with them, and this damn pain. I was hoping you could tell me where they come from, but I'm afraid this is going in the wrong direction."

The first meeting ended soberingly and openly about further contact. Ms. O. had to think twice about whether this would be of any use to her, because "talking alone like this is the wrong approach". Whatever her decision, she would get in touch by phone within the next week.

The therapist notes: "provisional diagnosis according to the tenth revision of the International Classification of Diseases (ICD-10): undifferentiated somatoform disorder (F45.1)".

1.1.2 The Sufferings of Mr. Z.

Mr. Z. is 54 years old, married for the second time and has two (as he says) "adorable" daughters aged 15 and 17. He is a successful businessman in a leading position in a small company (branch: food industry). His job means a lot to him and demands a lot of commitment.

He often works more than 60 h a week, is on the road a lot, sometimes even on weekends. He is glad that his family fully understands his situation and supports him where they can. Of course, he finds it sad that he doesn't get to see certain things in his family's everyday life and that he doesn't get to spend much time with his children. "But I guess that is the price I have to pay." Mr. Z says he is very physically active and enjoys playing badminton. He has been doing this for over 30 years and is a member of a club. So far he has always enjoyed good health: "I have never seen a hospital from the inside. Oh yes, as a visitor of course, but never as a patient."

A little more than 6 months ago, his health suddenly changed. "Out of nowhere" various gastro-intestinal symptoms had appeared: "Such a strange pulling. Sometimes just a massive feeling of pressure." After the symptoms had still not disappeared after 2 weeks, Mr. Z. consulted his primary care physician. He recommended to him seeing a gastroenterologist, which Mr. Z. did. The result of the examination was: "without pathological findings". Food intolerances were also ruled out as the cause of the symptoms. On the one hand, Mr. Z. was reassured, but on the other hand, the findings left him somewhat perplexed. "Well, and now? The symptoms are there after all. What should I do about it?" The family doctor in turn recommended Mr. Z. to ensure more relaxation in his everyday life and to pay attention to his "work-life balance". Mr. Z. could do little with this advice, but finally followed his wife's advice and tried a number of natural remedies. However, Mr. Z. did not change anything in his lifestyle. "Stress at work—that's just part of it. There's nothing I can do about it except make sacrifices." After a few weeks, the symptoms did indeed improve, so that Mr. Z. believed he was free of his suffering.

But now suddenly other, "very special and strange symptoms in his chest" appeared. He had never suffered a heart attack in his life and there had never been any "heart patients" in his family, but he was still massively unsettled every time by the sensations and wondered whether his heart could be damaged. Mr. Z. reported that he had always had to struggle with massive palpitations and feelings of tension in his chest in stressful situations. Because of his concerns about the health of his heart, he has seen several heart specialists, had various ECGs and other far more expensive tests, but each time he has been told, "Mr. Z, your heart is perfectly fine. Don't worry." Only in the short term could such statements reassure him. Doubts often arose as soon as he left the doctor's office.

Mr. Z. feels helpless again. He has temporarily stopped playing badminton "to avoid too much stress on my heart. It's exciting enough at work at the moment." In a bookshop, he stops briefly in front of a shelf of advice books from the field of psychology. His eyes roam over the offerings. The buzzwords "stress," "happiness," and "work-life balance" catch his interest for a moment. "Maybe I'll call that psychologist after all," Mr. Z. thinks to himself and rushes off to his next business appointment.

1.2 The Concept of "Somatization": Past—Present—Future

A wide variety of somatic symptom without a clear medical cause, as described in the two preceding case studies, form the core of the concept of somatoform disorders. This disorder concept is represented in the international classification system ICD-10. It was part of the former DSM-IV system (Diagnostic and Statistical Manual of Mental Disorders, DSM), but was abandoned there in 2013 during the transition to the DSM-5 system in favor of the more inclusive approach of "somatic symptom and related disorders." Somatic symptom and related disorders continue to include the disorders formerly referred to as somatoform, but also can include persistent somatic symptoms that can be medically explained, that are however associated with psychological distress (e.g., in myocardial infarction or diabetes mellitus). Thus, the concept of somatic symptom disorder according to DSM-5 no longer differentiates between symptoms with and without a somatic medical cause.

The different approaches make it clear that there is still no conclusive agreement on the nosological status of medically unclear physical symptoms. Criticism has been levelled at the concept of **"somatization"** or **"somatoform disorder"**, among other things. In the field of pain research in particular, the often unclear conceptualization of the phenomenon of somatization has been criticized, and the use of this term has been discouraged in favor of a more neutral term (e.g., somatic symptoms of unclear or medically unexplained etiology) (e.g., Crombez et al., 2009). Overall, many therapists and physicians fear that the term "somatization" or "somatoform" could be experienced by patients as stigmatizing and falsely associated with "imagination" or "simulation". In our view, this ambivalence towards the term "somatization" is primarily due to a confusion between the historical concept of somatization (in the sense of a psychodynamic conversion process) and the current conceptualization of somatoform disorders as an etiology-free and operational definition of somatic symptoms of unclear etiology (▶ Sect. 1.3.1). In order to better understand this development, we will briefly explain the historical basis of the term "somatization" or "somatoform" and its current use.

1.2.1 Past: History of the Term "Somatization"

The phenomenon of "medically unexplained symptoms" is by no means a phenomenon of modern times or Western industrialization (Eriksen et al., 2004), but is in all probability as old as humanity or medical doctrine itself. Morschitzky (2007), for example, outlines that descriptions of perceptual disorders and various inexplicable pain conditions, which we would call "somatoform" from today's perspective, can already be found in ancient Egyptian records.

In his article on the history of somatoform disorders, Kapfhammer (2001) points out that the term "somatization" was first used by Stekel (1908) and, from a psychodynamic perspective, meant the expression of mental conflicts at the organic level. However, Marin and Carron (2002) state that the term "somatization" is the product of an inaccurate translation of Stekel's book into English (by J. van Teslaar). Originally, Stekel himself used the term "organ language" to describe a conversion-like process of transforming strong emotions and psychological conflicts into bodily symptoms. Stekel himself did not explicitly use the term "somatization" until 1935 (Stekel, 1935, cited in Marin & Carron, 2002).

Hysteria (from Greek "**hystera**": uterus) is considered the most important and oldest precursor concept of somatoform disorders. As early as ancient Greece and Rome, "medically unexplained symptoms" were associated with abnormalities in the area of the uterus (e.g., dehydration due to lack of sexual activity or wandering of the uterus in the body) (Morschitzky, 2007). Inevitably, hysteria as a disorder was seen at this time as a purely female problem—a view that was not changed until later in the mid-nineteenth century by Briquet, Charcot and Janet's view of hysteria as a primary disease of the brain. In the Middle Ages, "hysterical complaints" were fatally associated with devil's work and the work of evil. Exorcisms and witch burnings resulted from this view (Morschitzky, 2007).

The decisive precursor concept of today's somatoform disorders (or somatization disorder in the narrower sense) was presented in the mid-nineteenth century by the French psychiatrist Pierre Briquet as the "**Briquet syndrome**" (Briquet, 1895). As Kapfhammer (2007) shows, Briquet's account is a remarkably modern multifactorial conceptualization of the contemporary phenomenon of somatization disorder, in which emotional influences, family experiences, and psychosocial stressors were already named as relevant influencing factors in the style of contemporary diathesis-stress models.

While Briquet was primarily concerned with the polysymptomatic variant of somatoform symptoms, at about the same time the French neurologist Jean-Martin Charcot and later his student Pierre Janet were primarily concerned with monosymptomatic, "pseudoneurological" (i.e. functional neurological) symptoms, which later found their way into the classification systems as "**conversion disorder**" and "**functional neurological disorder**". What was revolutionary here was the realization that the loss of certain physical functions (e.g., vision, hearing, or voluntary motor actions) is related to strong emotional states (e.g., as a result of trauma) and can also be actively induced under hypnosis (Kapfhammer, 2001). Janet coined the term "**dissociation**" in this context, which describes a disintegration of mental processes and contents such as experience, action or memory. The psychoanalytic concepts of Breuer and Freud on hysteria and conversion developed under the influence of the concepts of Charcot and Janet. However, Breuer and Freud's (1893) theorizing on conversion later focused less on the characteristics of external trauma and more on the individual's own interpretation of the experience in terms of aversiveness and threateningness and the degree of internal conflict subjectively experienced as a result. According to this approach, conversion symptoms serve to compromise a conflict between drives and psychological defensive reactions (Kapfhammer, 2001). Drive conflicts that can be traced back to traumatic experiences in biographically early life phases are initially successfully repressed in later life phases and can be updated again through analogous conflicts. Renewed repression can lead to "somatization", which means that the conflicts are felt "symbolically" in somatic symptoms. An exhaustive and appealing account of the history of somatoform disorders can be found in Morschitzky (2007).

In the presentation of R. J. Brown (2004), to which we will return below in the context of his cognitive-psychological model of somatoform symptoms (► Sect. 2.3), the two concepts of **dissociation** and **conversion** also form the two most important historical explanations of the current concept of somatization. It seems essential here that Janet (Janet, 1889, cited in Brown et al., 1990; Brown 2004) already conceptualized the disorder of hysteria as a consequence of a direct disturbance of the attentional system due to the experience of a traumatic event. Hypnosis and suggestion, according to Janet, represented effective interventions to modify the dysfunctions within the attentional system. Interestingly, even today, alterations in the attentional and working memory processes are considered central to explaining somatoform symptoms (corresponding current models are presented in ► Chap. 2).

One of the first "modern" approaches to operationally define somatization was by Bridges and Goldberg (1985). However, the authors define "somatization" as a concomitant of a primary mental disorder. Thus, Bridges and Goldberg (1985) list four necessary criteria for a diagnosis of somatization:

- a physician utilization pattern,
- a somatic attribution style of symptoms,
- the presence of a psychiatric illness and
- a response of the somatic symptoms to the treatment of the primary mental illness.

The much-cited work of Lipowski (1988), which already contains a multidimensional view of somatization and mentions perceptual (symptom experience), cognitive (primary somatic cause attribution) and, in particular, behavioral features (seeking medical help), had a decisive influence on today's view of somatization or on the conceptualizations of somatoform disorders. Thus Lipowski describes somatization as

> ... the tendency to experience and communicate physical distress and symptoms that cannot be explained by a pathological finding, to attribute them to an organic disease, and to seek medical help for them. (Lipowski, 1988)

1.2.2 Present: Current Diagnostic Concepts

Somatoform disorders are defined in the International Classification of Diseases ICD-10 (Dilling & Freyberger, 2000; World Health Organization, 1992) in largely etiology-free terms. In particular, there are no etiological inclusion criteria. For example, no psychological or psychosocial etiological factors need to be demonstrated for the diagnosis to be made. It is sufficient that physical symptoms of unexplained cause are present in the patient in question. However, because the concept of somatization originated in the psychodynamic tradition and is closely associated with a postulated conversion process, there is a discrepancy between the current etiology-neutral definition on the one hand and the broader conceptual meaning of "somatization" on the other (as in the diagnosis of somatization disorder, for example). This discrepancy is one of the main reasons for the growing resentment towards the term somatization. The generic term **somatoform disorders**, which expresses that there is not an actual somatic illness, but that the symptomatology only represents the "form" of such an illness, proves to be much more neutral in this context. In the ICD-10, somatoform disorders form a comparatively heterogeneous group of different disorders, ranging from the prototypical full-blown polysymptomatic somatoform disorder (based on Briquet's syndrome) with multiple symptoms and various organ systems affected (somatization disorder) to monosymptomatic variants (e.g., persistent somatoform pain disorder) and hypochondriasis (► Sect. 1.3.1).

The full picture of somatization disorder is formulated relatively restrictively by its diagnostic criteria, so that only a few of the patients affected by unsufficiently explained somatic symptoms receive this diagnosis. Therefore, complementary diagnostic concepts have been developed in research to which larger patient groups can be assigned. Probably the best known concept in this respect is the "**Somatic Symptom Index (SSI) 4/6**" by Escobar et al. (1989). According to the SSI-4/6, a somatoform disorder is present if 4 (in men) or 6 symptoms (in women) are reported. A similar concept as an alternative to the diagnosis of undifferentiated somatoform disorder was formulated by Kroenke et al. (1997) in the presence of at least 3 symptoms under the name "**multisomatoform disorder**". Within the German version of the "Patient Health Questionnaire" (PHQ-D; Kroenke et al., 2002), a "**somatoform syndrome**" is spoken of if a total of 3 out of 13 somatic symptoms are reported as strongly impairing during the last 4 weeks (Löwe et al., 2002). In the field of hypochondriasis, a less restrictive concept was presented by Fink et al. (2004).

An attempt to differentiate between different types of somatization in terms of content was made by Kirmayer and Robbins (1991), who propose a distinction between "hypochondriacal somatization", "presenting somatization" and "functional somatization". "Functional somatization" means the occurrence of somatic symptom that cannot currently be fully explained medically and that cannot be better explained by another primary mental disorder (e.g. a panic disorder) ("presenting somatization") and which, in contrast to hypochondriasis, do not merely represent the increased perception of normal bodily sensations (e.g. one's own heartbeat) ("hypochondriacal somatization").

Another distinction made by Rief and Hiller (1999) relates to the separation of mono- vs. polysymptomatic somatoform disorders. As an example of a **monosymptomatic somatoform disorder**, the irritable bowel syndrome (or a corresponding somatoform autonomic dysfunction according to the ICD-10) can be cited, in which the symptoms are primarily related to the gastrointestinal tract. Irritable bowel syndrome is often also referred to as a "functional somatic syndrome". Other examples of such **functional somatic syndromes** focus on a particular symptom or organ system include chronic fatigue syndrome, fibromyalgia, premenstrual syndrome, idiopathic environmental intolerance (formerly called multiple chemical sensitivity), and noncardiac chest pain (for a review of functional somatic syndromes, see Wessely et al., 1999). We will return to specific features of the functional somatic syndromes in later chapters of this book, focusing on treatment (► Sect. 4.1.2). In **polysymptomatic somatoform disorders**, on the other hand, at least two different organ systems or body regions are affected. The prototype of a polysymptomatic somatoform disorder is somatization disorder according to ICD-10.

Various terms currently coexist to describe individual somatoform symptoms. Some authors vehemently advocate the term "complaint" as opposed to "symptom" in order to emphasize the subjective character of the phenomenon (as opposed to a disease symptom, for which physiological evidence exists). The term "medically unexplained [physical] symptoms" (MU[P]S) has become internationally accepted over decades. With the introduction of the DSM-5 however, the differentiation between medically explained and medically unexplained symptoms was abolished. Terminology that focuses on this differentiation has been replaced by more descriptive terms such as "persistent somatic symptoms" which will be also adopted as a central term in this book.

Since hypochondriasis is currently also considered to be part of somatoform disorders, we will sometimes refer to "symptom-related" somatoform disorders within the manual in order to make it clear that the respective statements refer to mono- and polysymptomatic disorders, but not to hypochondriasis.

1.2.3 The Disappearance of Somatoform Disorders as a Separate Category in the DSM-5

As already mentioned, the DSM-5 (American Psychiatric Association, 2013; Falkai et al., 2015) has abandoned the terms "somatoform" and "somatization" and integrated the related disorders into a comprehensive chapter called "somatic symptom and related disorders". Comprehensive means that in addition to medically unexplained symptoms, medically explained symptoms are also taken into account, i.e. there is no longer any distinction between these two forms of occurrence.

The diagnoses somatization disorder, undifferentiated somatoform disorder and persistent somatoform pain disorder were abolished. The DSM-5 now assigns all of these disorders to "somatic symptom disorder". Therefore, this new diagnosis encompasses a conglomerate of very different clinical manifestations. The only prerequisite is the presence of at least one somatic symptom that is experienced as stressful or leads to significant impairment of everyday life. Furthermore, at least one of three listed psychological symptoms is required for the diagnosis:

- exaggerated and persistent thoughts about the seriousness of the symptoms,
- persistently high level of anxiety related to health or symptoms,
- excessive time and energy spent on symptoms or health concerns.

The symptom burden must also have persisted for at least 6 months. If pain symptoms are in the foreground, this can be highlighted as an additional specification of the diagnosis.

In addition to the core category of somatic symptom disorder, the new DSM-5 chapter lists the following additional diagnoses: Functional Neurological Symptom Disorder (Conversion Disorder), the diagnosis of Psychological Factors Affecting Other Medical Conditions, Factitious Disorder (with falsified or self-induced physical or psychological symptoms), and the obligatory residual categories of Other Specified or Unspecified Somatic Symptom and Related Disorder. Some patients previously diagnosed with hypochondriasis may be assigned to the new category of "Illness Anxiety Disorder." However, this diagnosis may only be made if the illness anxiety is accompanied by physical symptoms of at most low intensity. If the somatic symptoms are more severe, the diagnosis should be somatic symptom disorder rather than illness anxiety disorder. Here it becomes clear once again that somatic symptom disorder is by no means a homogeneous group of disorders, but rather a kind of "potpourri" for highly diverse manifestations and courses of symptoms.

The new DSM-5 chapter on somatic symptom and related disorder has been criticized in many respects (Rief & Martin, 2014; Hiller & Rief, 2014) and it is questionable whether it will ever be scientifically and clinically accepted. More generally, the lack of distinction between medically explained and unexplained bodily symptoms is questionable, if only because of the different conditions in which they arise. Criticisms further include that the new logic has not been consistently followed through, as conversion disorder is also defined in DSM-5 by symptoms that are "inconsistent with known neurological and physical disorders" (Falkai et al., 2015). It is also unclear how to delineate between somatic symptom disorder and the diagnosis of "psychological factors affecting other medical conditions," as both diagnoses include medically explained symptoms. Ultimately, the delimitation of hypochondriasis (illness anxiety disorder) to forms without or at most with mild physical symptoms also corresponds neither to the state of scientific knowledge nor to the requirements of clinical practice (Rief & Martin, 2014). Strictly speaking, the definition of illness anxiety disorder proposed in the DSM-5 does not fit into the chapter on somatic symptom and related disorders (due to the exclusion of somatic symptoms), and would therefore have found a more appropriate place in the chapter on anxiety disorders.

For the forthcoming introduction of the revised ICD-11 system, it is probably to be expected that the concept of somatoform disorders will be maintained, but possibly under the new designation Bodily Distress Syndrome (Budtz-Lilly et al., 2015a; Gureje, 2015).

1.3 Diagnostics

In practice, the diagnostic classification or the diagnostic process for persistent somatic symptoms is often not easy. On the one hand, this is due to the fact that there is an enormous variety of terms and classification attempts relating to persistent somatic symptoms, as was made clear in ► Sect. 1.2. Secondly, persistent somatic symptoms often occur in conjunction with other mental disorders (such as mood or anxiety disorders) or in addition to somatic diagnoses and are sometimes difficult to distinguish from these. The first problem mentioned will be addressed in the following two sections. Regardless of the various conceptual proposals for persistent somatic symptoms, the internationally recognized classification system **ICD-10** (Dilling & Freyberger, 2000; World Health Organization, 1992) is authoritative in therapeutic practice. It is used in particular by the German health insurance funds as the basis for coding mental illnesses for the application for psychotherapy. Accordingly, ► Sect. 1.3.1 provides an insight into how persistent somatic symptoms can be classified within the framework of the ICD-10 (or DSM-5) classification criteria. ► Section 1.3.2 refers to special features of the diagnostic process for persistent somatic symptoms. ► Section 1.3.3 deals with the second problem—differential diagnosis. Finally (► Sect. 1.3.4), various diagnostic aids and instruments are presented.

1.3.1 Diagnostic Classification Criteria According to ICD-10 and DSM-5

Persistent somatic symptoms are assigned to the category "F4 Neurotic, stress and somatoform disorders" according to ICD-10 and to "Somatic Symptom and Related Disorders" according to DSM-5. The term somatoform disorder was first introduced in 1980 by the then DSM-III and was incorporated into the then tenth revision of the ICD in 1994. In the previous versions of these classification systems, the corresponding term had been "functional disorders of mental origin" (category 306 in ICD-9).

Table 1.1 Comparison of somatoform disorders and disorders with physical symptoms in ICD-10 and DSM-5

ICD-10	DSM-5
Somatization disorder	Somatic symptom disorder
Undifferentiated somatoform disorder	
Somatoform autonomic dysfunction	
Persistent somatoform pain disorder	
Dissociative and conversion disorders[a]	Conversion disorder (Functional neurological symptom disorder)
Hypochondriacal disorder[b]	Somatic symptom disorder/Illness anxiety disorder
Other/unspecified somatoform disorder	Other specified and unspecified somatic symptom and related disorder

[a]Do not belong to the somatoform disorders in the ICD-10, but represent a separate disorder category

[b]Hypochondriacal disorder according to ICD-10 is represented within the DSM-5 in the two diagnoses "somatic symptom disorder" and "illness anxiety disorder". The illness anxiety disorder is conceived here as a "residual category", which is to be diagnosed only in the case of severe illness anxiety with missing or only slightly pronounced somatic symptoms. In the far more frequent case of serious illness anxiety and simultaneous clear somatic symptoms, the DSM-5 diagnosis of "somatic symptom disorder" should be selected

Table 1.1 compares the individual disorders (diagnoses) of somatoform disorders in the ICD-10 and the DSM-5. Hypochondriasis (illness anxiety disorder) will not be discussed further here, as this disorder is not primarily defined by somatic symptoms, but by the preoccupation with having or acquiring a serious illness.

The diagnoses in Table 1.1, which are primarily defined by the presence of somatic symptoms, can be roughly divided into poly- and monosymptomatic disorders. In polysymptomatic disorders, multiple somatic symptoms from different body regions and organ systems are present, whereas monosymptomatic disorders are limited to a specific symptom type, namely exclusively pain symptoms in persistent somatoform pain disorder and exclusively neurological symptoms in conversion disorder. In the following, the individual disorders will be briefly characterised.

▪ Somatization Disorder (ICD-10: F45.0)

For somatization disorder, at least 6 symptoms from a predefined list of symptoms that cannot or not suffi-

1

Fig. 1.1 Somatization disorder according to ICD-10 (F45.0)

A.	A history of at least 2 years of persistent complaints of multiple and changing physical symptoms that cannot be explained by any diagnosable medical condition. The presence of any known medical condition does not explain the severity, variety and duration of the physical symptoms or the associated social disability. If some vegetative symptoms are present, they are not the main feature of the disorder, i.e. they are not particularly persistent or distressing.	
B.	The constant worry about the symptoms leads to persistent suffering and to patients seeking multiple (three or more) consultations or additional examinations by primary care or specialists, and when medical facilities are inaccessible for financial or geographical reasons, to persistent self-medication or multiple consultations with local lay healers.	
C.	Persistent refusal to accept the medical determination that there is no sufficient physical cause for the physical symptoms. Acceptance of the physician's explanation of symptoms for only short periods of time at most, up to a few weeks, or immediately after a medical examination.	
D.	A total of six or more symptoms from the following list, with symptoms from at least two different groups:	
	Gastrointestinal symptom:	
	1.	Abdominal pain
	2.	Nausea
	3.	Flatulence bloating
	4.	Bad taste in the mouth or extremely coated tongue
	5.	Complaints of frequent diarrhea or leakage of fluid from the anus
	6.	Complaints of frequent diarrhea or leakage of fluid from the anus
	Cardiovascular symptoms:	
	7.	Breathlessness despite lack of physical exertion
	8.	Chest pain
	Urogenital symptoms:	
	9.	Dysuria or changed micturition frequency
	10.	Unpleasant sensations in or around the genital area
	11.	Complaints of unusual or increased vaginal discharge
	Skin and pain symptoms:	
	12.	Complaints about blotchy skin or colour changes of the skin
	13.	Pain in the limbs, extremities or joints
	14.	Unpleasant numbness or tingling sensation
E.	Most common exclusion criterion: the disorder does not occur exclusively during schizophrenia or a related disorder (F3) or panic disorder (F41.0).	

ciently be explained by a medical cause must be present. The symptoms must have lasted for at least 2 years and symptoms of vegetative agitation must not be the main feature of the disorder. Figure 1.1 shows the criteria for somatization disorder according to the ICD-10.

Somatoform Autonomic Dysfunction (ICD-10: F45.3)

Somatoform autonomic dysfunction has not gained sustained acceptance in the international research literature. According to the diagnostic criteria, at least three symptoms from a list of vegetative and other somatoform symptoms must be present that the patient in question attributes to a physical illness (Fig. 1.2). When choosing this diagnosis, particular care should be taken to distinguish it from anxiety disorders, since the latter are also mainly characterized by symptoms of the autonomic nervous system.

Undifferentiated Somatoform Disorder (ICD-10: F45.1)

Undifferentiated somatoform disorder is in principle a residual category for polysymptomatic disorders that cannot be classified either as somatization disorder or as somatoform autonomic dysfunction. The duration of the disorder must be at least 6 months. In the literature, the term "abridged somatization disorder" has been proposed as an alternative term in order to be able to include disorders that do not meet the strict inclusion criteria of somatization disorder. The Somatic Symptom Index SSI-4/6 introduced by Escobar et al. (1989), for example, specifies that at least 4 somatoform symptoms must be present in men and at least 6 in women.

Persistent Somatoform Pain Disorder (ICD-10: F45.4)

In this disorder, the somatoform symptomatology consists exclusively of one or more pain symptoms. A minimum duration of 6 months is required. Patients with a clinical diagnosis of fibromyalgia usually meet the criteria for this disorder. Complementary to the persistent somatoform pain disorder, a coding for "pain disorder with related psychological factors" (Nilges & Rief, 2010) has been introduced. It enables the coding of pain in which a somatic disease factor is present or very likely to be present as a trigger and often also as a maintaining factor. This makes it possible to classify pain syndromes within the framework of the F category of the ICD-10 that cannot be classified within the framework of a persistent somatoform pain disorder, such as migraine, tension-type headache or chronic regional pain syndrome (CRPS), which is also known as Sudeck's disease.

Conversion Disorder (ICD-10: F 44)

Conversion disorder is limited to neurological symptoms of the voluntary motor or sensory system. A con-

A.	Symptoms of autonomic (vegetative) excitation attributed by the patient to a physical illness in one or more of the following systems or organs:	
	1.	Heart and cardiovascular system
	2.	Upper gastrointestinal tract (esophagus and stomach)
	3.	Lower gastrointestinal tract
	4.	Respiratory system
	5.	Urogenital system
B.	Two or more of the following vegetative symptoms:	
	1.	Palpitations
	2.	Sweating (hot or cold)
	3.	Dry mouth
	4.	Hot flushes or or facial skin turns red
	5.	Feeling of pressure in the epigastrium, tingling or restlessness in the abdomen
C.	One or more of the following symptoms:	
	1.	Chest pain or a feeling of pressure in chest (area around heart)
	2.	Dyspnea or hyperventilation
	3.	Abnormal fatigue after light exertion
	4.	Aerophagia, singultus or burning sensation in the chest or epigastrium
	5.	Increased frequency of bowel movement
	6.	Increased micturition frequency or dysuria
	7.	Flatulence or bloating
D.	No evidence of disruption of structure or function of organs or systems complained of by patients.	
E.	Common exclusion criterion: the symptoms are not exclusively associated with a phobic disorder (F40.0-F40.3) or panic disorder (F41.0).	

Fig. 1.2 Somatoform autonomic dysfunction according to ICD-10 (F45.3)

nection to psychological factors is assumed, for example when conflicts or stressful experiences precede the onset or exacerbation of symptoms.

Somatoform Disorder, Unspecified (ICD-10: F45.9)

A residual category in ICD-10 is the diagnosis of unspecified somatoform disorder. As with all other mental disorders, such a residual category is necessary to allow the clinicians to make a diagnosis even in cases where a person has clinically significant symptomatology but clinicians have not obtained sufficient information about the patient's condition yet.

Functional Somatic Syndromes

In a broader sense, somatoform disorders also include the so-called functional somatic syndromes, which, however, are not defined in the ICD-10. However, they are frequently encountered in clinical usage. The most common terms are presented in the following overview:

Functional Syndromes

- **Chronic Fatigue Syndrome** (CFS; Fukuda et al., 1994) with a range of persistent somatic symptoms based around the main symptom of chronic fatigue.
- **Fibromyalgia**, a type of generalized pain syndrome with increased pain sensitivity that usually meets the criteria for persistent somatoform pain disorder.
- **Irritable bowel syndrome** (Drossman, 2006), a monosymptomatic manifestation of gastrointestinal symptoms with abdominal pain or discomfort and changes in bowel habits.
- Environmental symptoms with terms such as **multiple chemical sensitivity (MCS)** or **idiopathic** environmental intolerance (IEI), which summarises somatic symptoms that are attributed to environmental pollution or pollutants.
- Non-specific and **non-cardiac chest pain** as well as **somatoform vertigo** with the corresponding leading symptoms.
- **Premenstrual syndrome (PMS)**, characterized by both affective and physical symptoms during the luteal phase of the female menstrual cycle.

There are no internationally binding criteria for these diagnostic terms or concepts, nor are they rationally integrated into the context of the other somatoform or somatic stress disorders. Diagnostic criteria have been developed for some syndromes in the relevant research literature, e.g., the Rome criteria for irritable bowel syndrome (Drossman, 2006; Thompson et al., 1999), the Center for Disease Control and Prevention criteria (Fukuda et al., 1994) for CFS or the criteria for a particularly severe form of premenstrual syndrome—premenstrual dysphoric disorder (PMDD)—in the mood disorders chapter of the DSM-5. These diagnoses can therefore be made systematically, but must then be coded according to the ICD-10 (or DSM-5) criteria. According to the ICD-10, one can select the category of other specified or unspecified somatoform disorder or additionally check whether the criteria for autonomic somatoform dysfunction are fulfilled, which, for example, provides a subcategory for predominantly gastrointestinal symptoms, as is characteristic of irritable bowel syndrome.

1.3.2 Diagnostic Process and Special Features of Persistent Somatic Symptoms

The somatoform disorders described in ICD-10 and the somatic symptom and related disorders described in DSM-5 are typically diagnosed on the basis of a free clinical exploration or with the aid of structured interviews. Questionnaires may also be used (► Sect. 1.3.4) to screen for the presence of somatoform disorders or to assess associated psychopathological features (e.g., dysfunctional cognitions or illness behaviors). Questionnaires are also used to quantify the degree of severity of a somatoform disorder and to determine changes in the spontaneous course or during therapy.

▪ Structured Diagnostic Procedures

The diagnosis should always be based on an external exploration and not on questionnaire data. The prototype of the clinical interview is the "**Structured Clinical Interview**" (SCID), which, however, in its DSM-5-related form (First et al., 2015) was not yet available in German when this text was written. In the DSM-IV version of the SCID (Wittchen et al., 1997), there was a separate section for the group of somatoform disorders. Health burdens and physical symptoms could be inquired about according to the diagnostic criteria of the DSM-IV. The SCID has the disadvantage that diagnoses according to the ICD-10 are not provided. Some clinicians make do by assigning the corresponding ICD-10 codes to diagnoses made according to the DSM-IV (◘ Table 1.1).

Other well-known structured interviews are the "**Composite International Diagnostic Interview**" (CIDI; German version: Wittchen et al., 1998) and the "Diagnostic Interview for Mental Disorders" (DIPS), of which a short version also exists (Margraf et al., 1994). Based on the CIDI, a computerized version, the DIA-X (Wittchen & Pfister, 1997), was developed, with the help of which the patient's answers can be entered into the computer directly during the interview. Due to the programmed diagnostic algorithms, the applicable diagnoses can be identified immediately after the interview. A certain disadvantage of CIDI and DIA-X is that both procedures are not designed as clinical assessment procedures, but take over the patient's answers unfiltered. Therefore, discrepancies must be expected in comparison to clinical interviews such as the SCID.

A good alternative to the somewhat cumbersome interviews are the "**International Diagnostic Checklists**" (IDCL) developed by Hiller et al. (1997c), which are available for making diagnoses according to ICD-10. These are handy DIN A-5 sheets in the sense of a single-sheet collection, with all diagnostic criteria and decision rules included in a very clear form. In contrast to the above-mentioned interviews, there are no questions to be asked of the patient, which is not a disadvantage for experienced clinicians. A clinician familiar with the SCID can usually use the IDCL in a very reliable and straightforward manner.

For more specific somatoform and functional syndromes not listed in the ICD-10, such as chronic fatigue syndrome or irritable bowel syndrome, there are, to our knowledge, no structured procedures for diagnosis.

▪ Symptom—Syndrome—Diagnosis

The basic principle of any diagnostic examination—the careful distinction between symptom, syndrome and diagnosis—plays a special role especially in the diagnosis of persistent somatic symptoms. First of all, it must be determined whether somatic symptoms are present in the person examined or were present in the past. The longitudinal view is important because it is possible that individual symptoms occur only temporarily and therefore the longer-term course is characterized by a coming and going of different somatic symptoms. The assessment "medically explained" or "medically unexplained" should definitely be made already at the symptom level. Of course, a patient can have both somatic diseases and medically unclear symptoms at the same time. For the diagnosis of a **somatoform disorder**, however, only the latter may be evaluated.

> It should be noted that somatoform symptoms do not necessarily lead to a corresponding diagnosis.

It is known from epidemiological studies that more or less medically explained somatic symptoms of any degree of severity represent a ubiquitous phenomenon (e.g., temporary mild headaches, low back pain, digestive problems). In a study by Hiller et al. (2006), around 80% of representative respondents from a German general population sample reported current somatoform symptoms. In fact, however, only about 10–15% of them could be diagnosed with a somatoform disorder due to the severity of the symptomatology or the resulting impairments. To avoid false positive diagnoses based on (harmless) symptoms without pathological value, only clinically significant symptoms should be considered. As a rule of thumb, we recommend that clinical relevance be assumed if the person concerned has consulted a doctor, taken medication or changed his or her lifestyle because of the symptom.

> If several clinically significant somatoform symptoms are present, they constitute a somatoform syndrome in the sense of a "symptom bundle".

For example, a pain syndrome exists when a patient complains of head, back, joint and abdominal pain (i.e. several individual pain symptoms). We speak of a "multiple somatoform syndrome" when several individual symptoms from different body regions and organ systems are present (Rief, 1995).

> In order to be able to make a diagnosis, further characteristics must be identified (e.g., a certain duration or course characteristics, impairments in everyday life, differential diagnoses).

In the case of somatoform disorders, a syndrome is not mandatory, but a diagnosis may already be justified in the case of a severe and distressing individual symptom (e.g., pain disorder in the case of severe back pain, if this is associated with illness behavior and psychosocial impairment).

The overview of symptoms of somatoform disorders according to the ICD-10 and the former DSM-IV lists symptoms that can be specifically checked in the clarification of a possible somatoform disorder. These are all symptoms that are or were listed in the diagnostic categories of the ICD-10 or the former DSM-IV.

Symptoms of Somatoform Disorders According to ICD-10 and the Former DSM-IV

- Headache or facial pain
- Abdominal pain
- Back pain
- Joint pain
- Pain in the extremities
- Chest pain
- Rectal pain
- Pain during sexual intercourse
- Pain when urinating
- Nausea
- Fullness
- Feeling pressure in the epigastrium, tingling or restlessness in the abdomen
- Vomiting (outside pregnancy)
- Increased belching
- Aerophagia, hiccups, or burning in the chest or stomach area.
- Intolerance of different foods
- Bad taste in the mouth or a very clogged tongue
- Dry mouth
- Frequent diarrhea
- Anal leakage
- Frequent urination
- Palpitations
- Cardiac stress
- Sweating (hot or cold)
- Flushing or blushing
- Breathlessness without effort
- Hyperventilation
- Unusual fatigue with light exertion
- Patches or changes in the colour of the skin
- Sexual indifference
- Unpleasant sensations in or around the genital area
- Coordination or balance disorders
- Paralysis or muscle weakness
- difficulty swallowing or a lumpy feeling in the throat
- Whispered voice or loss of voice
- Urinary retention or difficulty urinating
- Sensory delusions
- Sensory deprivation
- Paresthesias
- Seeing double images
- Blindness
- Hearing loss
- Seizures
- Amnesia
- Loss of consciousness (different from simple fainting)
- For women:
  - Painful menstruation
  - Irregular menstruation
  - Very heavy menstruation
  - Vomiting throughout pregnancy
  - Unusual or increased vaginal discharge
- For men:
  - Erectile or ejaculatory dysfunction

1.3.3 Differential Diagnosis

Most carefully, somatoform disorders must be distinguished from medical conditions and anxiety disorders. A differential classification should already take place at the symptom level. It is possible that physical symptoms of different types are present and, as a result, the disorders or diseases may also be comorbid.

> The first most important differential diagnostic consideration concerns whether an organic disease is present.

The appropriate somatic-medical clarification is the task of the general practitioner or specialist. The interpretation of medical findings depends on the specialist knowledge, experience and special assessment of the doctors. In addition, the borderline area of what can be medically explained is constantly being changed and expanded by new research findings. In practice, it proves useful to assume somatoform symptoms when the symptoms cannot be regarded as a component of a medical condition that is currently known and generally recognized in medicine.

The **dichotomy** of **"somatic" vs. "no somatic" causes** should not be overestimated in its importance, since according to ICD-10 a somatoform disorder can be diagnosed in certain cases even if the symptom(s) in question is (are) co-caused somatically. For example, according to ICD-10, symptoms are considered "somatoform" even if the underlying medical condition does not explain "the severity, extent, variety, and duration of the somatic symptoms or the associated social disability." For example, back pain that has developed due to a herniated disc may be considered somatoform in this sense if the extent of the pain cannot be explained by the orthopedic findings alone and excessive psychosocial impairment has developed.

Anxiety Disorders

The differentiation from anxiety disorders is of particular importance insofar as physical symptoms can also occur as physiological correlates of anxiety. If, for example, symptoms such as palpitations or sweating only occur during panic attacks or phobic reactions, they are not to be considered part of a somatoform disorder. Due to the temporal limitation of the anxiety attacks, physical anxiety correlates and somatoform symptoms can usually be easily distinguished from each other. It is somewhat more difficult to distinguish them from generalized anxiety disorder, as this, like somatoform disorders, lasts for a longer period of time. However, in contrast to somatoform disorders, generalized anxiety disorder must be accompanied by persistent worries and fears about various aspects of everyday life.

Depressive Disorders

It is sometimes suspected that somatic symptoms may also occur as a component of another mental disorder, e.g., in the context of a depressive disorder (keyword "somatized depression"). In order to differentiate, it should first be carefully checked whether the somatic symptoms present are actually listed in the criteria catalogues of the disorders concerned. For example, exhaustion is part of a typical depressive syndrome, but other somatic symptoms are not found in the definition of major depression (corresponding to depressive episode and recurrent depressive disorder in the ICD-10) or in dysthymic disorder. In addition, the course of somatic and mood symptoms should be carefully compared. For example, if exhaustion occurs even during depression-free periods, this symptom cannot be interpreted solely as part of a depressive disorder. In most cases, there is no clear parallelism between the physical and depressive symptoms, so that several diagnoses should be assigned in accordance with the principles of comorbidity (see also Rief et al., 1992).

Psychotic Disorders

Occasionally, the differentiation of somatoform disorders from psychotic disorders such as schizophrenia can be important, especially when patients' hallucinations and delusions are related to their own bodily functions. These are usually bizarre perceptions such as feeling a snake in the gut or sensations of cold in the brain, which are often accompanied by experiences of external influence. Such phenomena are described in psychiatric parlance as cenesthetic (coenesthetic) hallucinations. They should not be considered as somatoform symptoms. However, this does not exclude comorbidity between a psychotic and a somatoform disorder.

Malingering and Factitious Disorder

Somatic symptoms must also be distinguished from those that occur in the context of a malingering or a factitious disorder. In the context of malingering, the person invents a symptom that is not actually present in order to gain an advantage (e.g., a balance disorder in order to be discharged for military service). In factitious disorder, a symptom is intentionally created in order to be able to take the sick role (e.g., secretly taking heparin to feign a bleeding disorder). In its chronic form, factitious disorder is often referred to as Münchausen syndrome.

Psychosomatic Diseases

Finally, the differential diagnosis between somatoform and the "classical" psychosomatic diseases should be mentioned. These include chronic inflammatory bowel diseases (Crohn's disease and ulcerative colitis), bronchial asthma, rheumatoid arthritis and neurodermatitis. A guiding feature in the differentiation can be that, in contrast to somatoform disorders, tissue or organ damage is present in these diseases, even if the causes of the disease are unknown or multifactorial. Separate categories exist for these disorders in both ICD-10 (F54: Psychological and behavioral factors associated with disorders and diseases classified elsewhere) and DSM-5 (Psychological factors affecting other medical conditions). However, these diagnoses are not limited to the "classical" diseases listed above, but may also include other diseases whose development, course and treatment may be influenced by psychological conditions (e.g., migraine, myocardial infarction, cancer, diabetes mellitus, hearing disorders such as hearing loss or Meniere's disease, epilepsy).

1.3.4 Further Diagnostic Procedures

The diagnostic clarification of somatoform disorders should not end with the diagnosis. A number of instruments are now available with which various **affective, cognitive and behavioral aspects** can be examined in greater detail. This allows a kind of differentiated **psychopathological profile** to be drawn up for the person under investigation. The procedures listed in ◘ Table 1.2

◘ **Table 1.2** Some questionnaire procedures for the extended diagnosis of somatoform disorders

	Subscales	Characteristics collected	Authors
Symptom lists			
Screening for somatoform disorders (SOMS)	Somatization index according to DSM-IV and ICD-10	Somatic symptoms	Rief and Hiller (2008)
Patient health questionnaire (PHQ-15), somatization scale	–	Somatic symptoms	Kroenke et al. (2002)
Symptom checklist (SCL-90-R), somatization scale	–	Somatic symptoms	Derogatis (1983)
Instruments for special disorders			
Fatigue scale (FS) (German version of the Chalder fatigue scale)	1. Mental exhaustion 2. Physical exhaustion	Fatigue	Chalder et al. (1993); Martin et al. (2010)
Whiteley index (WI)	1. Fear of illness 2. Somatic symptoms 3. Illness beliefs	Illness anxiety	Hiller and Rief (2004)
Illness attitude scales (IAS)	1. Illness anxiety 2. Illness behavior	Illness anxiety	Hiller and Rief (2004)
Multidimensional inventory of hypochondriacal traits (MIHT)	1. Hypochondriacal alienation 2. Hypochondriacal reassurance 3. Hypochondriacal worry 4. Hypochondriacal absorption	Illness anxiety	Longley et al. (2005); Witthöft et al. (2010)
Recording of associated characteristics			
Cognitions about body and health questionnaire (FKG)	1. Catastrophizing interpretation of bodily complaints 2. Intolerance of physical discomfort 3. Physical weakness 4. Autonomic sensation 5. Health behavior	Dysfunctional cognitions	Hiller et al. (1997a)
Scale for the assessment of illness behaviour (SAIB)	1. Diagnosis verification 2. Expression of symptoms 3. Medication 4. Illness consequences 5. Scanning	Illness behavior	Rief et al. (2003)
Coping with chronic pain scales (FESV)	1. Cognitive pain coping 2. Behavioral pain coping 3. Symptom distress	Pain coping and emotional distress	Geissner (2001)
Pain disability index (PDI)	–	Symptom disability	Dillmann et al. (1994); Modified version of Mewes et al. (2009).

have proven to be reliable and valid in scientific studies. The procedures can be roughly divided into

- Symptom lists,
- Procedures for the recording of special disturbance patterns and
- Instruments that capture associated clinical characteristics.

The "**Screening for Somatoform Disorders**" (SOMS) is suitable as a supplement to the classificatory diagnosis, as it contains all 55 physical symptoms listed in the ICD-10 and the former DSM-IV. The person completing the form is instructed to indicate only those symptoms for which no sufficient medical explanation was found during medical examinations. The SOMS exists in two versions: The SOMS-2 asks for the presence of individual symptoms for the period of the past 2 years, whereas the SOMS-7T asks for the past 7 days. However, in the SOMS-7T, the intensity/stress level can be specified for each symptom. This version is therefore suitable for measuring progress. The Patient Health Questionnaire (PHQ-15) consists of only 15 items and is often used because of its brevity. However, neither the PHQ-15 nor the somatization scale of the SCL-90-R differentiate between symptoms with and without medical causes in the instruction.

As instruments for **specific disorders**, only the "Fatigue Scale" (FS) and some instruments aiming at the assessment of hypochondriacal features are listed as examples. Important **associated characteristics** are dysfunctional cognitions with regard to the perception and interpretation of physical signals, causal symptom interpretations, illness fears and beliefs, illness and safety behavior, coping strategies and the degree of psychosocial impairment.

Symptom diaries represent another diagnostic option. They can be used for differentiated behavioral diagnostics, for example to record the daily or weekly course of symptom intensity and unpleasantness. An example of a standardized version is the SOMS Sensitivity Diary as part of the SOMS (Rief & Hiller, 2008). It contains visual analogue scales to assess one's own physical well-being, mood, subjectively experienced state of health, illness anxiety and other relevant characteristics. Triggers for symptom changes as well as consequences (e.g., own reactions or coping attempts) can also be entered and thus made accessible for systematic observation. However, a symptom diary can also be easily tailored to the individual patient using self-designed visual analogue scales. Examples of corresponding scales are illustrated in ◘ Fig. 1.3.

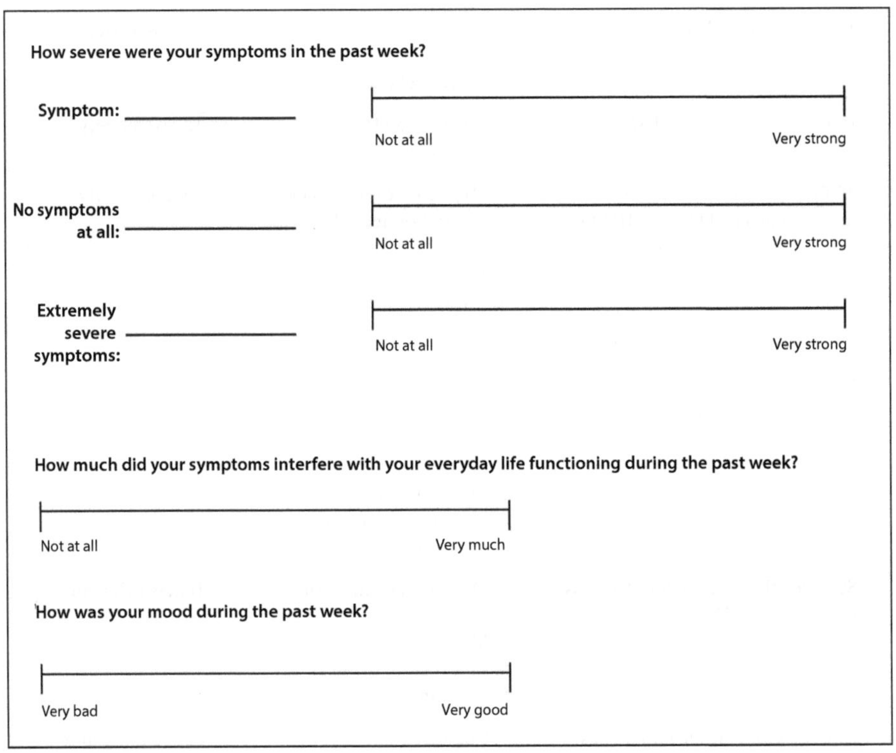

◘ **Fig. 1.3** Suggestions for visual analogue scales in a symptom diary

1.4 Epidemiology

1.4.1 Prevalence

▪ General Population

Persistent somatic symptoms represent a frequent phenomenon in the general population. In an epidemiological study by Hiller et al. (2006), the point prevalence of somatoform symptoms was determined in a German representative sample. It was found that 81.6% of the persons examined perceived at least one symptom associated with a slight degree of impairment and 0.7% perceived at least one symptom with a high degree of impairment at the time of the examination. In addition, there was an average frequency of seven symptoms per participant. Various pain symptoms (mainly back pain, headache, joint pain and pain in the extremities) as well as food intolerance, sexual indifference, menstrual pain and erectile or ejaculatory dysfunction were the most common. Including mild to severe levels of impairment, these symptoms had a prevalence number of over 20%. Furthermore, there was a trend for the individuals studied to have multiple somatic symptoms rather than single symptoms. Finally, the authors examined the frequency of syndromes of somatoform symptoms. This showed that a significantly larger proportion of the sample studied had symptoms from the pain cluster compared with the gastrointestinal symptom cluster or pseudoneurological symptoms. Comparable data can also be demonstrated in other European countries. In a representative population study by McAteer et al. (2011) in the United Kingdom, the most common symptoms reported over the past 2 weeks were feeling tired, headache, joint pain, back pain, and sleep disturbance. The average number of somatic symptoms over the past 2 weeks was just under four symptoms.

Determining the prevalence of clinically relevant somatoform symptoms is complicated by various aspects. As was made clear in ▶ Sect. 1.2, there are very different diagnostic concepts for the classification of persistent somatic symptoms. Accordingly, prevalence figures can only be considered in connection with the underlying diagnostic criteria. In addition, the determination of prevalence is complicated by the fact that somatoform symptomatology is often not recognized as such and thus the appropriate diagnosis cannot be made. This problem can be attributed to the fact that the primary point of contact for patients with somatoform symptoms is not so much psychosocial institutions as general practitioners and specialists. In addition, it must be assumed that patients with somatoform symptoms often make use of alternative medical services.

In recent years, several studies on the frequency of persistent somatic symptoms based on the diagnostic criteria of the DSM-IV (American Psychiatric Association, 2000; Saß et al., 2003), the ICD-10 (Dilling & Freyberger, 2000; World Health Organization, 1996) or the extended diagnostic concepts such as the SSI-4/6 (▶ Sects. 1.2.2 or 1.3.1) have been conducted in representative population samples using standardized clinical interviews. These include the 1998/1999 Federal Health Survey, a national survey of the prevalence of mental and physical disorders in a German adult sample (Jacobi et al., 2004). Prevalence figures are based on DSM-IV diagnoses collected through structured clinical interviews. A lifetime prevalence of 16.2%, a 12-month prevalence of 11% and a 4-week prevalence of 7.5% were determined for the total group of somatoform disorders. Regarding DSM-IV pain disorder, Jacobi et al. (2004) reported a 12-month prevalence of 8.1%. Almost one third of the patients reported at least 2 or more pain symptoms; excessive headache, lower abdominal pain and back pain were most frequently reported (Fröhlich et al., 2006). For undifferentiated somatoform disorder, a point prevalence of 19.7% was found in another German general population study (Grabe et al., 2003). The somatization disorder, as a diagnostic entity comprising extremely strictly defined criteria, was investigated in terms of its prevalence in the "Epidemiologic Catchment Area Study" for an American representative sample (Robins & Regier, 1991). Here a lifetime prevalence of less than 1% was found. In summary, across Europe, somatoform disorders are among the fourth most common mental disorders (after anxiety disorders, insomnia and depressive disorders) (Wittchen et al., 2011). Patients who meet the criteria of simplified diagnostic concepts of persistent somatic symptoms are much more common. Jacobi et al. (2004) report a lifetime prevalence for SSI-4/6 of 5.6%, a 12-month prevalence of 4.3%, and a 4-week prevalence of 3.1%. For an American sample, a lifetime prevalence of 11.6% was identified for somatoform syndromes that did not meet the strict criteria for somatization disorder. The prevalence of multisomatoform disorder (Kroenke et al., 1997; ▶ Sect. 1.2.2) was investigated using a structured clinical interview in a Norwegian population sample. A 6-month prevalence of 14% was found (Leiknes et al., 2007b).

As mentioned above, multiple persistent somatic symptoms also occur in the context of specific functional syndromes. The point prevalence varies considerably depending on the type of such syndrome or the underlying syndrome criteria. Classic functional syndromes include chronic fatigue syndrome, for which point prevalences of 0.2–0.4% have been found in two representative population samples (Jason et al., 1999; Reyes et al., 2003). Fibromyalgia represents another common functional syndrome. In the large-scale London Fibromyalgia Epidemiology Study, a point prevalence of 3.3% was found for this syndrome (White et al., 1999). Another epidemiological study of various European countries found a point prevalence of between 2.9% and 4.7%, depending on the criteria used (Branco et al., 2010). In studies of women of childbearing age, approximately 4.8–6.3% met DSM-IV research criteria for premenstrual dysphoric disorder, a particularly severe form of premenstrual syndrome (PMS; Soares et al., 2001; Rivera-Tovar & Frank, 1990). In irritable bowel syndrome (IBS), the point prevalence varies enormously depending on the underlying disorder criteria. According to recent reviews, prevalence can range from 2.1% to 22% (Grundmann & Yoon, 2010; Rey & Talley, 2009). A systematic review that only considered studies of patients who met Rome criteria for IBS found a pooled prevalence of 7%. The main prevalence data are summarized in ◘ Table 1.3. Prevalence data on the new disorder category of somatic symptom and related disorders in the DSM-5 (American Psychiatric Association, 2013) are not yet available at this time.

◘ Table 1.3 Prevalence of persistent somatic symptoms in the general population

	Lifetime prevalence (%)	Point prevalence (%)	12-month prevalence (%)
Syndromes of multiple persistent somatic symptoms			
Somatization disorder (according to DSM-IV/ICD-10)	0.1		
Pain disorder (according to DSM-IV)			8.1
Undifferentiated somatoform disorder (according to DSM-IV)		19.7	
SSI-4/6, other concepts of somatization disorder	5.6–11.6		
Specific functional somatic syndromes			
Chronic fatigue syndrome		0.2–0.4	
Fibromyalgia		2.9–4.7	
Premenstrual dysphoric disorder		4.8–6.3	
Irritable bowel syndrome		2.1–22.0	

▪ **Primary Care**

Particularly in primary care—primary care physician practices and general hospitals—a high proportion of patients present with persistent somatic symptoms. Burton (2003) showed in a systematic review that in 15–19% of cases somatic symptoms without a medical cause are the main reason for a consultation with the primary care physician. In a meta-analysis (Haller et al., 2015) of several high quality epidemiological studies in which DSM-IV or ICD-10 somatoform disorders were assessed using clinical structured interviews in primary care practice patients, point prevalences for somatization disorder were 0.8% and 5.9% respectively, for undifferentiated somatoform disorder 27.0% and 8.9% and for pain disorder 7.3% and 9.3%. Similar to the general population samples, the problem arises again that the prevalence rates vary greatly depending on the diagnostic criteria used. In a study by Nimnuan et al. (2001), a sample of consecutively admitted patients from a general hospital was examined, in which a point prevalence of 52% regarding somatoform symptoms was determined. The authors based their participant recruitment on a very broad definition of symptoms as somatic symptoms for which no defined medical diagnosis could be found in the context of an adequate medical examination. In comparison, Verhaak et al. (2006) included only patients in their analyses who had had at least four medical consultations regarding their somatic symptoms over the past year. In this sample, a point prevalence of somatoform symptoms of 2.5% was found. The prevalences of functional somatic syndromes do not appear to be necessarily elevated in the context of consultations with the primary care physician. Functional gastrointestinal disorder (including irritable bowel syndrome), for example, occurred in 3.6% of patients in primary care (Thompson et al., 2000), and chronic fatigue syndrome in 0.2% (Nacul et al., 2011).

A problem already mentioned is that somatoform symptoms are often not recognized as such by the general practitioner. Frequent referrals to other medical specialists are the rule. Accordingly, it is not surprising that also in specialist practices or specialist wards in general hospitals the prevalence of somatoform symptoms is significantly increased. In a previously cited study by Nimnuan et al. (2001), patients were assessed separately for the number of somatoform symptoms according to the specialist department from which they were referred. Patients referred from gynaecology (66%) and neurology (62%) departments had the highest prevalence rates, followed by patients from gastroenterology (58%) and cardiology (53%) wards. Another important finding of this study is that a healthcare system based on specialist clinics increases the likelihood that patients with somatoform symptoms present to many different clinics. Thus, it was shown that specific syndromes were not necessarily diagnosed more frequently in only one department, but in other departments as well. Noncardiac chest pain, for example, had an increased prevalence in cardiology departments (27.2%), but occurred with comparable prevalence in respiratory (39.0%), neurological (21.4%), gastrointestinal (13.5%) or rheumatology departments (14.3%). Patients with somatoform symptoms are also frequently encountered in the emergency department. In one study (Mehl-Madrona, 2008), among patients who frequently use the emergency department (>5 visits/year), 16.5% had a diagnosis of pain disorder and 11.0% of somatization disorder according to DSM-IV criteria. Also among patients who regularly visited an emergency department, the prevalences were significantly increased with 8.0% of a somatoform pain disorder and 6.0% of a somatization disorder. Current studies show that future diagnostic concepts, such as the Bodily Distress Syndrome, which will play an important role for the ICD-11, are associated with comparably high prevalence figures (14.6%; Budtz-Lilly et al., 2015b) in the primary care setting.

1.4.2 Socio-Demographic and Transcultural Characteristics

▪ Gender

Several epidemiological studies show that women suffer more frequently from somatoform symptoms than men. This finding is considered to be relatively stable and is evident not only for symptoms that are associated with only a low degree of stress (Hiller et al., 2006), but also for clinically relevant syndromes. In the study by Jacobi et al. (2004), the lifetime prevalence of SSI-4/6 criteria was almost twice as high in women as in men. In a Norwegian population sample, about 3.7 times more women fulfilled the criteria for multisomatoform disorder (Kroenke et al., 1997) in the past 6 months (Leiknes et al., 2007b). In samples from primary care, similar but not as pronounced gender differences emerge. In the study by Nimnuan et al. (2001), the point prevalence of somatoform symptoms was about 1.4 times higher in women than in men. In the study by Verhaak et al. (2006), the proportion of women with somatoform symptoms in a primary care sample was 66%.

▪ Age

The correlations between age and the frequency of somatoform symptoms are not as clear-cut as the gender-related effects. On the one hand, studies available to date show that in the general population older people appear to experience more somatoform symptoms in both mild and severe forms. In a study by Hiller et al. (2006), 87% and 27% of participants over 45 years of age reported at least one mild or severe somatoform symptom, respectively. In contrast, 70% and 13% of those under 45 years of age reported experiencing at least one somatoform symptom of mild or severe severity, respectively. In a study by Rief et al. (2001), comparable results were found. In addition, however, it was shown that the symptoms that occurred more frequently in old age were primarily symptoms that are possibly caused by non-specific age-related changes (e.g., numbness, erectile dysfunctions, joint pain, pain in the extremities, urological problems, palpitations). In contrast to the prevalence of somatoform symptoms in general, interestingly, the diagnosis of somatization disorder or subsyndromal somatization symptoms seems to be clustered in younger age groups. In a study by Leiknes et al. (2007b), the highest 6-month prevalence of a multisomatoform disorder (15.7%) was in the age group between 18 and 34 years. The prevalence systematically decreased over the subsequent age range to 9.8% in those over 66 years of age. In a study by Nimnuan et al. (2001), it was found that patients referred to a general hospital by outpatient specialists for somatoform tended to be younger. The highest prevalence was in the 16–25 years old group. However, differences must be made here depending on the nature of the symptoms. For example, while patients referred by gynaecological specialists tended to be younger, patients from cardiology practices tended to be older. In a Dutch primary care study (de Waal et al., 2004), the highest prevalence of somatoform disorders in general occurred in the 25–44 years old subsample (21.8%) and decreased significantly to 5.4% in the 65–79 years old sample.

▪ Cultural Characteristics

Existing epidemiological studies on transcultural differences show that "somatization" is a cross-cultural phenomenon. In studies in primary health care facilities in various Asian countries (Khoo et al., 2012), comparable point prevalences for somatization disorder (according to ICD-10: 2.1–5.8%; according to DSM-IV: 0.06%) were found as in epidemiological studies in Western countries. However, at the same time, differences in frequency between different cultures are apparent. In an epidemiological study conducted by the WHO in primary care (Üstun & Sartorius, 1995), in which almost 5500 patients were examined in 15 different centres (Ankara, Athens, Mainz, Berlin, Bangalore, Groningen, Ibadan, Manchester, Nagasaki, Paris, Rio de Janeiro, Santiago, Seattle, Shanghai, Verona) in 14 countries, high somatization tendencies were found in all centres. However, considerable variation in overall prevalence occurred, e.g., with respect to SSI-4/6 ranging from 7.6% to 36.8%. Particularly elevated prevalence rates were seen in the two South American centers. In the Epidemiologic Catchment Area study cited earlier (Robins & Regier, 1991), the overall prevalence of somatization disorder was 0.01%, but increased prevalences were seen in African American women (0.8%) and men (0.4%). In a study by Farooq et al. (1995), patients in UK general practices were assessed with an inventory of somatoform symptoms. There was a significantly higher number of somatoform symptoms in the Asian compared to a European sample, which was primarily explained by ethnicity rather than education and employment status.

A general problem of existing epidemiological studies on transcultural differences in the frequency of somatoform symptoms is that measurement instruments are used which are relatively insensitive to culture-specific symptoms. This is problematic because the nature and frequency of specific somatoform symptoms, as in Üstun and Sartorius's (1995) study, can vary widely between cultures. Unfortunately, many transcultural epidemiological studies conducted to date have neglected so-called cultural concepts of distress (Kohrt et al., 2014). Cultural concepts of distress influence how a person experiences, understands and classifies their symptoms or communicates them to others. A typical example is represented by symptoms related to male reproduction, which are, for example, more common in cultures where a "concern about sperm loss" is widespread (e.g., Dhat syndrome). In addition to Dhat syndrome, there are other cultural concepts of distress related to somatic symptoms, which are summarized in ◘ Table 1.4 (for more information, see e.g. Falkai et al., 2015; Kohrt et al., 2004; Min & Suh, 2010). Cultural factors are also thought to influence the sex ratio of somatoform symptoms. For example, it was shown in a study examining somatic symptoms in 15 different nations that while in Western countries women have significantly higher somatization scores than men, in countries such as Chile or Nigeria, on the other hand, the genders tend to be equally distributed (Piccinelli & Simon, 1997). Furthermore, transcultural epidemiological studies show only contradictory findings concerning correlations between the level of economic development of the

◘ Table 1.4 Cultural concepts of distress with somatic symptoms

Cultural concepts of distress/origin	Symptoms/postulated etiological factors
Nervios ("nerves"; Latin America and Latin Americans in USA) Nevra (Greeks in North America) Nierbi (Sicilian in North America) Nerves (whites in Newfoundland)	Headaches, "brain aches" (pain in the back of the neck and head), irritability, stomach problems, insomnia, agitation, tearfulness, concentration problems, tremors, tingling, "mareos" (lightheadedness with occasional dizzy spells) Etiological factors: stressful life events/circumstances
Shenjing shuairuo ("weakness of the nervous system"; China) Ashaktapanna (India) Shinkei-suijaku (Japan)	Weakness/mental fatigue, emotions (e.g., being angry), excitement, nervous pain (e.g., headaches), sleep disturbances Etiological factors: work and family related stressors, loss of face, sense of failure, imbalance in vital essences (e.g., loss of "qi" as vital energy)
Susto ("terror", "horror", Latin American in USA, Mexico, Central-/South America) Espanto (Andean region)	No specific symptoms defined; commonly observed: Appetite disturbances, sleep disturbances, sadness, low self-esteem, interpersonal sensitivity, listlessness, muscle pain, coldness in extremities, pallor, headache, stomach pain, diarrhea Etiological factors: due to a highly stressful event (e.g., natural disaster, interpersonal situation) the soul "leaves the body"
Hwa-byung ("trouble disorder", "fire disease"; Korea)	Emotional, cognitive, and somatic symptoms (e.g., anger, hot flashes, feelings of hatred) Etiological factors: long-term accumulation of "anger fire" caused by repeated unfair social situations
Yadargaa ("tiredness", "lack of strength"; Mongolia)	Fatigue, sleep disturbances, physical weakness, headaches, dizziness, concentration problems, increased blood pressure, slowing down, hair loss, sweating of the hands and legs, spasms, cold sweat Etiological factors: post-socialist economic changes

respective country and the frequency of somatic However, a stable moderate correlation between subjective stress experience and somatic symptoms seems to be demonstrable transculturally (Simon et al., 1996).

Finally, special features of the structure of the respective medical care system of the country and social stigmas must also be taken into account when interpreting the findings. In transcultural psychiatry, for example, it has become an established assumption that people in Southeast Asia tend to experience stress on a physical rather than a psychological level. One explanatory hypothesis is that in Southeast Asian countries, somatic symptoms are more likely to be seen as justifying seeing a doctor than depressive or other emotional problems. Accordingly, psychiatric hospitals primarily see depressed patients with pronounced body symptoms (Kawanishi, 1992). However, the empirical evidence on this assumption is very scanty and contradictory. Other research tends to suggest that somatization tendencies in Asia may be an artifact of a trend toward "psychologization" in Western nations. Ryder et al. (2008), for example, were able to show that differences between subjects in Asian and Canadian countries in the expression of physical versus psychological symptoms can be explained in part by differences in thinking styles between the countries. Whereas in Western countries more internally oriented thinking has been demonstrated, in Asian cultures an external style of thinking is more frequently found. In countries where psychiatric care is only available to the extremely ill, it is often the case that sufferers place a strong emphasis on their somatic symptoms in order to receive sufficient attention or adequate treatment (Kirmayer & Young, 1998).

Dhat Syndrome

The word "Dhat" is derived from the ancient Indian Sanskrit word "dhatu", meaning "elixir of life". This syndrome was first described in Western psychiatric writings as a complex of vague somatic symptoms such as fatigue, exhaustion, loss of appetite, and sexual dysfunction that are attributed by the patient to semen loss in the context of nocturnal ejaculation, urination, and masturbation, respectively. These symptoms of "semen loss anxiety" are ancient. Their description is found in Indian historical writings. It is based on the idea that semen loss is associated with a loss of vital energy. However, this phenomenon is reported not only in India but also, for example, in Sri Lanka or other areas of the subcontinent. While on the one hand Dhat is referred to as a specific "sexual neurosis of the Orient", other scholars such as Sumathipala et al. (2004) assume that it is not a culturally specific phenomenon. Historical writings show that comparable semen loss anxiety also occurred in Europe, the United States, and Australia in the nineteenth century. In these countries, the syndrome may have disappeared in response to industrialization and urbanization and accompanying social and economic changes. It is possible that this effect of the syndrome's decline will also occur in the long term in South (East) Asia.

▪ Socioeconomic Status

The results concerning the correlation between the level of education or social class and prevalence rates of persistent somatic symptoms are partly contradictory. In a high-quality German epidemiological study by Jacobi et al. (2004), the highest prevalence rates of somatoform disorders are found in people who live in the lowest social class (13.5%), who are unemployed (16%) or who are divorced, widowed or separated (15%).

1.4.3 Comorbidity

Patients with exclusively somatoform symptoms are rather rare. However, a distinction must be made here between mild somatoform symptoms, which represent frequent everyday phenomena (Hiller et al., 2006), and somatic symptoms with a higher degree of severity and greater functional impairment. Affected individuals suffering from the latter symptoms often have comorbid mental illnesses. This is not surprising, as somatoform symptoms can be associated with massive impairments in quality of life. In particular, patients with chronic and polysymptomatic somatoform syndromes often experience a decline in daily activity levels, work performance, social role functioning, and quality of life (Barsky et al., 2005; de Waal et al., 2004; Grabe et al., 2003). In a study of a German sample of inpatients (Hiller et al., 1997b) who met criteria for the diagnoses of pain disorder, somatization disorder, and SSI-4/6, respectively, comparably high levels of impairment in various social functioning domains were demonstrated as in patients with other mental illnesses (e.g., anxiety disorders or depression). A German study (Wiborg et al., 2013) in primary care also found increased suicidality rates in a subsample of patients diagnosed with somatoform disorders: 23.9% reported active suicidal ideation in the past 6 months and 17.6% had attempted suicide in the past (in the majority of cases, this attempt occurred after the onset of somatoform symptoms).

▪ Axis I Disorders

In the previously cited health survey by Jacobi et al. (2004), a good third of the patients who met the criteria of SSI-4/6 had only one diagnosis of somatoform symptoms. 22.1% met criteria for one other mental disorder, 19.2% met criteria for two other diagnoses, and 24.5% met criteria for three or more than three other mental disorders. The most common comorbid disorders observed were anxiety disorders, mood disorders, and substance use disorder for patients who met SSI-4/6 (Jacobi et al., 2004) and for patients who met criteria for somatoform pain disorder (Fröhlich et al., 2006). Similar findings emerged in American (Kroenke et al., 1994) and Dutch samples (de Waal et al., 2004).

It is important to consider that the comorbid disorders do not necessarily have to occur at the same time as the somatoform symptoms, but also with a time lag of weeks to years between the respective first occurrence. It also happens that the individual disorders do not overlap at all. This means that one disorder has already subsided before the other begins. Appropriately, a study of the lifetime prevalence of comorbid mental disorders in a sample of primary care patients (Brown et al., 1990) who met criteria for somatization disorder according to DSM-III (American Psychiatric Association, 1980) showed the highest prevalences for mood disorders (major depression: 54.6%), anxiety disorders (generalized anxiety disorder: 33.6%; phobic disorders: 31.1%; panic disorder: 26%), and alcohol use disorder or dependence (21%), with lifetime prevalence values significantly higher than the point prevalences in the previously cited studies. The comorbidity between somatoform disorders and mood and anxiety disorders is thus shown to be very stable across different studies in different populations, which rightly raises the question of the extent to which somatoform, anxiety and depressive symptoms overlap. Löwe et al. (2008) were able to demonstrate in a primary care sample that the overlap of somatization, anxiety and depressive symptoms was significantly more strongly related to patients' limitations in everyday life (variance explanation: 24.5%) than the individual syndromes (variance explanation: 0–7.1%). Nevertheless, it can be seen that the three different syndromes for themselves make a syndrome-specific contribution to the everyday impairment of the patients that is independent of the comorbidity.

▪ Physical Illness

Only a few studies have assessed the comorbidity of physical illness in somatoform disorders. One study showed that 42% of patients with somatoform disorders reported a circulatory disorder, 29% reported a musculoskeletal disorder, 20% reported a respiratory disorder, and 18% reported an endocrine or metabolic disorder (Hanel et al., 2009). In another study, 58% of patients with somatoform symptoms were found to have two or more chronic physical illnesses, primarily cardiovascular disease (Kolk et al., 2004). These study findings illustrate that somatoform disorders are more likely to co-occur with a diagnosed physical illness. At the same time, it appears that patients with somatoform symptoms have a significantly higher risk of developing a mood disorder (13.5%) or an anxiety disorder (19.0%) than patients without somatoform symptoms (7.4% and 13.3%, respectively; van Eck van der Sluijs et al., 2015). Substance misuse, interestingly, occurs most frequently in patients with both physically explained and unexplained symptoms (8.4%) compared to patients with only medically explained symptoms (4.6%) or only unexplained symptoms (7.1%).

> The consideration of comorbidity, the connection of comorbid disorders with the somatoform symptoms as well as the temporal course and the mutual condition of the respective syndromes plays a decisive role for the therapy planning.

▪ Axis II Disorders

However, high comorbidities of somatoform symptoms exist not only with Axis I but also with Axis II disorders. In a Danish study (Fink, 1995), a sample of patients with chronic somatoform symptoms was examined. A concomitant personality disorder according to the DSM-III criteria (American Psychiatric Association, 1980) could be diagnosed in 48% of the persons examined. The most common diagnoses were unspecified personality disorder (40.7%) and borderline personality disorder (37.0%), with patients with the former diagnosis primarily characterized by cluster B characteristics (antisocial, borderline, histrionic, and narcissistic personality disorder). In an American study (Rost et al., 1992), in a sample of patients who met the strict criteria for somatization disorder, as many as 60.6% had a comorbid personality disorder. Two or more comorbid personality disorders could be diagnosed in 37.2%. Self-insecure-avoidant personality disorder (26.7%), paranoid personality disorder (21.3%), self-injurious personality disorder (19.1%), and obsessive-compulsive personality disorder (17%) were the most common. The criteria of histrionic personality disorder were met by 12.8% of the sample and antisocial personality disorder by 7.4%. In another study, patients diagnosed with chronic fatigue syndrome had comparable point prevalences (16.3%) to a general population sample (16.3%) and significantly lower prevalences than a psychiatric sample (58.7%) (Kempke et al., 2013).

> The presence of a comorbid personality disorder has a decisive influence on therapy planning. As a rule, the somatoform symptoms or, if applicable, comorbid Axis I disorders should be the focus of treatment first. In the case of these, a rapid therapeutic success can be expected, which also has a stabilising effect on the patient-therapist relationship. Only then should the treatment of the personality disorder be considered, which in turn requires a stable therapeutic relationship.

1.4.4 Course of Persistent Somatic Symptoms

Research on the spontaneous course of somatoform disorders shows the stability of a somatoform diagnosis or other diagnostic concepts of persistent somatic symptoms and thus an increased risk of chronicity of the symptoms over different follow-up time intervals. For example, Jackson and Kroenke (2008) demonstrated 21% of patients diagnosed with multisomatoform disorder still had this diagnosis 5 years later. Steinbrecher and Hiller (2011b) showed a stability rate of 56.8% after 1 year for DSM-IV somatoform disorders. Budtz-Lilly et al. (2015b) showed stability of Bodily Distress Syndrome in 56.8% of the studied patients after 2 years. In a Dutch primary care study (Arnold et al., 2006), the authors reported that only 30 of 99 patients with somatoform disorders had remission after 6 months. In contrast, the remaining 69 patients still had persistent symptoms after 6 months, regardless of whether some of them had already received professional psychotherapeutic or psychiatric treatment. In a Norwegian study, a diagnostic survey was conducted on a general population sample specifically with regard to somatoform symptoms (Leiknes et al., 2007a). Sufferers were re-interviewed after 10–11 years following a baseline survey. 33.6% of those who had reported somatoform pain in the first survey still did so in the follow-up survey and were also exclusively women. A study by Speckens et al. (1996) also showed that women in particular, as well as patients with a high number of somatic symptoms, were at risk of developing a negative course. Interestingly, at the same time it is shown that despite the relatively high temporal stability of somatoform diagnoses, the individual somatic symptoms show only a low stability (Steinbrecher & Hiller, 2011b). This confirms the clinical impression that symptoms within a patient can fluctuate greatly over time.

Research has also provided insight into predictors of adverse and persistent symptom course. Thus, the following predictive variables for a negative course emerged:

- Number of symptoms (e.g. Tomenson et al., 2013) or number of body regions affected by pain (e.g. Mallen et al., 2007),
- Duration of symptoms (e.g. Olde Hartman et al., 2009),
- Diversity of symptoms (e.g. Budtz-Lilly et al., 2015b),
- Symptom severity (e.g., Olde Hartman et al., 2009),
- Anxiety and depressive symptoms (e.g., Steinbrecher & Hiller, 2011b),
- Illness concerns (e.g., Tomenson et al., 2013),
- Attribution style (e.g., Hilbert et al., 2010),
- Fear avoidance and catastrophizing (e.g., Chou & Shekelle, 2010),
- Critical life events (e.g., Steinbrecher & Hiller, 2011a),
- Early childhood abuse experiences (e.g., Creed et al., 2012) or parental neglect (e.g., Craig et al., 1993); and
- Severe symptom-related disability in everyday life (e.g. Steinbrecher & Hiller, 2011b).

Single studies have shown that physical illness in parents during patients' childhood or somatic illness in patients' own childhood (e.g., Craig et al., 1993), social aspects such as withdrawal from key attachment figures (e.g. Hilbert et al., 2010) or unmarried relationship status (e.g., Creed et al., 2012) and demographic variables such as older age (e.g., Creed et al., 2012) and low educational level (e.g., Creed et al., 2012) are important negative predictors of symptom progression. According to the disorder criteria defined in the DSM-IV, somatic symptoms must first appear before the age of 30. Typically, however, affected individuals meet the diagnostic criteria by the age of 25, with the first symptoms usually appearing in adolescence (Saß et al., 2003). With increasing chronic manifestation, the chances of achieving a complete remission of the symptoms decrease, even with professional treatment. Thus, it becomes clear how important an early adequate diagnosis is, so that, if possible, an appropriate treatment can be initiated at an early stage of the disease history.

The findings regarding the influence of comorbid disorders on the course of multiple somatoform symptoms are ambiguous. On the one hand, correlations between depressive and anxiety symptoms and symptom chronification have been demonstrated (Leiknes et al., 2007a; Steinbrecher & Hiller, 2011a; Creed et al., 2012). On the other hand, in a study by B. Leibbrand et al. (1998), patients with comorbid anxiety and depressive disorder or comorbid personality disorder did not show a stronger symptom expression with regard to various psychopathological dimensions and also no higher impairment in the psychosocial level of functioning compared to somatoform patients with a low degree of comorbidity. The findings on the predictive value of comorbid disorders at the beginning of treatment on the course of therapy are also rather contradictory (Kolk et al., 2004; Rief et al., 1995; Leibbrand et al., 1999; Bleichhardt et al., 2005; Nakao et al., 2001).

Irrespective of this, however, Rief and Hiller (2011) rightly emphasize that in clinical practice a more complex psychopathology is to be expected when a larger number of comorbid disorders are present. The authors emphasize that when comorbidity is low, it is usually easier to clearly define treatment goals. They postulate that in certain cases, however, a comorbid disorder may also facilitate the treatment of somatoform symptoms. As an example, they list anxiety disorders, which are usually well treatable with cognitive behavior therapy and make it easier for patients to understand the psychophysiological connections of their somatic symptoms.

1.4.5 Health Economic Relevance: Persistent Somatic Symptoms and Healthcare Costs

Studies on health economic aspects show that the treatment of patients with multiple somatoform symptoms is very cost-intensive. This problem can be attributed to various factors. First of all, it must be taken into account that somatoform patients have often somatic perceptions of their symptoms. Accordingly, the negative results are often at odds with the perceptions of those affected (Murray et al., 2016). A relationship between an insecure attachment style and increased utilization behavior in somatoform patients has also been demonstrated (Taylor et al., 2012). Patients often insist that an organic cause must be found or they report their symptoms in a sometimes very emotional and complaining manner, which can put therapists and physicians under pressure and causes them to prescribe a medical intervention (Ring et al., 2004). In many cases, this problem puts enormous strain on the doctor-patient relationship (Wileman et al., 2002). Accordingly, it is not surprising that in a study by Hahn et al. (1996) it was shown that treating physicians categorize their patients with multisomatoform symptoms as "difficult". Moreover, the data from this study demonstrate very graphically that, conversely, patients are also dissatisfied and more frequently make use of various medical interventions.

Furthermore, a study by Anderson et al. (2008) showed that physicians of patients with multiple somatoform symptoms more often use unhelpful strategies, such as unnecessary diagnostic tests or symptom-contingent appointments. These behaviors are often the only way to reassure patients. However, these strategies also motivate an increased use of medical services, which drives up treatment costs. Moreover, it seems particularly problematic in light of the fact that patients with multiple somatoform symptoms who are frequently referred on are psychologically and physically more distressed than patients who are referred less frequently (McGorm et al., 2010). Thus, repeated referral to other specialists does not appear to be a particularly appropriate treatment strategy. While it may be important for the final clarification of a diagnosis, it does not help patients to better manage their symptoms. Moreover, it leads to little continuity of care. In a previously cited American study (Barsky et al., 2005), it was shown that primary care patients with multiple somatoform symptoms were 2–3 times more likely to have hospitalizations, outpatient examinations, and emergency department visits per year compared to patients without somatoform symptoms. In addition, somatoform patients were 1.5 times more likely to have primary care physician visits and 1.7 times more likely to have specialist consultations. The **total costs for medical services** were 2.3 times higher. Comparable findings were obtained in a study of a German sample (Hiller et al., 2003).

Furthermore, it must be taken into account that increased health care costs do not only result directly from increased utilization behavior—also called "doctor shopping"—but also from **indirect costs**, such as increased absenteeism at the workplace, frequent sick leave and early retirement. In a German study (Larisch et al., 2005), it was shown that 42.6% of patients with somatization symptoms had been unable to work in the last 3 months before the start of data collection. In a Danish study (Rask et al., 2015), patients with acute somatoform symptoms versus persistent somatoform disorder versus clearly defined physical illness were compared in terms of their disability pension. The sample with persistent somatoform disorder had the highest rate of disability pension (19.1%) and the highest risk of receiving a disability pension in the future.

> From these results, it appears that addressing the use of healthcare systems plays an important role in the psychotherapy of those affected.

At the same time, it must of course be emphasized that not all patients with multiple somatoform symptoms belong to the group of these "high-utilizers". On the contrary, somatoform patients show great heterogeneity in their utilization behavior (Weiß et al., 2016). However, in order to do justice to these patients as well, this treatment manual provides instructions on how patients can reduce their utilization behavior to an appropriate level (► Sect. 9.4). Good cooperation and consultation between the treating clinical psychologist and the responsible physician are crucial prerequisites for this.

References

American Psychiatric Association. (1980). *Diagnostic and statistical manual of mental disorders (DSM III)* (3rd ed.). American Psychiatric Press.

American Psychiatric Association. (2000). *Diagnostic and statistical manual for mental disorders. Fourth edition, text revision*. American Psychiatric Press.

American Psychiatric Association. (2013). *Diagnostic and statistical manual of mental disorders. Fifth edition. DSM-5*. APA.

Anderson, M., Hartz, A., Nordin, T., Rosenbaum, M., Noyes, R., James, P., et al. (2008). Community physicians' strategies for patients with medically unexplained symptoms. *Family Medicine, 40*(2), 111–118.

Arnold, I. A., de Waal, M. W. M., Eekhof, J. A. H., & van Helmert, A. M. (2006). Somatoform disorder in primary care: Course and need for cognitive-behavioral treatment. *Psychosomatics, 47*(6), 498–503. https://doi.org/10.1176/appi.psy.47.6.498

Barsky, A. J., Orav, E. J., & Bates, D. W. (2005). Somatization increases medical utilization and costs independent of psychiatric and medical comorbidity. *Archives of General Psychiatry, 62*(8), 903–910. https://doi.org/10.1001/archpsyc.62.8.903

Bleichhardt, G., Timmer, B., & Rief, W. (2005). Predictors for short- and long-term outcome in patients with somatoform disorders after cognitive-behavioral therapy. *Zeitschrift für Klinische Psychologie, Psychiatrie und Psychotherapie, 53*(1), 40–58.

Branco, J. C., Bannwarth, B., Failde, I., Carbonell, J. A., Blotman, F., Spaeth, M., et al. (2010). Prevalence of fibromyalgia: A survey in five European countries. *Seminars in Arthritis and Rheumatism, 39*(6), 448–453. https://doi.org/10.1016/j.semarthrit.2008.12.003

Breuer, J., & Freud, S. (1893). Über den Mechanismus hysterischer Phänomene. Vorläufige Mitteilung. *Neurologisches Zentralblatt, 12*(4–10), 43–47.

Bridges, K. W., & Goldberg, D. P. (1985). Somatic presentation of DSM-III psychiatric-disorders in primary care. *Journal of Psychosomatic Research, 29*(6), 563–569. https://doi.org/10.1016/0022-3999(85)90064-9

Briquet, P. (1895). *Traité de l'hystérie*. Bailliere et Fils.

Brown, R. J. (2004). Psychological mechanisms of medically unexplained symptoms: An integrative conceptual model. *Psychological Bulletin, 130*(5), 793–812. https://doi.org/10.1037/0033-2909.130.5.793

Brown, F. W., Golding, J. M., & Smith, G. R., Jr. (1990). Psychiatric comorbidity in primary care somatization disorder. *Psychosomatic Medicine, 52*(4), 445–451. https://doi.org/10.1097/00006842-199007000-00006

Budtz-Lilly, A., Schröder, A., Rask, M. T., Fink, P., Vestergaard, M., & Rosendal, M. (2015a). Bodily distress syndrome: A new diagnosis for functional disorders in primary care? *BMC Family Practice, 16*, 180. https://doi.org/10.1186/S12875-015-0393-8

Budtz-Lilly, A., Vestergaard, M., Fink, P., Carlsen, A. H., & Rosendal, M. (2015b). The prognosis of bodily distress syndrome: A cohort study in primary care. *General Hospital Psychiatry, 37*(6), 560–566. https://doi.org/10.1016/j.genhosppsych.2015.08.002

Burton, C. (2003). Beyond somatisation: A review of the understanding and treatment of medically unexplained physical symptoms (MUPS). *British Journal of General Practice, 53*(488), 231–241.

Chalder, T., Berelowitz, G., Pawlikowska, T., Watts, L., Wessely, S., Wright, D., et al. (1993). Development of a fatigue scale. *Journal of Psychosomatic Research, 37*(2), 147–153. https://doi.org/10.1016/0022-3999(93)90081-P

Chou, R., & Shekelle, P. (2010). Will this patient develop persistent disabling low back pain? *Journal of the American Medical Association, 303*(13), 1295–1302. https://doi.org/10.1001/jama.2010.344

Craig, T. K. J., Boardman, A. P., Mills, K., Dalyjones, O., & Drake, H. (1993). The South London somatization study I: Longitudinal course and the influence of early-life experiences. *British Journal of Psychiatry, 163*, 579–588. https://doi.org/10.1192/bjp.163.5.579

Creed, F. H., Davies, I., Jackson, J., Littlewood, A., Chew-Graham, C., Tomenson, B., et al. (2012). The epidemiology of multiple somatic symptoms. *Journal of Psychosomatic Research, 72*(4), 311–317. https://doi.org/10.1016/j.jpsychores.2012.01.009

Crombez, G., Beirens, K., van Damme, S., Eccleston, C., & Fontaine, J. (2009). The unbearable lightness of somatisation: A systematic review of the concept of somatisation in empirical studies of pain. *Pain, 145*(1–2), 31–35. https://doi.org/10.1016/j.pain.2009.04.006

de Waal, M. W., Arnold, I. A., Eekhof, J. A., & van Hemert, A. M. (2004). Somatoform disorders in general practice: Prevalence, functional impairment and comorbidity with anxiety and depressive disorders. *British Journal of Psychiatry, 184*(6), 470–476. https://doi.org/10.1192/bjp.184.6.470

Derogatis, L. R. (1983). *The SCL-90-R manual. Scoring and adminstration procedures for SCL-90-R*. John Hopkins University School of Medicine.

Dilling, H., & Freyberger, H. J. (2000). *Taschenführer zur Klassifikation psychischer Störungen*. Huber.

Dillmann, U., Nilges, P., Saile, H., & Gerbershagen, H. U. (1994). Assessing disability in chronic pain patients [Behinderungseinschatzung bei chronischen Schmerzpatienten]. *Schmerz, 8*(2), 100–110. https://doi.org/10.1007/BF02530415

Drossman, D. A. (2006). The functional gastrointestinal disorders and the Rome III process. *Gastroenterology, 130*(5), 1377–1390. https://doi.org/10.1053/j.gastro.2006.03.008

Eriksen, H. R., Hellesnes, B., Staff, P, & Ursin, H. (2004). Are subjective health complaints a result of modern civilization? *International Journal of Behavioral Medicine, 11*(2), 122–125. https://doi.org/10.1207/s15327558ijbm1102_9

Escobar, J. I., Rubio-Stipec, M., Canino, G., & Karno, M. (1989). Somatic symptom index (SSI): A new and abridged somatization construct. Prevalence and epidemiological correlates in two large community samples. *Journal of Nervous and Mental Disease, 177*(3), 140–146. https://doi.org/10.1097/00005053-198903000-00003

Falkai, P., Wittchen, H.-U., Döpfner, M., Gaebel, W., Maier, W., Rief, W., et al. (2015). *Diagnostisches und Statistisches Manual Psychischer Störungen. DSM-5*. Hogrefe.

Farooq, S., Gahir, M. S., Okyere, E., Sheikh, A. J., & Oyebode, F. (1995). Somatization: A transcultural study. *Journal of Psychosomatic Research, 39*(7), 883–888. https://doi.org/10.1016/0022-3999(94)00034-6

Fink, P. (1995). Psychiatric illness in patients with persistent somatisation. *British Journal of Psychiatry, 166*(1), 93–99. https://doi.org/10.1192/bjp.166.1.93

Fink, P., Ornbol, E., Toft, T., Sparle, K. C., Frostholm, L., & Olesen, F. (2004). A new, empirically established hypochondriasis diagnosis. *American Journal of Psychiatry, 161*(9), 1680–1691. https://doi.org/10.1176/appi.ajp.161.9.1680

First, M. B., Williams, J. B. W., Karg, R. S., & Spitzer, R. L. (2015). *Structured clinical interview for DSM-5 disorders, clinician version (SCID-5-CV)*. American Psychiatric Association.

Fröhlich, C., Jacobi, F., & Wittchen, H. U. (2006). DSM-IV pain disorder in the general population – An exploration of the structure and threshold of medically unexplained pain symptoms.

European Archives of Psychiatry and Clinical Neuroscience, 256(3), 187–196. https://doi.org/10.1007/s00406-005-0625-3

Fukuda, K., Straus, S. E., Hickie, I., Sharpe, M. C., Dobbins, G. J., et al. (1994). The chronic fatigue syndrome: A comprehensive approach to its definition and study. *Annals of Internal Medicine, 121*(12), 953–959. https://doi.org/10.7326/0003-4819-121-12-199412150-00009

Geissner, E. (2001). *Fragebogen zur Erfassung der Schmerzverarbeitung FESV*. Hogrefe.

Grabe, H. J., Meyer, C., Hapke, U., Rumpf, H. J., Freyberger, H. J., Dilling, H., et al. (2003). Specific somatoform disorder in the general population. *Psychosomatics, 44*(4), 304–311. https://doi.org/10.1176/appi.psy.44.4.304

Grundmann, O., & Yoon, S. L. (2010). Irritable bowel syndrome: Epidemiology, diagnosis and treatment: An update for health-care practitioners. *Journal of Gastroenterology and Hepatology, 25*(4), 691–699. https://doi.org/10.1111/j.1440-1746.2009.06120.x

Gureje, O. (2015). Classification of somatic syndromes in ICD-11. *Current Opinion in Psychiatry, 28*(5), 345–349. https://doi.org/10.1097/Yco.0000000000000186

Hahn, S. R., Kroenke, K., Spitzer, R. L., Brody, D., Williams, J. B., Linzer, M., et al. (1996). The difficult patient: Prevalence, psychopathology, and functional impairment. *Journal of General Internal Medicine, 11*(1), 1–8. https://doi.org/10.1007/BF02603477

Haller, H., Cramer, H., Lauche, R., & Dobos, G. (2015). Somatoform disorders and medically unexplained symptoms in primary care. *Deutsches Ärzteblatt International, 112*(16), 279–287. https://doi.org/10.3238/arztebl.2015.0279

Hanel, G., Henningsen, P., Herzog, W., Sauer, N., Schaefert, R., Szecsenyi, J., et al. (2009). Depression, anxiety, and somatoform disorders: Vague or distinct categories in primary care? Results from a large cross-sectional study. *Journal of Psychosomatic Research, 67*(3), 189–197. https://doi.org/10.1016/j.jpsychores.2009.04.013

Hilbert, A., Martin, A., Zech, T., Rauh, E., & Rief, W. (2010). Patients with medically unexplained symptoms and their significant others: Illness attributions and behaviors as predictors of patient functioning over time. *Journal of Psychosomatic Research, 68*(3), 253–262. https://doi.org/10.1016/j.jpsychores.2009.09.012

Hiller, W., & Rief, W. (2004). *Internationale Skalen für Hypochondrie. Deutschsprachige adaptation des Whiteley-index (WI) und der illness attitude scales (IAS) (Manual)*. Huber.

Hiller, W., & Rief, W. (2014). Abolishing the somatoform disorders by DSM-5 – An academic piece of bungling? [Die Abschaffung der somatoformenStörungen durch DSM-5 – Ein akademischer Schildbürgerstreich?]. *Psychotherapeut, 59*(6), 448–455. https://doi.org/10.1007/s00278-014-1081-1

Hiller, W., Rief, W., Elefant, S., Margraf, J., Kroymann, R., Leibbrand, R., et al. (1997a). Dysfunctional cognitions in patients with somatization syndrome. *Zeitschrift für Klinische Psychologie – Forschung und Praxis, 26*(3), 226–234.

Hiller, W., Rief, W., & Fichter, M. M. (1997b). How disabled are patients with somatoform disorders? *General Hospital Psychiatry, 19*(6), 432–438. https://doi.org/10.1016/S0163-8343(97)00071-6

Hiller, W., Zaudig, M., & Mombour, W. (1997c). *IDCL – Internationale Diagnosen Checklisten für DSM-IV und ICD-10*. Hogrefe.

Hiller, W., Fichter, M. M., & Rief, W. (2003). A controlled treatment study of somatoform disorders including analysis of healthcare utilization and cost-effectiveness. *Journal of Psychosomatic Research, 54*(4), 369–380. https://doi.org/10.1016/S0022-3999(02)00397-5

Hiller, W., Rief, W., & Brähler, E. (2006). Somatization in the population: From mild bodily misperceptions to disabling symptoms. *Social Psychiatry and Psychiatric Epidemiology, 41*(9), 704–712. https://doi.org/10.1007/s00127-006-0082-y

Jackson, J. L., & Kroenke, K. (2008). Prevalence, impact, and prognosis of multisomatoform disorder in primary care: A 5-year follow-up study. *Psychosomatic Medicine, 70*(4), 430–434. https://doi.org/10.1097/PSY.0b013e31816aa0ee

Jacobi, F., Wittchen, H. U., Holting, C., Hofler, M., Pfister, H., Muller, N., et al. (2004). Prevalence, co-morbidity and correlates of mental disorders in the general population: Results from the German Health Interview and Examination Survey (GHS). *Psychological Medicine, 34*(4), 597–611. https://doi.org/10.1017/S0033291703001399S0033291703001399

Janet, P. (1889). *L'automatisme psychologique*. Alcan.

Jason, L. A., Richman, J. A., Rademaker, A. W., Jordan, K. M., Plioplys, A. V., Taylor, R. R., et al. (1999). A community-based study of chronic fatigue syndrome. *Archives of Internal Medicine, 159*(18), 2129–2137. https://doi.org/10.1001/archinte.159.18.2129

Kapfhammer, H. P. (2001). Somatoforme Störungen – Historische Entwicklungen und moderne diagnostische Konzeptualisierung. *Nervenarzt, 72*(7), 487–500.

Kapfhammer, H. P. (2007). Pierre Briquet (1796–1881) – Von der polysymptomatischen Hysterie zur Somatisierungsstörung der modernen psychiatrischen Klassifikationssysteme. *Psychosomatik und Konsiliarpsychiatrie, 1*(2), 81–84.

Kawanishi, Y. (1992). Somatization of Asians: An artifact of Western medicalization? *Transcultural Psychiatric Research Review, 29*(1), 5–36. https://doi.org/10.1177/136346159202900101

Kempke, S., Van den Eede, F., Schotte, C., Claes, S., Van Wambeke, P., Van Houdenhove, B., et al. (2013). Prevalence of DSM-IV personality disorders in patients with chronic fatigue syndrome: A controlled study. *International Journal of Behavioral Medicine, 20*(2), 219–228. https://doi.org/10.1007/s12529-012-9273-y

Khoo, E. M., Mathers, N. J., McCarthy, S. A., & Low, W. Y. (2012). Somatisation disorder and its associated factors in multiethnic primary care clinic attenders. *International Journal of Behavioral Medicine, 19*(2), 165–173. https://doi.org/10.1007/s12529-011-9164-7

Kirmayer, L. J., & Robbins, J. M. (1991). Three forms of somatization in primary care: Prevalence, co-occurrence, and sociodemographic characteristics. *Journal of Nervous and Mental Disease, 179*(11), 647–655. https://doi.org/10.1097/00005053-199809000-00006

Kirmayer, L. J., & Young, A. (1998). Culture and somatization: Clinical, epidemiological, and ethnographic perspectives. *Psychosomatic Medicine, 60*(4), 420–430. https://doi.org/10.1097/00006842-199807000-00006

Kohrt, B. A., Hruschka, D. J., Kohrt, H. E., Panebianco, N. L., & Tsagaankhuu, G. (2004). Distribution of distress in post-socialist Mongolia: A cultural epidemiology of yadargaa. *Social Science & Medicine, 58*(3), 471–485. https://doi.org/10.1016/S0277-9536(03)00216-8

Kohrt, B. A., Rasmussen, A., Kaiser, B. N., Haroz, E. E., Maharjan, S. M., Mutamba, B. B., et al. (2014). Cultural concepts of distress and psychiatric disorders: Literature review and research recommendations for global mental health epidemiology. *International Journal of Epidemiology, 43*(2), 365–406. https://doi.org/10.1093/ije/dyt227

Kolk, A. M. M., Schagen, S., & Hanewald, G. J. F. P. (2004). Multiple medically unexplained physical symptoms and health care utilization. Outcome of psychological intervention and patient-related predictors of change. *Journal of Psychosomatic Research, 57*(4), 379–389. https://doi.org/10.1016/j.jpsychores.2004.02.012

Kroenke, K., Spitzer, R. L., Williams, J. B., Linzer, M., Hahn, S. R., deGruy, F. V., et al. (1994). Physical symptoms in primary care. Predictors of psychiatric disorders and functional impairment. *Archives of Family Medicine, 3*(9), 774–779.

Kroenke, K., Spitzer, R. L., deGruy, F. V., 3rd, Hahn, S. R., Linzer, M., Williams, J. B., et al. (1997). Multisomatoform disorder. An alternative to undifferentiated somatoform disorder for the somatizing patient in primary care. *Archives of General Psychiatry, 54*(4), 352–358. https://doi.org/10.1001/archpsyc.1997.01830160080011

Kroenke, K., Spitzer, R. L., & Williams, J. B. W. (2002). The PHQ-15: Validity of a new measure for evaluating the severity of somatic symptoms. *Psychosomatic Medicine, 64*(2), 258–266. https://doi.org/10.1097/00006842-200203000-00008

Larisch, A., Fisch, V., & Fritzsche, K. (2005). Kosten-Nutzen-Aspekte psychosozialer Interventionen bei somatisierenden Patienten in der Hausarztpraxis. *Zeitschrift für Klinische Psychologie und Psychotherapie, 34*(4), 282–290.

Leibbrand, B., Schröder, A., Hiller, W., & Fichter, M. (1998). Komorbide Persönlichkeitsstörungen: Ein negativer Prädiktor für den Therapieerfolg bei somatoformen Störungen. *Zeitschrift für Klinische Psychologie und Psychotherapie, 27*(4), 227–233.

Leibbrand, R., Hiller, W., & Fichter, M. (1999). Influence of personality disorders on therapy outcome in somatoform disorders at 2-year follow-up. *Journal of Nervous and Mental Disease, 187*(8), 509–512. https://doi.org/10.1097/00005053-199908000-00008

Leiknes, K. A., Finset, A., Moum, T., & Sandanger, I. (2007a). Course and predictors of medically unexplained pain symptoms in the general population. *Journal of Psychosomatic Research, 62*(2), 119–128. https://doi.org/10.1016/j.jpsychores.2006.08.009

Leiknes, K. A., Finset, A., Moum, T., & Sandanger, I. (2007b). Current somatoform disorders in Norway: Prevalence, risk factors and comorbidity with anxiety, depression and musculoskeletal disorders. *Social Psychiatry and Psychiatric Epidemiology, 42*(9), 698–710. https://doi.org/10.1007/s00127-007-0218-8

Lipowski, Z. J. (1988). Somatization – The concept and its clinical application. *American Journal of Psychiatry, 145*(11), 1358–1368.

Longley, S. L., Watson, D., & Noyes, R., Jr. (2005). Assessment of the hypochondriasis domain: The multidimensional inventory of hypochondriacal traits (MIHT). *Psychological Assessment, 17*(1), 3–14. https://doi.org/10.1037/1040-3590.17.1.3

Löwe, B., Spitzer, R. L., Zipfel, S., & Herzog, W. (2002). *PHQ-D Gesundheitsfragebogen für Patienten, 2. Auflage, Manual Komplettversion und Kurzform, Autorisierte deutsche Version des Prime MD Patient Health Questionnaire (PHQ)*. Pfizer.

Löwe, B., Spitzer, R. L., Williams, J. B. W., Mussell, M., Schellberg, D., & Kroenke, K. (2008). Depression, anxiety and somatization in primary care: Syndrome overlap and functional impairment. *General Hospital Psychiatry, 30*(3), 191–199. https://doi.org/10.1016/j.genhosppsych.2008.01.001

Mallen, C. D., Peat, G., Thomas, E., Dunn, K. M., & Croft, P. R. (2007). Prognostic factors for musculoskeletal pain in primary care: A systematic review. *British Journal of General Practice, 57*(541), 655–661.

Margraf, J., Schneider, S., & Ehlers, A. (1994). *DIPS – Diagnostisches Interview bei Psychischen Störungen* (Bd. 2). Springer.

Marin, C., & Carron, R. (2002). The origin of the concept of somatization. *Psychosomatics, 43*(3), 249–250. https://doi.org/10.1176/appi.psy.43.3.249

Martin, A., Staufenbiel, T., Gaab, J., Rief, W., & Brähler, E. (2010). Messung chronischer Erschöpfung – Teststatistische Prüfung der Fatigue Skala (FS). *Zeitschrift für Klinische Psychologie und Psychotherapie, 39*(1), 33–44.

McAteer, A., Elliott, A. M., & Hannaford, P. C. (2011). Ascertaining the size of the symptom iceberg in a UK-wide community-based survey. *British Journal of General Practice, 61*(582), e1–e11. https://doi.org/10.3399/bjgp11X548910

McGorm, K., Burton, C., Weller, D., Murray, G., & Sharpe, M. (2010). Patients repeatedly referred to secondary care with symptoms unexplained by organic disease: Prevalence, characteristics and referral pattern. *Family Practice, 27*(5), 479–486. https://doi.org/10.1093/fampra/cmq053

Mehl-Madrona, L. E. (2008). Prevalence of psychiatric diagnoses among frequent users of rural emergency medical services. *Canadian Journal of Rural Medicine, 13*(1), 22–30.

Mewes, R., Rief, W., Stenzel, N., Glaesmer, H., Martin, A., & Brahler, E. (2009). What is "normal" disability? An investigation of disability in the general population. *Pain, 142*(1–2), 36–41. https://doi.org/10.1016/j.pain.2008.11.007

Min, S. K., & Suh, S. Y. (2010). The anger syndrome hwa-byung and its comorbidity. *Journal of Affective Disorders, 124*(1–2), 211–214. https://doi.org/10.1016/j.jad.2009.10.011

Morschitzky, H. (2007). *Somatoforme Störungen: Diagnostik, Konzepte und Therapie bei Körpersymptomen ohne Organbefund*. Springer.

Murray, A. M., Toussaint, A., Althaus, A., & Löwe, B. (2016). The challenge of diagnosing non-specific, functional, and somatoform disorders: A systematic review of barriers to diagnosis in primary care. *Journal of Psychosomatic Research, 80*, 1–10. https://doi.org/10.1016/j.jpsychores.2015.11.002

Nacul, L. C., Lacerda, E. M., Pheby, D., Campion, P., Molokhia, M., Fayyaz, S., et al. (2011). Prevalence of myalgic encephalomyelitis/chronic fatigue syndrome (ME/CFS) in three regions of England: A repeated cross-sectional study in primary care. *BMC Medicine, 9*, 91. https://doi.org/10.1186/1741-7015-9-91

Nakao, M., Myers, P., Fricchione, G., Zuttermeister, P. C., Barsky, A. J., & Benson, H. (2001). Somatization and symptom reduction through a behavioral medicine intervention in a mind/body medicine clinic. *Behavioral Medicine, 26*(4), 169–176.

Nilges, P., & Rief, W. (2010). F45.41 Chronic pain disorder with somatic and psychological factors. A coding aid [F45.41 Chronische Schmerzstörung mit somatischen und psychischen Faktoren]. *Schmerz, 24*(3), 209–212. https://doi.org/10.1007/s00482-010-0908-0

Nimnuan, C., Hotopf, M., & Wessely, S. (2001). Medically unexplained symptoms: An epidemiological study in seven specialities. *Journal of Psychosomatic Research, 51*(1), 361–367. https://doi.org/10.1016/s0022-3999(01)00223-9

Olde Hartman, T. C., Borghuis, M. S., Lucassen, P. L. B. J., van de Laar, F. A., Speckens, A. E., & van Weel, C. (2009). Medically unexplained symptoms, somatisation disorder and hypochondriasis: Course and prognosis. A systematic review. *Journal of Psychosomatic Research, 66*(5), 363–377. https://doi.org/10.1016/j.jpsychores.2008.09.018

Piccinelli, M., & Simon, G. (1997). Gender and cross-cultural differences in somatic symptoms associated with emotional distress. An international study in primary care. *Psychological Medicine, 27*(2), 433–444. https://doi.org/10.1017/S0033291796004539

Rask, M. T., Rosendal, M., Fenger-Gron, M., Bro, F., Ornbol, E., & Fink, P. (2015). Sick leave and work disability in primary care patients with recent-onset multiple medically unexplained symptoms and persistent somatoform disorders: A 10-year follow-up of the FIP study. *General Hospital Psychiatry, 37*(1), 53–59. https://doi.org/10.1016/j.genhosppsych.2014.10.007

Rey, E., & Talley, N. J. (2009). Irritable bowel syndrome: Novel views on the epidemiology and potential risk factors. *Digestive and Liver Disease, 41*(11), 772–780. https://doi.org/10.1016/j.dld.2009.07.005

Reyes, M., Nisenbaum, R., Hoaglin, D. C., Unger, E. R., Emmons, C., Randall, C., et al. (2003). Prevalence and incidence of chronic fatigue syndrome in Wichita, Kansas. *Archives of Internal Medicine, 163*(13), 1530–1536. https://doi.org/10.1001/archinte.163.13.1530

Rief, W. (1995). *Multiple somatoforme Symptome und Hypochondrie*. Huber.

Rief, W., & Hiller, W. (1999). Toward empirically based criteria for the classification of somatoform disorders. *Journal of Psychosomatic Research, 46*(6), 507–518. https://doi.org/10.1016/S0022-3999(99)00023-9

Rief, W., & Hiller, W. (2008). *SOMS – Das Screening für Somatoforme Störungen. Manual zum Fragebogen* (4. Aufl.). Huber.

Rief, W., & Hiller, W. (2011). *Somatisierungsstörung* (Bd. 1, Fortschritte der Psychotherapie). Hogrefe.

Rief, W., & Martin, A. (2014). How to use the new DSM-5 somatic symptom disorder diagnosis in research and practice: A critical evaluation and a proposal for modifications. *Annual Review of Clinical Psychology, 10*, 339–367. https://doi.org/10.1146/annurev-clinpsy-032813-153745

Rief, W., Schaefer, S., Hiller, W., & Fichter, M. M. (1992). Lifetime diagnoses in patients with somatoform disorders: Which came first? *European Archives of Psychiatry and Clinical Neuroscience, 241*(4), 236–240.

Rief, W., Hiller, W., Geissner, E., & Fichter, M. M. (1995). A two-year follow-up study of patients with somatoform disorders. *Psychosomatics, 36*(4), 376–386. https://doi.org/10.1016/S0033-3182(95)71647-4

Rief, W., Hessel, A., & Brähler, E. (2001). Somatization symptoms and hypochondriacal features in the general population. *Psychosomatic Medicine, 63*(4), 595–602. https://doi.org/10.1007/BF02190259

Rief, W., Ihle, D., & Pilger, F. (2003). A new approach to assess illness behaviour. *Journal of Psychosomatic Research, 54*(5), 405–414. https://doi.org/10.1016/S0022-3999(02)00401-4

Ring, A., Dowrick, C., Humphris, G., & Salmon, P. (2004). Do patients with unexplained physical symptoms pressurise general practitioners for somatic treatment? A qualitative study. *British Medical Journal, 328*(7447), 1057–1060. https://doi.org/10.1136/bmj.38057.622639.EE

Rivera-Tovar, A. D., & Frank, E. (1990). Late luteal phase dysphoric disorder in young women. *American Journal of Psychiatry, 147*(12), 1634–1636. https://doi.org/10.1176/ajp.147.12.1634

Robins, L. N., & Regier, D. A. (Eds.). (1991). *Psychiatric disorders in America: The epidemiological catchment area study*. The Free Press.

Rost, K. M., Akins, R. N., Brown, F. W., & Smith, G. R. (1992). The comorbidity of DSM-III-R personality disorders in somatization disorder. *General Hospital Psychiatry, 14*(5), 322–326. https://doi.org/10.1016/0163-8343(92)90066-J

Ryder, A. G., Yang, J., Zhu, X. Z., Yao, S. Q., Yi, J. Y., Heine, S. J., et al. (2008). The cultural shaping of depression: Somatic symptoms in China, psychological symptoms in North America? *Journal of Abnormal Psychology, 117*(2), 300–313. https://doi.org/10.1037/0021-843x.117.2.300

Saß, H., Wittchen, H.-U., Zaudig, M., & Houben, I. (Eds.). (2003). *Diagnostische und Statistisches Manual Psychischer Störungen. Textrevision. DSM-IV-TR*. Hogrefe.

Simon, G., Gater, R., Kisely, S., & Piccinelli, M. (1996). Somatic symptoms of distress: An international primary care study. *Psychosomatic Medicine, 58*(5), 481–488. https://doi.org/10.1097/00006842-199609000-00010

Soares, C. N., Cohen, L. S., Otto, M. W., & Harlow, B. L. (2001). Characteristics of women with premenstrual dysphoric disorder (PMDD) who did or did not report history of depression: A preliminary report from the Harvard Study of Moods and Cycles. *Journal of Womens Health & Gender-Based Medicine, 10*(9), 873–878. https://doi.org/10.1089/152460901753285778

Speckens, A. E., van Hemert, A. M., Spinhoven, P., & Bolk, J. H. (1996). The diagnostic and prognostic significance of the whitely index, the illness attitude scales and the somatosensory amplification scale. *Psychological Medicine, 26*(5), 1085–1090. https://doi.org/10.1017/S0033291700035418

Steinbrecher, N., & Hiller, W. (2011a). Course and prediction of somatoform disorder and medically unexplained symptoms in primary care. *General Hospital Psychiatry, 33*, 318–326. https://doi.org/10.1016/j.genhosppsych.2011.05.002

Steinbrecher, N., & Hiller, W. (2011b). Examination of the stability of medically unexplained symptoms and somatoform disorders over time within the context of different diagnostic concepts. *Psychotherapie Psychosomatik Medizinische Psychologie, 61*(8), 356–363. https://doi.org/10.1055/s-0031-1277167

Stekel, W. (1908). *Nervöse Angstzustände und ihre Behandlung*. Urban & Schwarzenberg.

Stekel, W. (1935). *Fortschritte und Technik der Traumdeutung*. Weidmann.

Sumathipala, A., Siribaddana, S. H., & Bhugra, D. (2004). Culture-bound syndromes: The story of dhat syndrome. *British Journal of Psychiatry, 184*(3), 200–209. https://doi.org/10.1192/bjp.184.3.200

Taylor, R. E., Marshall, T., Mann, A., & Goldberg, D. P. (2012). Insecure attachment and frequent attendance in primary care: A longitudinal cohort study of medically unexplained symptom presentations in ten UK general practices. *Psychological Medicine, 42*(4), 855–864. https://doi.org/10.1017/S0033291711001589

Thompson, W. G., Longstreth, G. F., Drossman, D. A., Heaton, K. W., Irvine, E. J., & Muller-Lissner, S. A. (1999). Functional bowel disorders and functional abdominal pain. *Gut, 45*(Suppl. 2), 43–47. https://doi.org/10.1136/gut.45.2008.ii43

Thompson, W. G., Heaton, K. W., Smyth, G. T., & Smyth, C. (2000). Irritable bowel syndrome in general practice: Prevalence, characteristics, and referral. *Gut, 46*(1), 78–82. https://doi.org/10.1136/Gut.46.1.78

Tomenson, B., Essau, C., Jacobi, F., Ladwig, K. H., Leiknes, K. A., Lieb, R., et al. (2013). Total somatic symptom score as a predictor of health outcome in somatic symptom disorders. *British Journal of Psychiatry, 203*(5), 373–380. https://doi.org/10.1192/bjp.bp.112.114405

Üstun, T., & Sartorius, N. (1995). *Mental illness in primary care: An international study*. Wiley.

van Eck van der Sluijs, J. V., Ten Have, M., Rijnders, C., van Marwijk, H., de Graaf, R., & van der Feltz-Cornelis, C. (2015). Medically unexplained and explained physical symptoms in the general population: Association with prevalent and incident mental disorders. *PLoS One, 10*(4), e0123274. https://doi.org/10.1371/journal.pone.0123274

Verhaak, P. F., Meijer, S. A., Visser, A. P., & Wolters, G. (2006). Persistent presentation of medically unexplained symptoms in general practice. *Family Practice, 23*(4), 414–420. https://doi.org/10.1093/fampra/cml016

Weiß, F. D., Rief, W., Gottschalk, J.-M., Schwarz, J., & Kleinstäuber, M. (2016). Health care use and the role of health anxiety and disability in an outpatient sample of patients with somatoform disorders. *International Journal of Behavioral Medicine, 23*(Suppl. 1), S244. https://doi.org/10.1007/s12529-016-9586-3

Wessely, S., Nimnuan, C., & Sharpe, M. (1999). Functional somatic syndromes: One or many? *Lancet, 354*(9182), 936–939. https://doi.org/10.1016/S0140-6736(98)08320-2

White, K. P., Speechley, M., Harth, M., & Ostbye, T. (1999). The London Fibromyalgia Epidemiology Study: Comparing the demographic and clinical characteristics in 100 random community cases of fibromyalgia versus controls. *Journal of Rheumatology, 26*(7), 1577–1585.

Wiborg, J. F., Gieseler, D., Fabisch, A. B., Voigt, K., Lautenbach, A., & Löwe, B. (2013). Suicidality in primary care patients with somatoform disorders. *Psychosomatic Medicine, 75*(9), 800–806. https://doi.org/10.1097/Psy.0000000000000013

Wileman, L., May, C., & Chew-Graham, C. A. (2002). Medically unexplained symptoms and the problem of power in the primary care consultation: A qualitative study. *Family Practice, 19*(2), 178–182. https://doi.org/10.1093/fampra/19.2.178

Wittchen, H.-U., & Pfister, H. (1997). *DIA-X-interviews. Manuale und Auswertungsprogramm*. Swets und Zeitlinger.

Wittchen, H.-U., Schramm, E., Zaudig, M., & Unland, H. (1997). *SKID – Strukturiertes klinisches Interview für DSM-IV, Achse I, deutsche Version*. Hogrefe.

Wittchen, H.-U., Pfister, H., & Garcynski, E. (1998). *CIDI – Composite International Diagnostic Interview nach ICD-10 und DSM-IV (der Weltgesundheitsorganisation). Deutsche Version*. Hogrefe.

Wittchen, H. U., Jacobi, F., Rehm, J., Gustavsson, A., Svensson, M., Jonsson, B., et al. (2011). The size and burden of mental disorders and other disorders of the brain in Europe 2010. *European Neuropsychopharmacology, 21*(9), 655–679. https://doi.org/10.1016/j.euroneuro.2011.07.018

Witthöft, M., Haaf, A., Rist, F., & Bailer, J. (2010). Erfassung von Krankheitsangst mit dem Multidimensional Inventory of Hypochondriacal Traits (MIHT). *Diagnostica, 56*(1), 2–12. https://doi.org/10.1026/0012-1924/a000005

World Health Organization. (1992). *International statistical classification of diseases. 10th revision (ICD-10)*. World Health Organization.

World Health Organization. (1996). *International statistical classification of diseases. 10th revision (ICD-10)*. World Health Organization.

Theories, Models and Concepts of Persistent Somatic Symptoms, Somatoform Disorders, and Somatic Symptom Disorders

Contents

M. Kleinstäuber et al., *Cognitive Behavior Therapy for Persistent Somatic Symptoms and Somatic Symptom Disorder*, https://doi.org/10.1007/978-3-662-69726-9_2

2.1 Concept of Somatosensory Amplification

The concept of somatosensory amplification was proposed by Barsky et al. (1990) and describes the tendency to perceive normal body sensations as intense, dangerous, and disturbing (◘ Fig. 2.1). Part of the concept is a catastrophizing evaluation of harmless and everyday body sensations (e.g., tingling in arms and legs) as signs of serious illness (e.g., degenerative nerve disease). Here it becomes clear that this concept has a closer relationship to the disorder pattern of illness anxiety disorder, which is increasingly defined as an anxiety disorder rather than a variant of somatoform disorders. Barsky himself was very early to point out closer references of the concept of somatosensory amplification to hypochondriasis or illness anxiety disorder as compared to symptom-related somatoform disorders (e.g., Barsky et al., 1990). It should additionally be critically noted that the concept of somatosensory amplification has so far been investigated and confirmed almost exclusively by questionnaire procedures. Unfortunately, only few experimental findings on objectively altered somatosensory perception and evaluation processes in patients with somatoform disorders are available so far. Overall, therefore, the concept of somatosensory amplification appears to be more descriptive than explicative in nature and, moreover, more relevant in individuals with illness anxiety compared to individuals with symptom-related somatoform disorders.

The somatosensory amplification model forms the core concept of the cognitive-behavioral models of somatoform disorders that we will outline below.

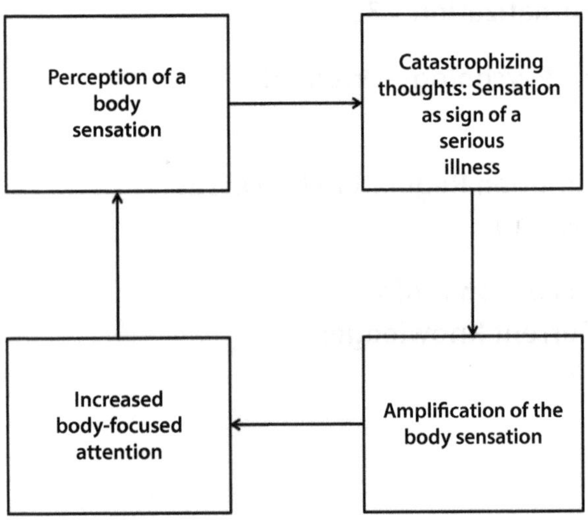

◘ **Fig. 2.1** Barsky's model of somatosensory amplification. (Based on Barsky et al. (1990))

2.2 Cognitive-Behavioral Models

The model of the development and maintenance of somatoform disorders formulated by Rief and Hiller (1998, 2011) takes up the mechanism of somatosensory amplification, but additionally addresses potential triggers and behavioral consequences of somatic symptoms. The model is illustrated in ◘ Fig. 2.2. As possible triggers for the development of somatoform symptoms, this model postulates increased physiological states of arousal (e.g., as a consequence of persistent psychosocial stressors), prolonged episodes of primarily somatic illnesses (e.g., infections) or also illness-related media reports, whereby the latter media factors in all probability assume a higher significance in the genesis of illness anxiety or special functional syndromes (such as the idiopathic environmental intolerances). As a consequence of these triggering conditions, physical changes may develop that are increasingly perceived with heightened attention and possibly (mis)interpreted in a catastrophizing manner. Following the approach of somatosensory amplification, amplification of the somatic sensations and thus an increased symptom experience occurs as a result of increased attention.

> In the relevant literature, there is an increasing differentiation between body sensations and body symptoms. A certain body sensation only becomes a symptom through a negative evaluation.

According to Rief and Hiller's model, consequences at the behavioral level in particular determine whether the vicious circle of symptom perception, catastrophizing misinterpretation and symptom amplification (i.e. somatosensory amplification) is maintained. In this sense, "maintaining behaviors" include, excessive scanning and checking of one's own body for signs of a possible illness ("**scanning**"), frequent repeated visits to the doctor, the initiation of many medical examinations as well as increased medication intake and a tendency toward **avoidance behavior**. Checking and avoidance behaviors can vary greatly from individual to individual. Examples of checking behaviors include excessive blood pressure checks, checking one's pulse rate, or excessive examinations of one's bowel movements (e.g., looking for signs of bleeding in the bowel). Typical avoidance behaviors include, for example, reducing physical activity or following certain diets in cases of functional gastrointestinal disorders (e.g., irritable bowel syndrome). The medium- and long-term dysfunctional effect of avoidance behaviors is mainly to be seen in an increasing sensitization of the organism, which in turn favors new symptom perceptions. For example, increased physical

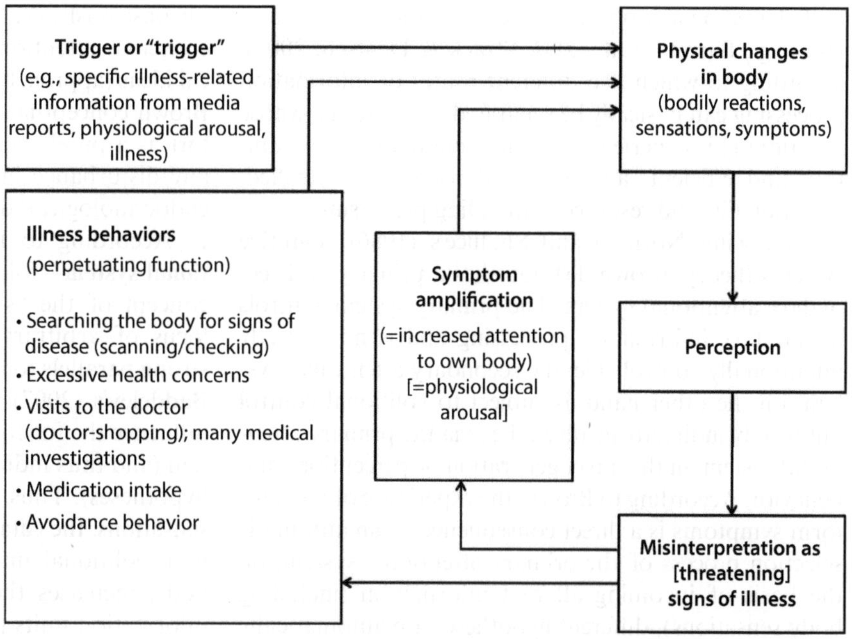

Fig. 2.2 Model of somatoform disorders. (Based on Rief and Hiller (2011))

inactivity leads to a decrease in physical fitness and thus to increased symptoms of stress and fatigue at a previously well-tolerated level of physical stress. In the case of the gastrointestinal symptoms mentioned, dietary behavior without a clear indication, e.g., due to an allergy, can cause an increasing sensitization of the gastrointestinal system, which subsequently reacts more and more strongly to "unfamiliar" foods.

It should be noted that the cognitive-behavioral model of somatoform disorders outlined in Fig. 2.2 shows great similarity to the model of panic disorder (Clark, 1986). In contrast to panic disorder, however, somatosensory amplification in the context of somatoform disorders typically does not lead to rapid-onset anxiety attacks, but rather to more sluggish, gradual amplification of somatic symptoms over time.

In the English-speaking context, a similar multifactorial model of the development and maintenance of somatoform symptoms was formulated by Kirmayer and Taillefer (1997). According to this model, physiological changes (either due to medical factors or due to strong emotional arousal) lead to an increase in body-focused attention, an increased risk of interpreting bodily sensations as signs of illness, as well as to increased worries and catastrophizing thoughts regarding a feared illness. On the behavioral level, this results in help-seeking behavior (from friends, physicians and relatives) and avoidance behavior with regard to physical activity. Within this model, neuroticism and absorption (in the sense of increased suggestibility) are also named as predisposing personality traits that increase the risk of entering the aforementioned vicious circle. In addition, this model names possible social maintaining factors (such as financial compensations, social attention and support), which are sometimes also referred to as "secondary gain".

It should be critically noted with regard to the cognitive-behavioral conceptualizations of somatoform disorders that they do not explicitly differentiate between different types of somatization (e.g., in the sense of Kirmayer & Robbins, 1991) (in particular, there is no clear differentiation between illness anxiety and somatoform symptoms; Brown, 2004). Moreover, in the approaches outlined, it remains open whether the perceptual and evaluative processes of body sensations and symptoms described are conscious processes subject to voluntary control, or whether processes of automatic, preconscious information processing may play a more central role in the development and maintenance of somatoform symptoms. The latter position is supported by cognitive psychology and constructivist considerations that have led to the formulation of innovative models of the genesis and maintenance of somatoform disorders (Brown, 2004; Van den Bergh et al., 2017), which we discuss in more detail below.

2.3 Integrative Conceptual Model

The model of the emergence of somatoform disorders proposed by Brown (2004) is based on the historical concepts of **dissociation** and **conversion** outlined above and also draws on the cognitive-behavioral model conceptions of somatoform symptoms outlined earlier. However, the focus of the model is on how exactly somatoform symptoms arise within the cognitive system, rather than on how to explain the behavioral consequences of increased symptom perception. Brown's model is essentially based on a two-process theory of the cognitive system (e.g., Barrett et al., 2004; Strack & Deutsch, 2004), according to which two different routes of information processing can basically be separated: a fast route, whose functioning is experienced as fast, unintentionally, intuitive, and efficient, and a second route of controlled, intentionally, and resource-demanding processing.

Following Norman and Shallice's (1986) cognitive systems theory, Brown distinguishes a primary and secondary attentional system. The primary system controls involuntary information processing and is not directly intentionally controllable; the secondary attentional system, on the other hand, is subject to volitional control but is only indirectly involved, i.e., via the primary attentional system, in the direct generation of perceptions and behavior. According to Brown, the experience of somatoform symptoms is a direct consequence of an automatic selection process of the primary attentional system: on the basis of incoming afferent information (including body sensations), different hypotheses are automatically generated in parallel by the cognitive system. The primary attentional system automatically selects one of these hypotheses and thus decides whether a bodily sensation becomes salient in the sense of a symptom experience at the conscious level. In this context, Brown speaks of "symptom representations" that exist within the cognitive system due to previous experiences (e.g., physical illness, traumatization, or even experience of severe illness in others) and are selected and activated by the **primary attentional system**. From this it is clear that Brown interprets the experience of bodily discomfort as the result of a constructive mental process within somatosensory information processing that operates essentially unconsciously, i.e., without necessary volitional effort or conscious attention. In contrast to other psychobiological ideas (approach of Rief & Barsky, 2005; ► Sect. 2.4), Brown conceptualizes the experience of bodily discomfort as a purely cognitive process that does not require any disturbance in the physiological (e.g., neuronal or endocrinological) domain.

According to Brown (2004), the **secondary attentional system**—following Norman and Shallice's (1986) concept of the "supervisory attentional system" as a locus of arbitrary decisions, which conceptually has strong parallels to the concept of the central executive in Baddeley's (2007) working memory model—is able to influence the functioning of the primary attentional system (and thus indirectly also the selection of perceptual hypotheses). Thus, a conscious, chronic focus on bodily sensations, the catastrophizing of which, in conjunction with volitional intense preoccupation with one's own body, increases the activation level of corresponding information units (e.g., symptom representations), may lay the base for the development of bodily sensations (through selection of symptom representations) by the primary attentional system. Deceptively, however, the final process of generating a symptom perception is completely automatic and involuntary, being directly controlled by the primary attentional system (accompanied by feelings of helplessness and lack of control). It follows from Brown's model that all cognitive and behavioral activities that focus on the subject of illness and possible bodily symptoms are indirectly involved in the development and maintenance of somatoform symptoms. The central components of Brown's model are shown in ◘ Fig. 2.3.

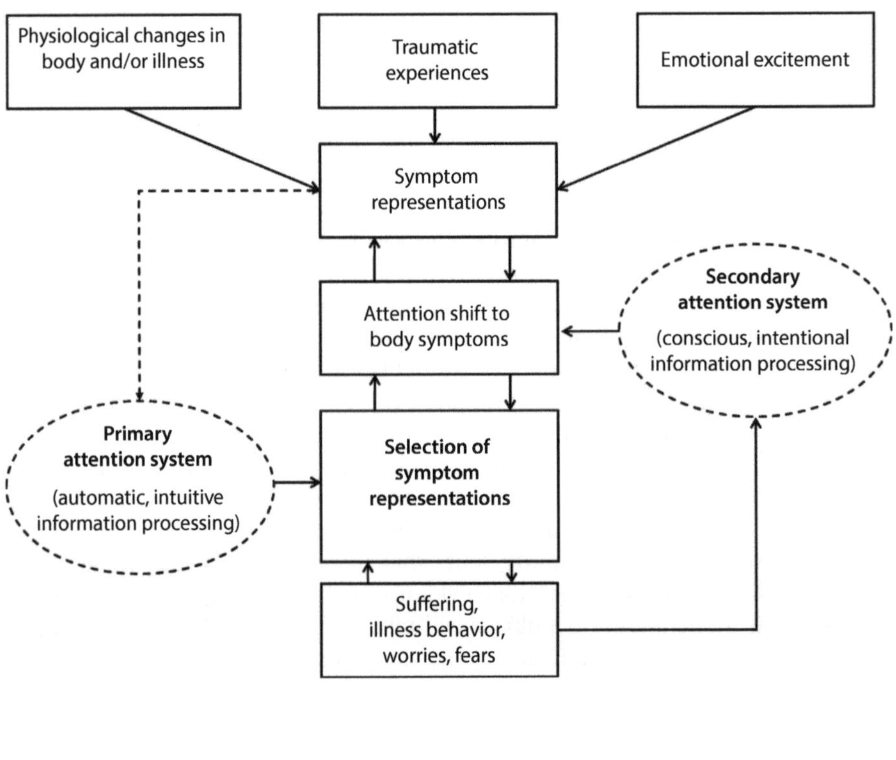

◘ **Fig. 2.3** The integrative conceptual model of somatoform symptoms according to Brown. (Based on Brown (2004))

A critical aspect of Brown's model is that aspects of learning theory, which could be involved in the maintenance of the symptoms, have not yet been taken into account. Also, the proposed model focuses mainly on the genesis of functional neurological symptoms and excludes adjacent phenomena, such as functional disorders (e.g., irritable bowel syndrome or fibromyalgia), for no apparent reason. In addition, empirical evidence to support the proposed model is unfortunately scarce to date.

The model of the emergence and maintenance of somatoform symptoms proposed by Brown differs fundamentally from previous concepts of symptom perception (e.g., somatosensory amplification model and cognitive-behavioral model) in that no peripheral physiological changes ("arousal") are assumed to be necessary conditions for the emergence of body sensations. This idea of symptom emergence based on constructive perceptual processes within the cognitive system has recently been taken up by Van den Bergh et al. (2017) and extended to a general model of symptom perception in the domain of persistent somatic symptoms. Based on Helmholtz's work, according to which perceptual processes do not represent a passive reception of environmental stimuli, but are based on active model-guided and inferential processes in the sense of hypothesis testing, this model conceptualizes the process of symptom generation as a probabilistic decision of the cognitive system, which is based on previous experiences and, based on these experiences, generates or interprets current sensations according to the principle of maximum likelihood. Crucial for the generation of symptom perceptions is thus an internal probabilistic model that is based on previous experiences and processes and categorizes current sensations against the background of this model. Similar principles of model-based inferential perception have been postulated for the domain of visual and auditory perception in both "healthy" and psychopathological phenomena (e.g., hallucinations and delusions in schizophrenia; Friston et al., 2016) and can be described mathematically using Bayesian models of the probability of conditional events. Discrepancies between subjective symptom perception and lack of pathological physical findings, characteristic of patients with somatoform disorders, can thus be attributed to idiosyncratic mental models and associated perceptual and evaluative processes. Neurobiological and neuroanatomical insights into cytoarchitecture and signal transmission within cortical structures are consistent with Bayesian models of active inference (Barrett & Simmons, 2015). Edwards et al. (2012) have recently outlined a corresponding neurobiological model (based on the principles of Bayesian active inference) for the domain of functional neurological symptoms (such as motor and sensory dysfunction).

Comprehensive empirical tests of these models as well as a derivation and testing of concrete therapeutic implications are still largely pending. However, there are already initial indications that central predictions of the models can be modified experimentally in the form of altered information processing processes (e.g., distorted and less accurate interoception) and are associated with a reduction in somatic symptom perceptions (Schäfer et al., 2014).

2.4 Psychobiological Filter Model

The filter model presented by Rief and Barsky (2005) shows a certain similarity to Brown's (2004) model (◘ Fig. 2.4). This model also assumes that the experience of somatic symptoms is the result of a selection process of the higher cognitive system. Cognitive processes thus mediate between bodily signals of somatic origin and the conscious experience or conscious perception of these signals (statistically speaking, this is a mediation between bodily signals and their experience due to a filtering process). The filter model is based on the central assumption that at any given moment a multitude of signals from all regions of the body inevitably arrive in the central nervous system and are processed. Because our cognitive resources for conscious processing are clearly limited, only a comparatively small proportion of bodily responses are normally experienced as conscious, while the majority of afferent bodily signals are filtered. A similar model has been postulated in the field of pain research as gate-control theory (Melzack & Wall, 1965). In contrast to Brown's model, within which symptom experiences can arise in a purely cognitive, cortical way (through the activation of symptom representations), the filter model assumes that "real" body signals are always involved in the experience of somatoform symptoms, which are not sufficiently filtered and thus come increasingly into the focus of attention.

Based on the filter model and its three central components (body sensations, filter and cortical perception), different mechanisms arise that can lead to the development of somatoform symptoms: For example, increased perception of bodily sensations (with unchanged filtering and perceptual processes) may result, as it were, "bottom-up," for example, from increased stress-related bodily signals (e.g., due to chronic overexcitation of the stress system in the form of the hypothalamic-pituitary-adrenocortical axis [HPA axis] or other factors illustrated in ◘ Fig. 2.4). Alternatively, it is conceivable that when the intensity of

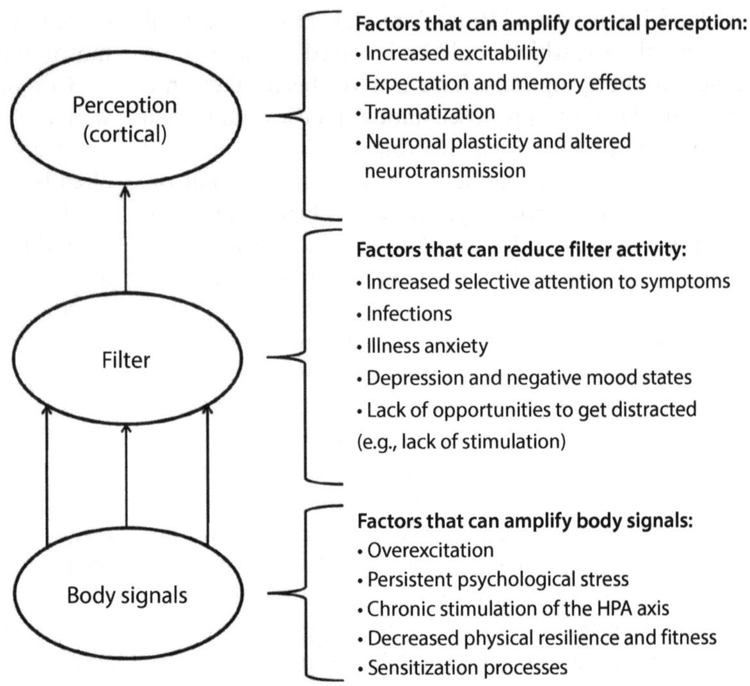

Fig. 2.4 Filter model of somatoform symptoms according to Rief and Barsky. (Based on Rief and Barsky (2005) and Rief and Broadbent (2007))

bodily signals is constant, altered filtering of somatosensory stimuli may lead to enhanced cortical perception of bodily signals. Finally, the model also opens the possibility that altered cortical processes ("top-down") in the form of expectancy and memory effects may be significantly responsible for the perception of bodily signals. Especially in this last point, the model by Rief and Barsky (2005) is very similar to the approach by Brown (2004).

2.5 Model of Classical Conditioning of Somatoform Symptoms

A theory that has been incomprehensibly little received in the context of cognitive behavior therapy was developed by **Van den Bergh et al.** (e.g. Van den Bergh et al., 2002) and states that somatoform symptoms can be relatively easily "learned" via the mechanism of classical conditioning and finally triggered by conditioned stimuli (in the complete absence of an organic pathology). In a series of experiments, Van den Bergh demonstrated that after only a few couplings between a negative odor and CO_2-enriched breath, the odor alone was able to trigger the nonspecific body symptoms of CO_2 (e.g., chest tightness, sweating, palpitations, dizziness). Interestingly, however, this conditioned response only worked for negative odors and not for positive odors, pointing to a key role of negative affect (both dispositional and situational) within this model, which we will discuss later in this section. Moreover, it was observed that the conditioned response generalized to other negative odors as well. The acquired conditioned response proved to be very stable over time, but could be reversed by an extinction phase in which the conditioned stimulus was applied several times without a symptom provocation.

The model outlined (Fig. 2.5), in which classically conditioned negative odors are capable of triggering bodily symptoms without organic cause (e.g., dizziness, fatigue, and feeling light-headed), has been used in particular to explain the phenomenon of multiple chemical sensitivity (MCS), in which those affected report strong olfactory intolerance reactions in conjunction with multiple bodily symptoms. The symptom pattern of MCS is now considered by most experts in psychology and medicine to be a functional syndrome or a somatoform disorder (Witthöft & Hiller, 2010). However, such a psychological or psychophysiological explanatory model is vehemently rejected by many of those affected.

However, Van den Bergh et al.'s mechanism of classical conditioning of somatic symptoms is not limited to olfactory triggers in the form of odors, but could also be demonstrated with virtual triggers in the form of mental images: In an interesting study, Stegen et al. (1999) asked subjects to imagine being in an oppressive situation in a confined space (e.g., in a sauna or in a stuck elevator). At the same time, the subjects were given CO_2-enriched breathing air, which was capable of provoking symptoms of anxiety such as shortness of breath and feelings of suffocation. Following this "learning phase", the subjects were asked to imagine themselves once again in the imagined oppressive situation. Even without the CO_2 provocation, the subjects experienced similar symptoms

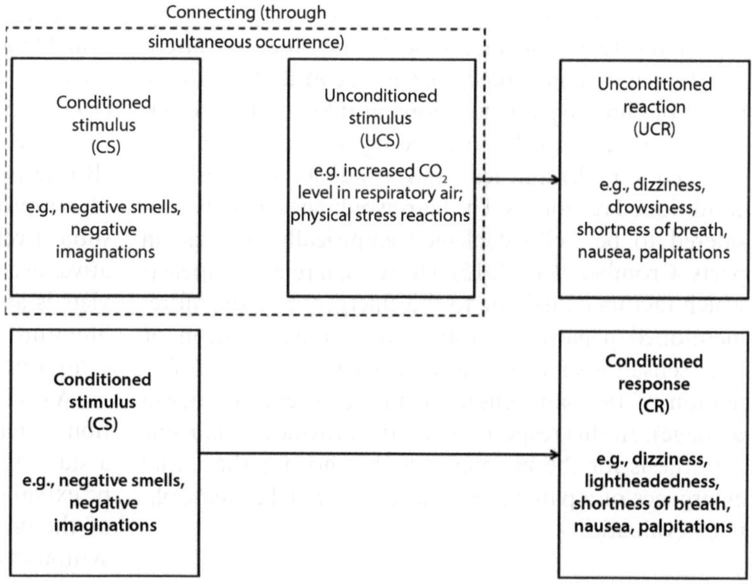

Fig. 2.5 Model of conditioning of somatoform symptoms. (Based on Van den Bergh et al. (2001))

as before under the direct influence of the CO_2. As with odors, however, this conditioning process only worked with negative mental images, not with positive ones (Van den Bergh et al., 2002).

As indicated above, negative affect plays a central role within this model. Van den Bergh et al. (2002) were able to show that individuals with higher neuroticism scores (i.e., dispositionally stronger negative affectivity) were better able to acquire conditioned responses and that in these individuals the acquired conditioned responses also generalized more strongly. If one considers the findings that only stimuli with a negative affective quality (e.g., images, smells, thoughts) are capable of functioning as conditioned stimuli, it seems plausible to assume that negative affective states per se can trigger somatoform symptoms as conditioned stimuli. The implication for a successful treatment of somatoform symptoms is that, among other things, a reduction of negative affective states should lead in a direct way to a reduction of somatoform symptoms. At the same time, exposure-oriented approaches such as systematic desensitization appear promising for changing existing conditioned reactions (e.g., body symptoms as a result of aversive odors).

All in all, it can be stated that the model of the classical conditioning of somatic symptoms represents one of the empirically best-evidenced approaches to explain somatoform symptoms. However, this conception is by no means limited to the area of somatoform symptoms, but is most likely also involved in primarily organ-medical disorders in which a clear association between pathological laboratory findings and subjective symptom experience is often lacking (such as in asthma). It is therefore all the more surprising that the described conditioning approach has received comparatively little attention in the international and German-language research and treatment landscape of somatoform disorders. The conditioning model outlined also appears compatible with the Bayesian models of symptom perception outlined earlier. In this respect, learning processes could be significantly involved in the formation of corresponding model parameters (in the sense of expectations or so-called priors), which in turn influence the symptom perception process (Van den Bergh et al., 2017).

2.6 Fear-Avoidance Model of Chronic Pain

Operant and associative learning processes are thought to play an important role in the development of persistent somatic symptoms. They represent a central element of the fear-avoidance model of chronic pain (Vlaeyen et al., 2016). The model borrows heavily from cognitive-behavioral models in the field of anxiety disorders and attempts to explain why and under what circumstances pain develops from acute and, from a survival perspective, meaningful and informative pain sensations to a persistent pain without any discernibly meaningful warning function. The core of the model is the assumption that the individual evaluation of a pain episode (as threatening or non-threatening or harmless) is significantly involved in the chronic manifestation of pain. In the case of a threatening and catastrophizing interpretation of a pain sensation, anxiety results as a conditioned response as well as the initiation of avoidance behavior to mitigate or avoid the pain sensation. Such avoidance behavior leads to a reduction of pain in the short term, but to a maintenance of the catastrophizing evaluation of pain sensations in the medium and long term. Similar to the models described previously, within the fear-avoidance model, body-focused attention (hypervigilance) functions as a central maintaining factor of chronic pain sensations, as it fosters the formation of associations between bodily sensations (as conditioned stimuli) and fear and avoidance responses as conditioned responses. The fear-avoidance model is considered to be well established empirically, at least in parts (Crombez et al., 2012). However, it remains unclear which factors contribute to the emergence of the aforementioned negative, catastrophizing interpretation of pain sensations and which factors per se favor the formation of the pain sensation (in the absence of organ damage). In this respect, the model provides a plausible hypothesis for the maintenance, but not for the initial emergence of a pain problem and associated catastrophizing evaluation.

2.7 Mechanism of Central Sensitization

Ursin (1997) proposed the mechanism of "**central sensitization**" to explain the development of persistent somatic symptoms that are not sufficientl medically explained. This primarily refers to sensitization at the central nervous, psychophysiological, and especially neurophysiological level (e.g., changes in synaptic efficiency due to increased neuronal activity in certain brain regions, especially within limbic structures, which are considered essential for emotional processing). The concept of sensitization is based on the concept of neuronal plasticity, according to which sustained neuronal activation patterns are capable of changing the central nervous system not only functionally but also structurally (e.g., through neuronal growth, establishment of new synaptic connections). The concept of sensitization originates from the field of pain research and has also been transferred to the field of functional syndromes such as irritable bowel syndrome or Multiple Chemical Sensitivities (e.g. Bell et al., 1992). In this context, sensitivity is held responsible for the fact that a certain organism reacts with a stronger response (e.g., an increased stress response) to an environmental stimulus that is usually tolerated without problems by the general population. In the context of MCS, for example, a sensitization in the area of olfactory-limbic signal transmission is held responsible for the mostly olfactory symptoms of the patients, but so far there is a lack of clear empirical evidence for this theoretical view.

In the context of his model, Ursin (1997) explicitly speaks of "subjective health complaints" and advocates dispensing with the term "symptom", since the complaints expressed are not yet proven signs of a clear disease process (in the sense of a symptom). In our opinion, this renunciation of the term "symptom" seems questionable at this point, since it again indirectly forces a dualistic conception of body and soul, which Ursin (1997) opposes elsewhere. In this respect, the proposal from the working group around Omer Van den Bergh (Bogaerts et al., 2010) seems more helpful to us to speak of symptoms when they are physical sensations that are subjectively interpreted by a person as problematic, negative, aversive and possibly as signs of a disease. This view is also in line with the current mainstream of the literature, which primarily speaks of persistent somatic symptoms.

A critical objection to the model of central sensitization is that it seems tautological in many respects, since a state (sensitization) in the sense of a phenomenon to be explained is equated with an explanation (in the form of the process of sensitization). In this respect, chronic symptoms are used as evidence for the phenomenon of sensitization. Independent empirical evidence for the process of sensitization as a causal factor in the development of persistent somatic symptoms is lacking to date.

2.8 Physiological and Psychophysiological Factors in Somatization

In addition to these possible biological influencing factors outlined within the model of central nervous synaptic sensitization processes, there are well-founded assumptions regarding the involvement of further biological factors in the development of somatoform symptoms. The role of altered endocrinological processes in connection with the body's own stress response has been best investigated to date. Thus, somatoform symptoms and functional somatic syndromes (such as chronic fatigue syndrome, fibromyalgia or irritable bowel syndrome) appear to be associated with a reduction in the stress hormone **cortisol (hypocortisolism)** or a reduced responsiveness in the range of cortisol levels in the blood (Heim et al., 2000). This reduced cortisol secretion and reactivity is in all probability the result of multiple altered processes in the hypothalamic-pituitary-adrenal axis, which can be triggered by chronic stress and trauma (Heim et al., 2000).

Since the glucocorticoid cortisol normally has a dampening effect on the immune system (immunosuppression), it is plausible to assume that the described hypocortisolism is involved in a dysfunctional activation of the immune system. Heim et al. (2000), for example, describe that a reduction in cortisol and its reactivity causes a disinhibition of immunological reactions and could promote various autoimmune diseases. In the area of somatoform disorders, correlations have indeed been demonstrated between an increased immunological response in the area of proinflammatory cytokines and a subjective feeling of being ill, as well as typical illness behaviors (e.g., rest, reduction in activity), although the cause-effect relationship remains unclear to date (Rief & Barsky, 2005). The altered immunological reaction could therefore also be a consequence of the somatoform disorder and the associated cognitive and behavioral processes.

It should be mentioned, however, that the outlined changes in the peripheral physiological stress response have not yet been consistently demonstrated in persons with somatoform symptoms (e.g., Houtveen & van Doornen, 2007). It is possible that stress-related psychophysiological dysregulations exist only in a subgroup of patients with somatoform symptoms.

Another psychophysiological mechanism is the phenomenon of **hyperventilation**, which is very likely responsible for some somatoform symptoms, especially in the cardiovascular area (Rief & Hiller, 2011) (e.g., chest pain and tightness, feelings of drowsiness, tingling sensations in the extremities). Hyperventilation is a change in breathing in which there is increased expiration of CO_2 through the breath. As a result, alkalosis results in the form of a reduction in the acidity of the arterial and venous blood (which is documented in a rising pH; e.g., Duzár et al., 1925). The decrease in the partial pressure of CO_2 in the blood causes vasoconstriction of the peripheral blood vessels and associated paraesthesias, such as pressure and tingling sensations in the head, arms, and legs. Because of the ability of hyperventilation to actively induce a series of harmless somatic symptoms within a short period of time that are reversible within a few minutes, this mechanism can be used for provocation testing in the course of treatment, similar to the treatment rationale for panic disorder, as part of behavioral experiments and symptom exposures. We will discuss this possibility in more detail in the treatment section (► Chaps. 8 and 9).

In addition to the changes outlined in the area of endocrinological, immunological and respiratory-chemical processes, possible **genetic predispositions** for the development of somatoform symptoms are also currently being discussed. For example, Rief et al. (2010) described that a certain polymorphism in the area of a serotonin transporter gene (5-HTTLPR) is associated with the report of persistent somatoform symptoms. However, this also raises the question to what extent the detected genotypes are specifically associated with somatoform symptoms. Overall, there appears to be a moderately increased heritability in somatoform disorders, suggesting an inherited vulnerability to develop somatoform symptoms (Rief et al., 2010). However, it should be borne in mind that (as with most psychological and psychophysiological disorders) the main part of the individual variability of symptomatology cannot be explained by genetic factors.

Regarding **biological factors** in somatoform disorders, the interested reader is referred to the more detailed accounts in Rief and Barsky (2005) and Rief et al. (2010).

2.9 Interpersonal Model of Somatization

Stuart and Noyes (1999) formulated an interpersonal model of somatoform disorders that focuses primarily on an assumed interpersonal functionality of somatoform symptoms. According to the authors, somatoform symptoms are primarily an expression of help-seeking behavior, as patients have developed an anxious, insecure attachment style due to unfavorable past attachment experiences and frequent emotional neglect. This dysfunctional attachment style provokes new, unfavorable relationship experiences (e.g., rejections), which in turn promote somatizing behaviors (especially excessive use of medical services). At the heart of this model, therefore, is a vicious circle of unmet need for closeness and affection and an inadequate attempt, based on somatization, to satisfy this need (◘ Fig. 2.6).

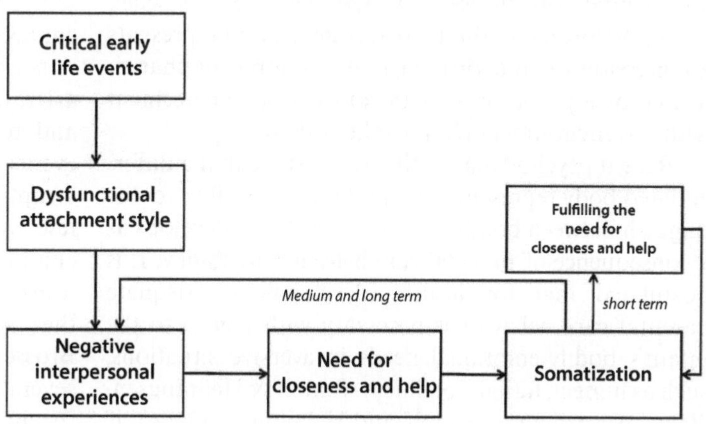

◘ **Fig. 2.6** The interpersonal model of somatization. (Based on Stuart and Noyes (1999))

Stuart and Noyes (1999) conceptualize somatization as a personality trait that has developed as a reaction to stressful life events as a result of unfavorable early attachment experiences and a particular family emphasis on the topic of illness or health. Whereas within the originally formulated model (Stuart & Noyes, 1999) there was no clear differentiation between hypochondriasis (or illness anxiety disorder) and polysymptomatic somatoform disorders, Noyes et al. provide an interesting overview of the differences between the two phenomena in a later paper (2006).

The lack of empirical evidence for the described model should be critically noted. Furthermore, it seems better able to provide an explanation for characteristic behaviors (e.g., safety behavior) in the context of hypochondriasis (or illness anxiety disorder), but less so of symptom-related somatoform disorders. Overall, Stuart and Noyes' (1999) interpersonal model focuses on the behavioral level, but not on the issue of symptom emergence and symptom perception. Thus, somatoform symptoms that are not accompanied by increased help-seeking behavior appear difficult to explain.

2.10 Psychoanalytic and Depth Psychology-Oriented Concepts

As described in ► Sect. 1.2.1, Freud's **conversion model** is probably the most influential psychoanalytic model for explaining somatic symptoms without an organic cause. The model postulates the development of somatoform symptoms as a consequence of repressed psychological conflicts. The presentation of symptoms serves here to resolve conflict and defend against affect (Kanwischer, 2006).

Another analytical concept, the theory of **de- or resomatization**, originates from Max Schur and is based on a developmental psychological perspective, according to which individual development in childhood is characterized by an increasing separation of physical and mental perceptions and experiences (Kanwischer, 2006). According to this theory, somatization represents a regression to an earlier stage of development characterized by a primarily somatic and sensory engagement with the environment (Kanwischer, 2006).

Recent psychodynamic theories assume that a differentiated body representation (and thus the ability to distinguish between bodily and affective states) develops as a consequence of **parental care behavior in infancy**. It is postulated that for healthy development, adequate parental care behavior is necessary with regard to the infant's bodily-emotional needs in aversive situations, such as hunger, fatigue, or illness (Rudolf & Henningsen, 2006). According to Rudolf and Henningsen (2006), if this is lacking or not adequately developed, characteristic disorders in later life result, such as the inability to distinguish between physical and affective events, to calm oneself or through support from others, and unfavorable cognitive appraisals characterized by a rigid biomedical explanatory models of illness. Overall, then, the current psychodynamic view of somatoform symptoms assumes an early disruption of the parent-child relationship—a view that is ultimately also contained in Stuart and Noyes' (1999) interpersonal model of somatization described earlier.

Deficits in emotional experience and behavior, which in the psychodynamic tradition represent the consequence of unfavorable attachment and relationship experiences, have been subsumed under the keyword "alexithymia". **Alexithymia** (going back to Sifneos, 1972; cited after Gündel et al., 2000) means here:

- Deficits in the ability to perceive one's own feelings and to relate them to psychosocial stressors,
- Lack of affective expression when describing stressful events, and
- A high degree of dependency and social conformity.

Overall, however, the empirical foundation of the alexithymia concept in the context of somatoform disorders is considered controversial, as alexithymia seems to be generally associated with increased psychopathology and not specifically with somatoform symptoms. An overview of the existing findings in alexithymia research can be found, for example, in Gündel et al. (2000).

2.11 Outlook: Dysfunctional Emotion Regulation Processes in Somatoform Symptoms

Processes of emotion regulation in somatoform disorders have so far been studied primarily within the framework of the psychodynamically based alexithymia concept described above and thus mostly on the basis of self-report data. Against the background of a probable connection between psychosocial stressors and the experience of somatoform symptoms, the question inevitably arises as to whether problems or dysfunctional strategies and regulatory processes in response to stressful life events could be involved in the genesis of somatoform symptoms. Interestingly, there have been comparatively few systematic studies of the relationship between emotion regulation processes and somatoform symptoms. An interesting approach is being investigated by the working group around Brosschot et al. (e.g. Brosschot et al., 2006; Verkuil et al., 2007). In their perseveration cognition hypothesis (Brosschot et al., 2006), the authors postulate that persistent mental preoccupation following a stressful life event (as well as anticipatory mental preoccupation with expected negative events and consequences) is capable of preserving negative effects of the stress reaction not only at the affective level, but also at the physiological level (e.g., cardiovascular and endocrinological, immunological), thereby promoting somatic symptoms. However, the extent to which patients with somatoform disorders are more prone to such perserverating cognitive processes is still unclear.

Current correlative findings within the general population suggest that both the experience of physical discomfort and the interpretation of physical discomfort as a sign of serious illness are associated with increased use of more dysfunctional and decreased use of more functional styles of emotion regulation. Thus, positive associations were found between habitual suppression of emotion expression and the experience of cardiopulmonary and fatigue-related bodily symptoms (Witthöft et al., 2013). Illness anxiety was found to be most strongly associated with more dysfunctional cognitive emotion regulation strategies, such as rumination and catastrophizing (Görgen et al., 2014). It should be mentioned that these are only correlative findings and do not allow any conclusions regarding possible causality. Future experimental studies in the area of cognitive-psychological and psychophysiological parameters therefore appear promising in order to systematically investigate a possible connection between altered emotion regulation processes and somatoform symptoms.

2.12 Etiology and Pathogenesis of Somatoform Disorders According to Current Knowledge: An Integrative Model

An extensive and detailed reflection of all known approaches would go beyond the scope of this treatment manual. The interested reader is referred here to relevant reviews in this field (e.g. Deary et al., 2007; Rief & Broadbent, 2007; Witthöft & Hiller, 2010; Van den Bergh et al., 2017).

A common feature of current models of somatoform symptoms is that the experience of somatic symptoms is regarded as the result of a complex, active, cognitive construction process and not as a passive and valid representation of a physiological event. As banal as this idea may sound after reading the models described, this view is experienced as new (and sometimes complicated and strange) by patients whose own model of illness often corresponds to a clear and direct relationship between organ damage and the perception of a symptom. However, it is now known that even in primarily organic diseases, there is considerable interindividual variability in symptom experience with similar physiological pathology (e.g., in the case of bronchial asthma or spinal deformities and degenerations). The comprehensive model of symptom perception based on Bayesian principles of active inference recently presented by Van den Bergh et al. (2017) perhaps currently best accounts for this.

It should also be noted that all the models presented implicitly or explicitly (e.g. Ursin, 1997) speak out against a body-soul dualism. Thus it seems not only scientifically but also therapeutically questionable to use the concepts "psychic" vs. "organic" or "psychogenic" vs. "biogenic" in contrast, even if this dichotomy is often still reflected in the subjective models of the patients. The new conceptualization of the chapter on somatoform disorders in the DSM-5 described in ▶ Sect. 1.2.3 takes this problem into account, at least in part, by removing the strict division between medically explained and medically unexplained physical symptoms as a diagnostic feature of somatoform disorders. Consequently, the elimination of a medical cause to explain symptoms is no longer a mandatory component of the diagnosis of somatic symptom disorder. At first, this may be viewed critically, but on closer examination it becomes clear that the abandonment of the principle of a diagnosis of exclusion is well justified: for example, the determination of an organic basis for a particular symptom often lacks any reliability (in the psychometric sense); descriptive research and pseudo-diagnoses with the most complex terms possible (e.g., vegetative dystonia) are no longer used. All too often, descriptive research and pseudo-diagnoses with the most complex terms possible (e.g., vegetative dystonia) suggest a clear organic genesis, initially satisfy the patient's need for a supposedly clear diagnosis (thus having a calming effect on patients in the short term), but in the long term maintain a vicious circle of increased self-observation, activity reduction and social isolation. At the same time, the criticism of the new conceptualization of somatoform disorders in the DSM-5 expressed in ▶ Sect. 1.2.3, particularly with regard to the separation of pathological fears of illness and other variants of somatic stress disorder, is legitimate and well-founded.

In addition to the cognitive factors described above (e.g., processes of attention control and evaluation), there has been increasing evidence in recent years for the involvement of physiological factors in the development and maintenance of somatoform symptoms. In particular, a reduction in the glucocorticoid cortisol (or its reactivity) as a result of traumatic experiences and chronic stress seems to play a significant role in some patients with somatoform symptoms. A connection between this hypocortisolism and a permanently harm-

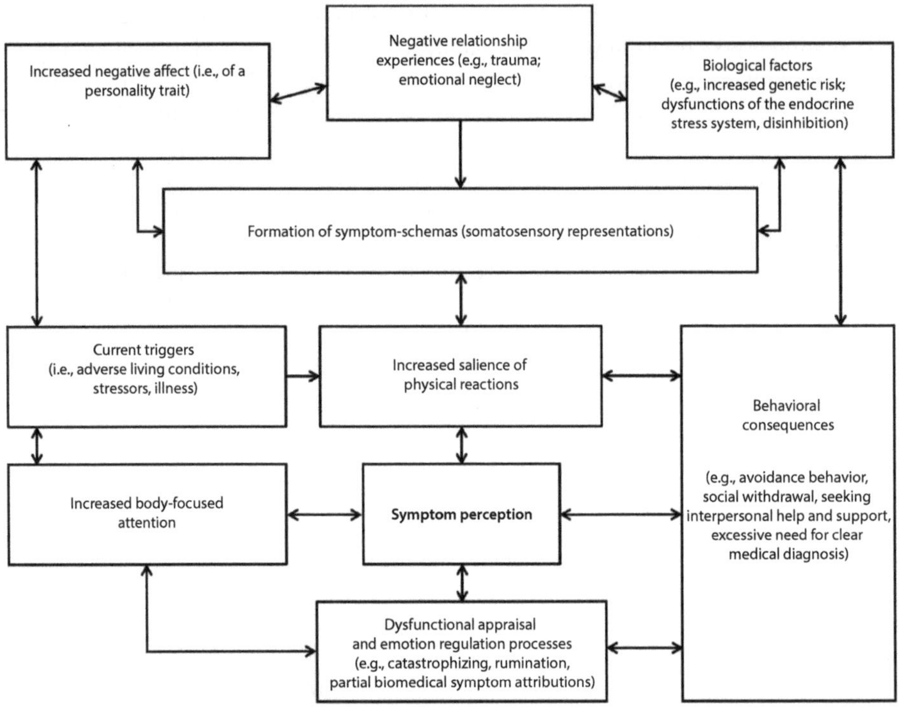

Fig. 2.7 Integrative model of the genesis and maintenance of somatoform symptoms

ful disinhibition of immunological processes is considered probable. Overall, however, it seems unlikely that biological processes are monocausally responsible for the development of somatoform disorders and that a diagnostically relevant biomarker can be identified in the foreseeable future.

> It can be assumed that somatoform symptoms and disorders result from a complex interaction of unfavorable life circumstances, beginning in childhood and adolescence (e.g., emotionally invalidating environment, trauma), from the resulting affective and physiological adaptation processes and current stressors.

If one considers the empirical foundation of individual explicative constructs with regard to the triggering of somatoform symptoms, which were named in this chapter, it can be stated that currently the **phenomenon of negative affectivity** represents the construct that has been best documented to date.

A corresponding multifactorial integrative model of conditions, which subsumes the most important aspects of the genesis and maintenance of somatoform symptoms, is outlined in Fig. 2.7. It should be noted here that the postulation of unidirectional relationships has been largely dispensed with, since according to current knowledge most of the factors involved influence each other reciprocally and are subject to continuous change, not least because of a neuronal plasticity that persists into old age.

References

Baddeley, A. (2007). *Working memory, thought and action*. Oxford University Press.

Barrett, L. F., & Simmons, W. K. (2015). Interoceptive predictions in the brain. *Nature Reviews Neuroscience, 16*(7), 419–429. https://doi.org/10.1038/nrn3950

Barrett, L. F., Tugade, M. M., & Engle, R. W. (2004). Individual differences in working memory capacity and dual-process theories of the mind. *Psychological Bulletin, 130*(4), 553–573. https://doi.org/10.1037/0033-2909.130.4.553

Barsky, A. J., Wyshak, G., & Klerman, G. L. (1990). The somatosensory amplification scale and its relationship to hypochondriasis. *Journal of Psychiatry Research, 24*(4), 323–334. https://doi.org/10.1016/0022-3956(90)90004-A

Bell, I. R., Miller, C. S., & Schwartz, G. E. (1992). An olfactory-limbic model of multiple chemical sensitivity syndrome: Possible relationships to kindling and affective spectrum disorders. *Biological Psychiatry, 32*(3), 218–242. https://doi.org/10.1016/0006-3223(92)90105-9

Bogaerts, K., van Eylen, L., Li, W., Bresseleers, J., van Diest, I., de Peuter, S., et al. (2010). Distorted symptom perception in patients with medically unexplained symptoms. *Journal of Abnormal Psychology, 119*(1), 226–234. https://doi.org/10.1037/A0017780

Brosschot, J. F., Gerin, W., & Thayer, J. F. (2006). The perseverative cognition hypothesis: A review of worry, prolonged stress-related physiological activation, and health. *Journal of Psychosomatic Research, 60*(2), 113–124. https://doi.org/10.1016/j.jpsychores.2005.06.074

Brown, R. J. (2004). Psychological mechanisms of medically unexplained symptoms: An integrative conceptual model. *Psychological Bulletin, 130*(5), 793–812. https://doi.org/10.1037/0033-2909.130.5.793

Clark, D. M. (1986). A cognitive approach to panic. *Behaviour Research and Therapy, 24*(4), 461–470. https://doi.org/10.1016/0005-7967(86)90011-2

Crombez, G., Eccleston, C., Van Damme, S., Vlaeyen, J. W. S., & Karoly, P. (2012). Fear-avoidance model of chronic pain the next generation. *Clinical Journal of Pain, 28*(6), 475–483. https://doi.org/10.1097/AJP.0b013e3182385392

Deary, V., Chalder, T., & Sharpe, M. (2007). The cognitive behavioural model of medically unexplained symptoms: A theoretical and empirical review. *Clinical Psychology Review, 27*(7), 781–797. https://doi.org/10.1016/j.cpr.2007.07.002

Duzár, J., Holló, J., & Weiß, S. (1925). Über die Wirkung der mechanisch hervorgerufenen Hyperventilation auf das Säurebasengleichgewicht. *Research in Experimental Medicine, 45*(1), 708–713. https://doi.org/10.1007/BF02626086

Edwards, M. J., Adams, R. A., Brown, H., Parees, I., & Friston, K. J. (2012). A Bayesian account of "hysteria". *Brain, 135*, 3495–3512. https://doi.org/10.1093/brain/aws129

Friston, K., Brown, H. R., Siemerkus, J., & Stephan, K. E. (2016). The dysconnection hypothesis (2016). *Schizophrenia Research, 176*(2–3), 83–94. https://doi.org/10.1016/j.schres.2016.07.014

Görgen, S. M., Hiller, W., & Witthöft, M. (2014). Health anxiety, cognitive coping, and emotion regulation: A latent variable approach. *International Journal of Behavioral Medicine, 21*(2), 364–374. https://doi.org/10.1007/s12529-013-9297-y

Gündel, H., Ceballos-Baumann, A. O., & von Rad, M. (2000). Aktuelle perspektiven der alexithymie. *Nervenarzt, 71*(3), 151–163.

Heim, C., Ehlert, U., & Hellhammer, D. H. (2000). The potential role of hypocortisolism in the pathophysiology of stress-related bodily disorders. *Psychoneuroendocrinology, 25*(1), 1–35. https://doi.org/10.1016/S0306-4530(99)00035-9

Houtveen, J. H., & van Doornen, L. J. P. (2007). Medically unexplained symptoms and between-group differences in 24-h ambulatory recording of stress physiology. *Biological Psychology, 76*(3), 239–249. https://doi.org/10.1016/j.biopsycho.2007.08.005

Kanwischer, H. (2006). Somatoforme Störungen. In F. Leichsenring (Hrsg.), *Lehrbuch der Psychotherapie für die Ausbildung zur/zum Psychologischen PsychotherapeutIn und für die ärztliche Weiterbildung* (3. Aufl., Bd. 2, S. 173–182). CIP-Medien.

Kirmayer, L. J., & Robbins, J. M. (1991). Three forms of somatization in primary care: Prevalence, co-occurrence, and sociodemographic characteristics. *Journal of Nervous and Mental Disease, 179*(11), 647–655. https://doi.org/10.1097/00005053-199809000-00006

Kirmayer, L. J., & Taillefer, S. (1997). Somatoform disorders. In S. M. Turner & M. Hersen (Eds.), *Adult psychopathology and diagnosis* (3rd ed., pp. 333–383). Wiley.

Melzack, R., & Wall, P. D. (1965). Pain mechanisms: A new theory. *Science, 150*(699), 971–979.

Norman, D. A., & Shallice, T. (1986). Attention to action: Willed and automatic control of behavior. In R. J. Davidson, G. E. Schwartz, & D. Shapiro (Eds.), *Consciousness and self-regulation: Vol. 4. Advances in research an therory* (pp. 1–18). Plenum Press.

Noyes, R., Stuart, S., Watson, D. B., & Langbehn, D. R. (2006). Distinguishing between hypochondriasis and somatization disorder: A review of the existing literature. *Psychotherapy and Psychosomatics, 75*(5), 270–281. https://doi.org/10.1159/000093948

Rief, W., & Barsky, A. J. (2005). Psychobiological perspectives on somatoform disorders. *Psychoneuroendocrinology, 30*(10), 996–1002. https://doi.org/10.1016/j.psyneuen.2005.03.018

Rief, W., & Broadbent, E. (2007). Explaining medically unexplained symptoms-models and mechanisms. *Clinical Psychology Review, 27*(7), 821–841. https://doi.org/10.1016/j.cpr.2007.07.005

Rief, W., & Hiller, W. (1998). *Somatisierungsstörung und Hypochondrie (Fortschritte der Psychotherapie Band 1)*. Hogrefe.

Rief, W., & Hiller, W. (2011). *Somatisierungsstörung* (Bd. 1, Fortschritte der Psychotherapie). Hogrefe.

Rief, W., Hennings, A., Riemer, S., & Euteneuer, F. (2010). Psychobiological differences between depression and somatization. *Journal of Psychosomatic Research, 68*(5), 495–502. https://doi.org/10.1016/j.jpsychores.2010.02.001

Rudolf, G., & Henningsen, P. (2006). Somatoforme Störungen. In C. Reimer & U. Rüger (Hrsg.), *Psychodynamische Psychotherapien: Lehrbuch der tiefenpsychologisch fundierten Psychotherapieverfahren*. Springer.

Schäfer, M., Egloff, B., Gerlach, A. L., & Witthöft, M. (2014). Improving heartbeat perception in patients with medically unexplained symptoms reduces symptom distress. *Biological Psychology, 101*, 69–76. https://doi.org/10.1016/j.biopsycho.2014.06.012

Sifneos, P. E. (1972). *Short-term psychotherapy and emotional crisis*. Harvard University Press.

Stegen, K., de Bruyne, K., Rasschaert, W., van de Woestijne, K. P., & van den Bergh, O. (1999). Fear-relevant images as conditioned stimuli for somatic complaints, respiratory behavior, and reduced end-tidal pCO2. *Journal of Abnormal Psychology, 108*(1), 143–152. https://doi.org/10.1037/0021-843X.108.1.143

Strack, F., & Deutsch, R. (2004). Reflective and impulsive determinants of social behavior. *Personality and Social Psychology Review, 8*(3), 220–247. https://doi.org/10.1207/s15327957pspr0803_1

Stuart, S., & Noyes, R. (1999). Attachment and interpersonal communication in somatization. *Psychosomatics, 40*(1), 34–43. https://doi.org/10.1016/S0033-3182(99)71269-7

Ursin, H. (1997). Sensitization, somatization, and subjective health complaints. *International Journal of Behavioral Medicine, 4*(2), 105–116. https://doi.org/10.1207/s15327558ijbm0402_1

Van den Bergh, O., Devriese, S., Winters, W., Veulemans, H., Nemery, B., Eelen, P., et al. (2001). Acquiring symptoms in response to odors: A learning perspective on multiple chemical sensitivity. *Role of Neural Plasticity in Chemical Intolerance, 933*(1), 278–290.

Van den Bergh, O., Winters, W., Devriese, S., & van Diest, I. (2002). Learning subjective health complaints. *Scandinavian Journal of Psychology, 43*(2), 147–152. https://doi.org/10.1111/1467-9450.00280

Van den Bergh, O., Witthöft, M., Petersen, S., & Brown, R. J. (2017). Symptoms and the body: Taking the inferential leap. *Neuroscience and Biobehavioral Reviews, 74*, 185–203. https://doi.org/10.1016/j.neubiorev.2017.01.015

Verkuil, B., Brosschot, J. F., & Thayer, J. F. (2007). A sensitive body or a sensitive mind? Associations among somatic sensitization, cognitive sensitization, health worry, and subjective health complaints. *Journal of Psychosomatic Research, 63*(6), 673–681. https://doi.org/10.1016/j.jpsychores.2007.08.010

Vlaeyen, J. W. S., Crombez, G., & Linton, S. J. (2016). The fear-avoidance model of pain. *Pain, 157*(8), 1588–1589. https://doi.org/10.1097/j.pain.0000000000000574

Witthöft, M., & Hiller, W. (2010). Psychological approaches to origins and treatments of somatoform disorders. *Annual Review of Clinical Psychology, 6*, 257–283. https://doi.org/10.1146/annurev.clinpsy.121208.131505

Witthöft, M., Loch, N., & Jasper, F. (2013). Somatoform symptoms and strategies of emotion regulation [Somatoforme Beschwerden und Stile der Emotionsregulation]. *Verhaltenstherapie & Verhaltensmedizin, 34*(4), 444–464.

Therapeutic Approaches for Persistent Somatic Symptoms, Somatoform Disorders, and Somatic Symptom Disorders

Contents

M. Kleinstäuber et al., *Cognitive Behavior Therapy for Persistent Somatic Symptoms and Somatic Symptom Disorder*, https://doi.org/10.1007/978-3-662-69726-9_3

3.1 Psychotherapy and Other Psychological Treatment Approaches

Multiple persistent somatic symptoms often pose a challenge in therapeutic practice. The patients are usually under a high level of suffering and bear the clear risk of chronicity and development of comorbid mental disorders. Both of these factors may have to be taken into account as negative influences on the course of the disease and therapeutic responsiveness. Furthermore, the often negative attitude of patients with persistent somatic symptoms towards psychological or psychiatric interventions as well as towards biopsychosocial disorder models can make it difficult to establish a stable doctor-patient or therapist-patient relationship. Studies show that patients with somatic symptoms are reluctant to seek psychological treatment because of a "mental illness stigma" (Freidl et al., 2007). It is also evident that on the part of the therapist or physician, the affected person often receives the stigma "difficult patient" (Hahn et al., 1996). In turn, patients often feel that they are not taken seriously as they experience the referral to psychotherapy as incongruent with their subjective perception of being physically ill (Murray et al., 2016). This challenging diagnosis has therefore inspired the development of various treatment approaches, particularly in the field of psychotherapy. Corresponding to current scientific knowledge, cognitive behavior therapy is the best evaluated approach for persistent somatic symptoms (Kleinstäuber et al., 2011; van Dessel et al., 2014). Accordingly, the following account will focus on cognitive behavior therapy. Furthermore, approaches in depth psychology-oriented as well as interpersonal systemic therapy for chronic somatic symptoms have developed. A brief insight into these will also be given.

Treatment Methods for Persistent Somatic Symptoms

- **Psychotherapy and psychological interventions**
  - Cognitive behavior therapy
  - Behavioral medicine interventions
  - Exposure-based pain management
  - Therapy methods of the "third wave" of cognitive behavior therapy
  - Relaxation techniques (e.g. progressive muscle relaxation, autogenic training, hypnotherapy)
  - Biofeedback
  - Reattribution training
  - Depth psychology-oriented therapy
  - Interpersonal therapy
  - Sports and exercise therapy
- **Pharmacotherapy**
  - Tricyclic antidepressants
  - Selective serotonin or norepinephrine reuptake inhibitors
  - Antiepileptic drugs

3.1.1 Cognitive Behavior Therapy and Behavioral Medicine Approaches

Cognitive behavior therapy for persistent somatic symptoms fundamentally assumes a complex interaction of emotional, cognitive, psychophysiological, and behavioral factors. This reciprocal, interactive interaction of different factors is illustrated in ◘ Fig. 3.1.

Furthermore, learning processes involved in the development and maintenance of persistent somatic symptoms represent an important basis for the application of cognitive behavior therapy techniques. In this context, social learning processes regarding reactions to somatic symptoms and responding learning processes regarding the linking of triggering external and internal stimuli with somatic symptoms play an important role. In addition, operant learning factors are significant in the positive and negative reinforcement of patients' dysfunctional behaviors by the social environment.

Based on a multifactorial model of disorders (▶ Sect. 2.12), various classical cognitive behavioral intervention strategies, which are usually derived from therapy approaches for other mental disorders, were transferred and adapted to persistent somatic symptoms and associated distress. The corresponding therapy elements were then often combined within the framework of multimodal, cognitive behavior therapy (Allen et al., 2006; Escobar et al., 2007; Kashner et al., 1995; Rief et al., 1995; Schilte et al., 2001; Speckens et al., 1995; Sumathipala et al., 2008) or behavioral medicine programs (Bleichhardt et al., 2004; Nickel et al., 2006). ◘ Table 3.1 contains a summary of the most important components of cognitive behavior therapy.

In therapy practice, the elements can be combined and varied depending on the individual problem situation. They can be used in individual as well as in group therapy, in outpatient as well as in inpatient therapy settings. The involvement of relatives can be individually important if the respective attachment figures have a reinforcing function with regard to the symptoms.

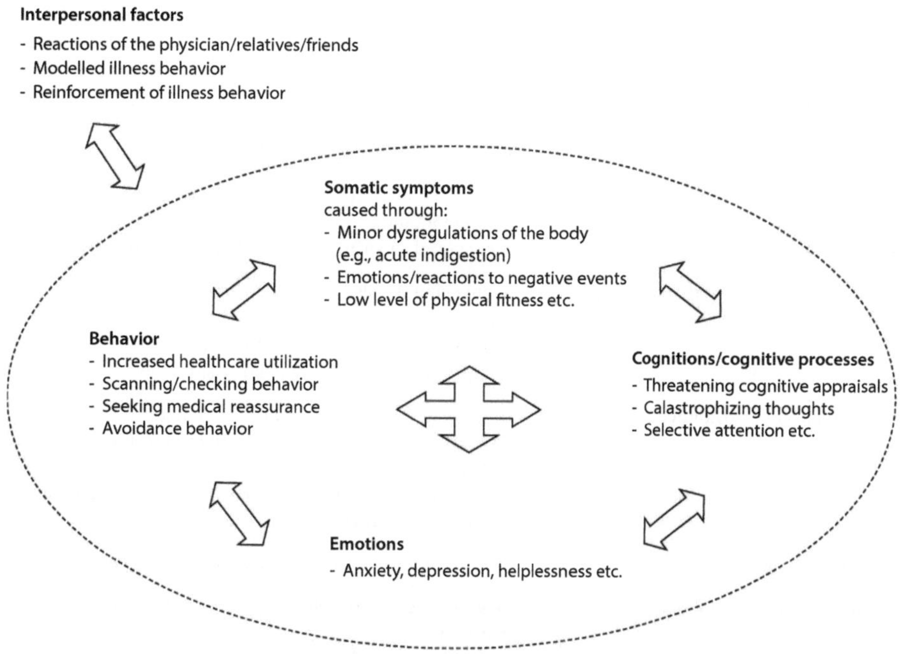

Fig. 3.1 The interaction of emotional factors, cognitive and behavioral processes, interpersonal factors with somatic symptoms

Table 3.1 Overview of the most important therapeutic elements of cognitive behavior therapy for multiple persistent somatic symptoms and associated distress

Therapy element	Brief description
Therapy initiation	Clarification of the reason of referral Clarification of the general conditions of a therapy Diagnostics and taking patient history Exploration of pre-treatments of the patient Exploration of the patients' subjective explanatory model of their symptoms
Functional assessment of behavior	Exploration of the behavioral, cognitive, emotional, and physiological components, possible reinforcement conditions and model experiences of the patient with regard to illness behavior Explaining to to patients how different components of problem behavior are related to each other
Clarification of therapy goals and building motivation for change	Conveying a realistic perspective on the success of treatment
Techniques for dealing with patients' bio-medical models	Providing information and psychoeducation Recording of associations situations and symptoms Use of journaling Exercises demonstrating the influence of attention control on perceptual processes Biofeedback
Relaxation techniques Stress management and coping techniques	E.g. progressive muscle relaxation, autogenic training Stress management/psychoeducation about stress and its effects Reactivation of other stress management techniques that have already been successful with the patient Building positive activities Problem solving therapy
Development of a realistic concept of health	Use of cognitive techniques to restructure the often narrow concept of health of affected people Behavioral experiments

(continued)

Table 3.1 (continued)

Therapy element	Brief description
Dealing with catastrophizing thoughts	Exploration of the catastrophizing thoughts Assessment of the credibility of the thoughts Collecting pro and con arguments regarding the thoughts and reassessment of the credibility of the thoughts Behavioral experiments to challenge thoughts
Dealing with reassurance behavior	Conveying the short-term positive consequences and the long-term, sustaining relationship between reassurancesurance and somatic symptoms Techniques to reduce reassurance behavior (e.g., agreeing on time-contingent rather than symptom-contingent physician visits)
Reduction of avoidance behavior	Building motivation for behavior change Hierarchy of goals and increasing level of physical exercise Self-rewarding techniques Preparation of cognitive exposure and exposure with response prevention to cope with avoidance behavior
Emotion regulation	Techniques to observe feelings, encouraging emotion expression, and accept feelings
Social skills training	Techniques to promote adequate communication of somatic symptoms or communication with the physician Role plays with video feedback Support patient in building a social network
Improvement of the subjective well-being and resilience	Cognitive strategies to improve self-image Exercises to promote positive body experiences (e.g., enjoyable physical activities, massage) Relaxation techniques Euthymic exercises Establishment/reactivation of positive activities
Improvement of sleep quality	Sleep hygiene and stimulus control techniques
Vocational reintegration	Therapeutic support for the return to work Motivational support of the patient Support in the perception of a sense of achievement Development of realistic goals for the professional re-entry Balance the advantages and disadvantages of early retirement
Relapse prevention	Teaching of rules of conduct for the prevention of or better handling of relapses Addressing the issue of excessive healthcare utilization behavior Agreement on rules concerning the patients' future healthcare utilization behavior

According to Rief and Hiller (2011)

▪ Exposure-Based Pain Management

Particularly in patients who experience long-lasting pain symptoms, we have already seen in the context of the fear-avoidance model in ► Sect. 2.6 that fears of physical activity can develop (Vlaeyen et al., 1995). Patients have the expectation that physical activity could lead to an aggravation of their somatic symptoms, especially pain, or (repeated) injury. As a result, these patients develop marked avoidance behavior. The fears can generalize and develop a phobic character. Severe restrictions in everyday life, deconditioning, bad posture, and depressive mood can be the result. In the context of exposure-based pain therapy, this subgroup of pain patients with pronounced fear-avoidance cognitions is treated with the help of exposure to physical exercise. Comparable to classical exposure therapy for anxiety (e.g. Margraf & Schneider, 1990), patients work out a hierarchy of avoided motions, ordered according to the severity of the accompanying anxiety. Subsequently, patients perform the motions and are exposed to their fears until a predetermined level of fear reduction is achieved (Vlaeyen et al., 2001).

▪ The "Third Wave" of Cognitive Behavior Therapy: Mindfulness-Based Therapy and Acceptance-Commitment Therapy

The "third wave" of cognitive behavior therapy techniques places a greater emphasis on the negative emotions associated with somatic symptoms. Of these procedures, **mindfulness-based therapy** and **acceptance-**

commitment therapy (ACT) have so far been adapted for patients with chronic somatic symptoms—especially in the field of therapy for chronic pain (Veehof et al., 2011) or other chronic conditions with psychosomatic features, such as tinnitus (Westin et al., 2011).

Fjorback et al. (2013) and van Ravesteijn et al. (2013) developed a mindfulness-based group therapy for patients with multiple persistent somatic symptoms. These therapy approaches complement cognitive behavior therapy with mindfulness-based strategies. Various forms of meditation, yoga exercises, and body journeys assist patients in mindfully noticing their bodies, feelings, and internal psychological processes. This mindfulness-based attitude is designed to help patients learn to accept their symptoms and develop more compassion for themselves.

ACT includes mindfulness-based interventions as well as acceptance strategies and commitment building and behavior change techniques. In the context of treating chronic pain syndromes, ACT is designed to help patients confront their pain and develop acceptance toward their discomfort (Veehof et al., 2011). This technique is intended to lead to the reduction of pain perception and maintenance or restoration of the sufferer's level of functioning. The inclusion of acceptance-based techniques in psychotherapy for persistent somatic symptoms may be of tremendous importance. A new treatment program that enriches cognitive behavior therapy for persistent somatic symptoms with acceptance-, mindfulness-based, and other emotion-regulation strategies is currently still under development and scientific evaluation (Kleinstäuber et al., 2016). This treatment approach focuses primarily on the negative feelings that accompany the somatic symptoms and on possible emotion regulation problems.

3.1.2 Relaxation Techniques and Biofeedback

Psychophysiology describes several mechanisms that can explain somatic symptoms in the absence of organic findings. These mechanisms include overactivity or dysregulation of the autonomic nervous system, smooth muscle contractions, endocrine hyperactivity, and hyperventilation (Rief et al., 1998). Accordingly, it seems reasonable to use techniques that focus on reducing physiological arousals in patients with persistent somatic symptoms. These include progressive muscle relaxation, autogenic training, hypnotherapy and biofeedback.

Relaxation techniques fulfil different functions at the same time:

- On the one hand, they should help the patient to recognize connections between relaxation and well-being.
- Furthermore, with the help of relaxation techniques, the increased activation level, which has been demonstrated in patients with persistent somatic symptoms, should be reduced. This can be accompanied by a reduction of the hyperactivation of the autonomous nervous system.
- At the same time, the positive experiences patients have during the initiation of a relaxation state support the process of reattribution of somatic symptoms in a sense of a biopsychosocial symptom model.

Progressive Muscle Relaxation

A particularly proven method is progressive muscle relaxation. This can also be used as a successful distraction method. By concentrating on the relaxation instruction and consciously noticing the differences between the state of tension and the state of relaxation, attention can be consciously diverted away from other bodily sensations.

Autogenic Training and Hypnotherapeutic Methods

Autogenic training or hypnotherapeutic exercises have been proven to be effective as alternative relaxation methods. However, these methods require sufficient mentalization abilities. Both relaxation methods are based on the basic concept of concentrative self-relaxation, in which patients can influence physical processes via autosuggestive ideas.

> Long-term training in a relaxation technique should help patients to cope better with stressful situations in general. Relaxation techniques are thus an important coping technique.

An improved sense of well-being as well as a more positive experience of the body can help in the long term to loosen dysfunctional, negative attitudes towards one's own body (e.g., as a "body burdened with symptoms").

Biofeedback

Biofeedback has various important functions in therapy (Nanke & Rief, 2003). Demonstrating that mental processes have an influence on physical reactions through feedback of psychophysiological parameters, can help to develop a psychobiological understanding of physical perceptions. Reattribution processes can thus be set in motion. At the same time, patients can learn to gain control over their bodily responses via feedback of physiological processes. In this way, patients not only acquire important coping strategies, they can also regain self-confidence in their bodies and develop internal control beliefs regarding their somatic symptoms. By establishing appropriate self-management skills, patients thus have the opportunity to overcome their feelings of helplessness and experience self-efficacy. For patients with persistent somatic symptoms, different types of biofeedback can be used depending on the symptoms, e.g. electromyographic, skin temperature, skin conductance or blood pressure biofeedback. More detailed information on the use of biofeedback can be found in Rief and Birbaumer (2006).

3.1.3 Reattribution Training

Since the primary care provider is usually the first point of contact for patients with persistent somatic symptoms, they play a crucial role in the treatment process. Therefore, it is important to train primary care providers or other treating physicians with regard to psychological interventions as well as an adequate handling of this special patient group. In the family practice, the way is usually already paved for later treatments. An inadequate handling of the patient by the physician (e.g., by wrong advice or reinforcement of catastrophizing cognitions by unnecessary diagnostic examinations) can weaken the patient's motivation for a possible psychological intervention at a very early stage. Therefore, appropriate trainings for GPs have been developed in recent years (Aiarzaguena et al., 2007; Blankenstein et al., 2002; Morriss et al., 2007; Larisch et al., 2004). These approaches are all based on an important basic concept: reattribution according to the three-stage **reattribution model of** Goldberg et al. (1989).

> The aim of these trainings is to train the primary care providers in how to provide the patient with a simple, psychobiological explanatory model (somatic symptom, psychosocial problem, establishing the link between somatic symptom and psychosocial problem) for their somatic symptoms.

The model is summarized in ◘ Table 3.2.

GPs are first trained to develop "bodily empathy" for the patient to accompany the physical examination. This is done by the physician taking a psychosocial history of the somatic symptoms before the actual physical examination. Patients feel more taken seriously and that they are being listened to. In addition, the clinician learns communication strategies through role-playing with video feedback to illustrate to the patient connections between negative emotions, cognitions, and psychophysiological processes. Successful reattribution training can thus greatly facilitate the patient's referral to psychotherapy. Fink et al. (2002) took the reattribution model and further elaborated it as the TERM model (The Extended Reattribution and Management Model). Important extensions of the original model include a guideline for continuation treatment or for the treatment of patients with persistent somatic symptoms.

◘ **Table 3.2** The three stages of the reattribution model according to Goldberg et al. (1989)

Stage	Contents
Building empathy and understanding for the somatic symptoms	Exploration of somatic symptoms, psychosocial problems, mood state, thoughts and evaluations regarding somatic symptoms Relevant physical examination
Broadening of perspectives regarding the somatic symptom	Summary and discussion of physiological and psychosocial findings
Establishing a link between somatic symptoms and psychosocial problems	Derivation of temporal and physiological relationships between somatic symptoms and psychosocial processes

Also in the case of reattribution training, it becomes clear that close cooperation and regular consultation between the treating physician and therapist is of enormous importance during the therapy of individuals with persistent somatic symptoms. A simple way to support this interdisciplinary cooperation is the use of so-called consultation letters (Rost et al., 1994; Wilkinson & Mynors-Wallis, 1994). These letters contain information on persistent somatic symptoms and their course, recommendations to the primary care providers in dealing with the patient (e.g., arranging time-contingent rather than symptom-contingent appointments, consultation with therapists regarding the initiation of further diagnostic measures or hospitalization), or information, for example, on communication strategies (e.g., avoiding expressions such as "It's all in your head.").

3.1.4 Depth Psychology-Oriented Therapy Approaches

As was made clear in ▶ Sect. 2.10, a variety of different psychoanalytic and depth psychology-oriented concepts for understanding somatoform phenomena have emerged. As a result, it is not possible to speak of a generally accepted model of disorders and an associated method of treatment in modern depth psychology-oriented therapy either. However, it can be stated that in depth psychology-oriented therapy the development of persistent somatic symptoms is no longer described monocausally, but is seen as an interaction of psychological, biological and social factors (Kanwischer, 2006).

> The special feature of depth psychology is that in its treatment methods it places an emphasis on the life-historical experiences of the patient—the influence of early object relations on the later handling of physical illness (Taerk & Gnam, 1994; Taylor, 1992). Against this background, this approach tries to make the disorder more understandable, which should enable the patients to "do without" their symptomatology in the long term.

Procedure Depending on the Structural Level of the Patient

The depth psychological approach is strongly oriented towards the patient's structural level of functioning. It is assumed that patients with persistent somatic symptoms are not homogeneous with regard to their structural level.

- In patients persistent somatic symptoms, in which a **more mature structural level is** expected, it is assumed that the disorder is based on a current, partly conscious experience of conflict, which is expressed by "somatization". Von Uexküll and Köhle (1996) postulate in their treatment model for "functional symptoms" that the somatic symptoms are based on a current triggering process (psychological or somatic) that leads to a functional change of the organism. If this is perceived by the affected person, it can be amplified by maladaptive emotional processing of the experience. In this case, the therapy is rather oriented towards the actual situation of the patient.
- In another group of patients with persistent somatic symptoms, a **neurotic personality organization** is assumed. The goal of taking the patient's history is to identify inner conflicts as well as a triggering situations. In this group of patients, the focus of treatment, after the establishment of a therapeutic relationship, is on illuminating the conflict that underlies the symptomatology.
- In a third group, persistent somatic symptoms are seen as an expression of a **personality disorder**. These patients are more likely to have a low level of structural functioning and an early childhood developmental disorder. In therapy in this case, the emphasis is accordingly placed on identifying the developmental deficits. A sufficiently stable therapy relationship is of enormous importance here before the interpretation of unconscious contents can flow into the therapy.

Special Features of Depth Psychology-Oriented Therapy of Persistent Somatic Symptoms

The **therapist's attitude and tasks** are characterized by absorbing ("containing") affects and emotions that are hard to bear for the patient and thus to take over a psychological processing of these affects and emotions. The therapist then later brings the previously unbearable affects and emotions back into the treatment.

Furthermore, the patients should be given sufficient space in therapy to develop their **explanatory model of illness** and to experience their therapist to be accepting, supportive attitude. Somatic symptoms should not be interpreted too quickly as a phenomenon of resistance. Patients' mourning and demonstratively helpless behavior should not be perceived primarily as an aggravation tendency, but should be viewed against the background of relational experiences in pretreatment. A too quick confrontation of patients with the psychogenesis of their symptoms is avoided.

Motivation for therapy usually has to be encouraged first and cannot be assumed. In the first stage of therapy, the therapeutic procedure is **less conducive to transfer**. Initially, work is done less biographically, but rather in the patient's current situation. In this therapy stage, an additional group therapy in the depth psychological understanding can be helpful. An adoption of alternative perspectives on the patient's symptomatology can be particularly encouraged by the other group participants. The focus on transference-related work is only helpful after the development of a sustainable therapeutic relationship.

3.1.5 Psychodynamic-Interpersonal Therapy Approaches

Interpersonal approaches to therapy for persistent somatic symptoms derive from assumptions of Sullivan's (1953) interpersonal theory and Bowlby's (1969) attachment theory. Based on these basic theories, Stuart and Noyes (1999) developed a concept of disorder according to which persistent somatic symptoms are seen as a combination of insecure attachment type and lack of medical reassurance (► Sect. 2.9). Due to their insecure attachment style and the associated inability to adequately express their problems, individuals with persistent somatic symptoms try to demand help and psychological support with regard to their symptoms by frequently complaining about their somatic symptoms and by their illness behavior. This communication style leads to rejection on the part of the respective caregiver and in turn confirms patients in their assumption that they are not receiving care and support regarding their somatic symptoms.

> The task of the treating physician or therapist is to break this vicious circle. The therapy focuses on the interactional behavior of the patient and their significant others and teaches them helpful methods for communicating their need for support.

To do this, the therapist applies a variety of therapeutic techniques (Stuart & Noyes Jr., 2006). In interpersonal therapy, the use of "bridging metaphors" avoids dichotomizing the problem as either medical or psychological, or discussing the existence of the symptoms or identifying their cause. Instead, the patients are motivated to improve their management of the symptoms. The therapy concept is based on the assumption that patients with persistent somatic symptoms in particular experience a pronounced power imbalance in relation to their therapist or physician. For this reason, a contract is established and written up together with the patient at the beginning of therapy, in which contacts between patient and physician are arranged as well as emergency contacts are specified. Another important element of therapy is to make patients aware of the effect their way of communicating has on the behavior and reactions of those around them. For this purpose, interpersonal contact situations are re-enacted in connection with the patient's search for support. Verbal as well as non-verbal aspects of communication are analyzed in detail for specific situations. The therapist works out together with the patient how and why the counterpart reacted in a certain way in specific situations.

As a basic therapeutic attitude, interpersonal therapy presupposes "authentic empathy". This is promoted by the therapist explaining the development of the patient's insecure attachment style and thus being able to better empathize with the patient's situation. In addition, the therapist can use targeted positive reinforcement in an authentic and realistic manner. Interpersonal therapy is based on the assumption that patients with persistent somatic symptoms find it difficult to cope with an abrupt end to therapy. They feel abandoned and may react negatively accordingly. In order to prevent this reaction, but at the same time to prevent a dependency between patient and therapist, the interpersonal treatment concept recommends a maintenance therapy with a gradual reduction of therapeutic contacts.

▪ Psychodynamic-Interpersonal Therapy for Somatoform Disorders (PISO)

The PISO intervention, developed by the PISO working group (2012), is a 12-h, phase-defined treatment concept for patients with pain-dominated somatoform disorder, which aims to work out connections between affect regulation and somatization, to clarify individual interpersonal processes of symptom development and maintenance, and to expand the patient's individual model of illness. The modification of patients' biomedical symptom attributions is to be achieved through the mediation of a biopsychosocial model. However, with its 12 sessions, this approach is not profound enough as an intervention for patients who usually come to psychotherapy for the first time after many years of unsuccessful attempts at treatment. PISO is therefore understood more as a "sensitization tool" for further subsequent psychological interventions (Arbeitskreis PISO, 2012).

3.1.6 Sport and Exercise Therapy

> It is scientifically proven that physical activity improves mood and sleep and can increase the perception threshold for pain (Minor, 1991; Weyerer & Kupfer, 1994).

Theories assume that exercise and sport strengthen the immune response by increasing the endorphin level and increase the level of the adrenocorticotropic hormone prolactin and the growth hormone (Harber & Sutton, 1984). Accordingly, several concepts already exist in which these positive effects of physical activity are used as therapeutic tools. The effectiveness of exercise therapy has been demonstrated in intervention studies on fibromyalgia and chronic fatigue syndrome (Busch et al., 2007; Edmonds et al., 2004).

Particular challenges in the treatment of patients with persistent somatic symptoms are the interindividual heterogeneity of the symptoms and the often low motivation to change. Since many of those affected have a pronounced tendency to avoid exercise, it is all the easier to explain why it is initially necessary to build up extensive motivation for exercise therapy.

▪ Aerobic Exercise

To date, there are very few published programs. In the group program of Peters et al. (2002), up to 10 affected persons receive aerobic training (including 2 appointments of 1 h per week) over 10 weeks, which was carried out by physical therapists. Accompanying the training, the patients receive a heart rate monitor to check their pulse. Before the training begins, a psychoeducational introduction to the effects of physical activity on persistent somatic symptoms takes place. Patients are provided with information to understand that an improved physical condition helps them to cope better with everyday life stressors. In addition, the participants' somatic symptoms and their symptom-related dysfunctional evaluations are repeatedly addressed during the training. During training, care is taken to maintain the participants' heart rate at 60–65% of the age-appropriate maximum heart rate. A training session will be initiated with 10 min of warm-up. This is followed by 40 min of aerobic exercise. The final 10 min is then used as a recovery period. Feedback is given to participants at regular intervals based on pulse measurements to improve their fitness. Patients will also be given homework, whereby they will be expected to perform specific exercises from the training 3 times per week for 20 min on their own. Exercise performance will be recorded in a training diary. The diary is evaluated weekly with the physical therapist and goals for the coming week are agreed. At the end of the training, an individual plan for the continuation of the exercises is worked out with the patient.

Although there are few specific exercise programs for patients with persistent somatic symptoms, increased activity exercises are an important component in multimodal behavioral medicine programs (Hiller et al., 2003; Leibbrand, 1997) and cognitive behavior therapies (Allen et al., 2006; Martin et al., 2007).

3.2 Psychopharmacotherapy

The administration of psychotropic drugs to patients with persistent somatic symptoms is not uncommon. A problem is the widespread use of medicines such as benzodiazepines and low-dose depot neuroleptics, for which no or only very few studies are available providing empirical evidence of efficacy (Rief & Hiller, 2011). This means that drugs such as benzodiazepines, which have a potential for dependence or significant side effects, are prescribed without evidence of efficacy. Furthermore, low potency opioids are promoted by the pharmaceutical industry for administration in somatoform pain disorders. However, their efficacy has not been proven by clinical case reports or controlled studies and is considered very critical due to the high dependence potential of these agents (Wambach et al., 2001). It is recommended that long-term opioid therapy in patients with nociceptive or neuropathic pain syndromes and comorbid mental disorders should only be undertaken under close monitoring by a psychiatrist or psychologist. Patients who already have a substance dependence should be treated in close cooperation between addiction and pain therapists (Wambach et al., 2001).

Psychotropic drugs for which there is already good empirical evidence of efficacy according to the current state of research are antidepressants (Kleinstäuber et al., 2014). There are various hypotheses on the mechanisms of action of antidepressants. Among others, it is assumed that their effect on somatic symptoms is based on their action on the neurotransmitters serotonin and noradrenaline. Serotonin and norepinephrine are thought to play an important role in the production of analgesic effects. Tricyclic antidepressants in particular (e.g., opipramol, doxepin, amitriptyline, desipramine, trimipramine) are thought to act on the gastrointestinal system due to anticholinergic effects and can be used in particular to treat diarrhoea (Jackson et al., 2006). However, due to side effects, high discontinuation rates of 20–30% have been shown, especially for the latter (Rief & Hiller, 2011). In the past 10 years, the efficacy of serotonin reuptake inhibitors (e.g. fluoxetine, sertraline), serotonin-norepinephrine reuptake inhibitors (e.g. venlafaxine) or other new generation antidepressants (e.g. tetracyclic antidepressants) has been increasingly investigated. The advantage of this group of psychotropic drugs is the lower rate of side effects. However, the effectiveness, especially with regard to somatic symptoms, seems to be rather low. Alternatively, the herbal antidepressant Hypericum perforatum, or St. John's wort has been used to treat persistent somatic symptoms (Kleinstäuber et al., 2014). In addition to antidepressants, low-dose antiepileptic drugs such as gabapentin or pregabalin are also administered for pain-dominated syndromes, such as fibromyalgia (Cooper et al., 2017; Moore et al., 2009; Derry et al., 2016).

3.3 Evidence of Effects of Different Therapeutic Approaches to Persistent Somatic Symptoms

As explained in ► Sects. 3.1 and 3.2, a variety of therapeutic approaches have been developed for the treatment of multiple forms and syndromes of persistent somatic symptoms. In order to assess their usefulness it is important to study the quality of evidence of how effective they are. A widely used four-level system of different levels of evidence developed by the Agency of Health Care Policy and Research (United States Department of Health and Human Services, 1993) can be applied for this purpose (◘ Table 3.3).

► Section 1.2.2 explained that the literature distinguishes polysymptomatic syndromes of persistent somatic symptoms and monosymptomatic syndromes. The following overview of the status quo of evidence on the treatment approaches discussed in ► Sects. 3.1 and 3.2 refers primarily to polysymptomatic syndromes. ◘ Figure 3.2 provides an overview of meta-analytic work that has examined the evidence of effectiveness of different treatment approaches for more specific syndromes such as fibromyalgia or chronic fatigue syndrome. In contrast to more specific syndromes, evidence of efficacy at the highest level of evidence is scarce for the treatment of polysymptomatic syndromes.

3

Table 3.3 Levels of evidence according to the Agency of Health Care Policy and Research (1993)

Level of evidence	
Ia	Evidence based on meta-analyses of randomized controlled trials
Ib	Evidence based on at least one randomized controlled trial
IIa	Evidence based on at least one well-designed controlled trial without randomization
IIb	Evidence based on at least one well-designed, quasi-experimental study
III	Evidence based on well-designed, non-experimental descriptive studies (e.g., case-control studies)
IV	Evidence based on reports/opinions of expert groups, consensus conferences and/or clinical experience of recognized authorities

In addition to previous meta-analyses (Kleinstäuber et al., 2011; van Dessel et al., 2014), there are at least a few narrative reviews of the effectiveness of various interventions for persistent somatic symptoms. These are summarized in Table 3.4.

However, the results of these reviews are challenging to interpret due to the subjectivity the qualitative data summary. Accordingly, the following presentation of the evidence of how effective the various therapeutic methods presented in ► Sects. 3.1 and 3.2 are, will focus on the highest level of evidence.

3.3.1 Psychological Interventions

Two meta-analyses are currently available (van Dessel et al., 2014; Kleinstäuber et al., 2011), which examined the effects various psychological interventions for persistent somatic symptoms. In their literature search, the authors primarily encountered studies on cognitive behavior therapy, behavioral medicine treatment approaches, reattribution training, and only a few stud-

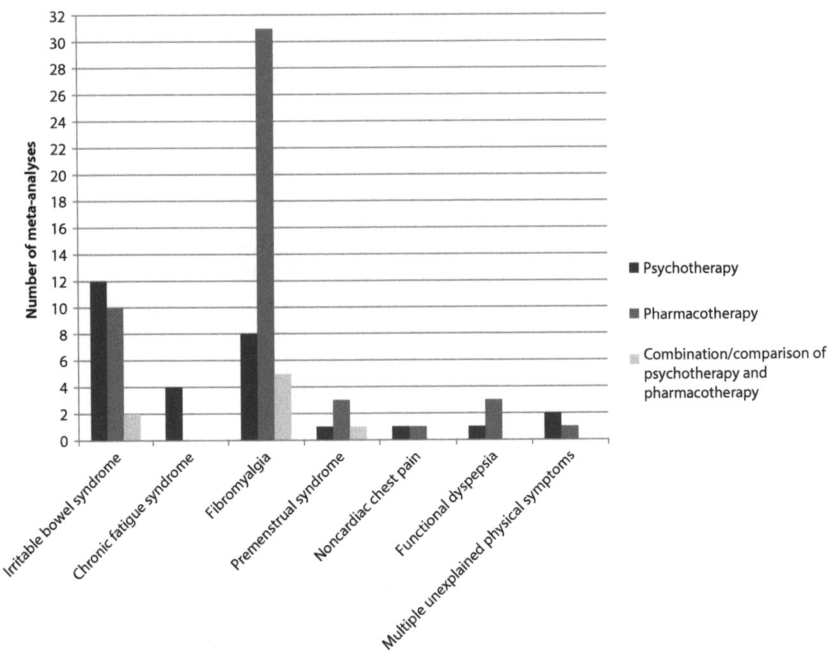

Fig. 3.2 Overview of the number of meta-analyses on various functional syndromes compared with polysymptomatic syndromes of persistent somatic symptoms in adults. (References to the meta-analyses in ► Sect. 3.6)

Table 3.4 Overview of narrative reviews on the effectiveness of various psychosocial interventions for multiple persistent somatic symptoms

Authors	Symptoms/Syndromes	Treatment approaches
Allen et al. (2002)	Somatization disorder, irritable bowel syndrome (IBS), chronic fatigue syndrome (CFS), fibromyalgia	Cognitive behavior therapy (CBT), cognitive therapy (CT), behavior therapy (BT), relaxation training, exercise therapy, biofeedback, hypnotherapy, depth psychology-oriented therapy,
Guthrie (1996)	Persistent somatic symptoms (PSS), CFS, functional dyspepsia, IBS, chronic headache or back pain, non-cardiac chest pain	CBT, depth psychology-oriented therapy, problem solving therapy
Kroenke (2007)	PSS, somatization disorder, somatoform autonomic dysfunction, hypochondriasis, body dysmorphic disorder, conversion disorder	CBT, reattribution training, psychiatric consultation letters, antidepressants, hypnosis, stress management, exercise therapy, paradoxical interventions,
Kroenke and Swindle (2000)	PSS, CFS, irritable bowel syndrome, chronic lower abdominal pain, back pain, headaches, non-cardiac chest pain, tinnitus, burning mouth syndrome, insomnia, fibromyalgia, hypochondria, temporomandibular dysfunction	CBT
Looper and Kirmayer (2002)	PSS, hypochondriasis, body dysmorphic disorder, conversion disorder, non-cardiac chest pain, CFS	Psychiatric consultation letters, CBT, psychoeducation, hypnosis
Nezu et al. (2001)	PSS, CFS, fibromyalgia, non-cardiac chest pain	CBT
Sumathipala (2007)	Somatization disorder, undifferentiated somatoform disorder, somatoform autonomic dysfunction, PSS, CFS, fibromyalgia	CBT, depth psychology-oriented therapy, family therapy, reattribution training, problem-solving therapy, psychiatric consultation letters, antidepressants

ies on other therapy methods (e.g., emotion-focused, depth psychology-oriented, and eclectic therapy). They summarized results for various outcome measures such as the severity of somatic symptoms, cognitive, emotional, and behavioral symptoms, depressiveness, general psychopathology, health-related quality of life, or health care utilization. The meta-analysis by van Dessel et al. (2014) includes a total of 21—exclusively randomized controlled—studies and the meta-analysis by Kleinstäuber et al. (2011) includes a total of 27—partly randomized controlled, partly uncontrolled—studies. To calculate effect sizes, Hedges g was calculated for the comparison between treatment and control groups. With regard to the interpretation of both effect size measures, the following conventions can be used: Values from 0.20 to 0.30 indicate small effects, values from 0.50 indicate medium effects, and values above 0.80 indicate large effects (Cohen, 1977).

- **Effectiveness of Cognitive Behavior Therapy and Behavioral Medicine Interventions, Reattribution Training, and Relaxation Techniques**

Across outcome measures, **cognitive behavior therapy** (including **biofeedback**) yield small to medium effects ranging from $g = 0.07$ to $g = 0.68$ (van Dessel et al., 2014) and from $g = 0.03$ to $g = 0.25$ (Kleinstäuber et al., 2011) with respect to comparisons of treatment and control groups (predominantly waiting control groups or treatment as usual). The effects appear to be stable. For 1–2 year follow-up, effect sizes were $g = 0.08$ and $g = 0.94$ (van Dessel et al., 2014) and $g = 0.12$ and $g = 0.33$ (Kleinstäuber et al., 2011), respectively. Kleinstäuber et al. (2011) separately evaluated behavioral interventions and reattribution training. For the former, small to large effects ($g = 0.17$ and $g = 0.85$) were found at the end of therapy compared to a wait-list control group. Long-term follow-ups were not available. Small to moderate effects were found for reattribution training at the end of therapy and at follow-up assessments after the end of therapy ($g = 0.10$ and $g = 0.78$, respectively). The data for reattribution training must be interpreted with caution as they show high levels of heterogeneity, are often based on very small numbers of included studies and small sample sizes. Van Dessel et al. (2014) separately evaluated the effectiveness of "third wave" cognitive behavior therapy. The meta-analysis includes two studies of **mindfulness-based therapy** for functional somatic syndromes (Fjorback et al., 2013; van Ravesteijn et al., 2013). The comparison of mindfulness-based therapy with treatment as usual showed only small or, in some cases, even null effects ($g = -0.10$ and $g = 0.31$; van Dessel et al., 2014) across different outcomes in both studies at the end of therapy as well as at 9 and 12 months follow-up, respectively. To date, there are no findings on **acceptance-commitment therapy** for syndromes of persistent somatic symptoms. However, conclusions can be drawn from study results on patients with chronic pain. In a meta-analysis by Veehof et al. (2011), small effect sizes were found for pain, depression, perceived status of physical health and quality of life ($0.25 \leq g \leq 0.43$) and moderate effect sizes for anxiety symptoms ($g = 0.55$). Furthermore, the results of this work show that ACT is not superior to cognitive behavior therapy for chronic pain, but can be considered a good alternative.

When interpreting the results of both meta-analyses (van Dessel et al., 2014; Kleinstäuber et al., 2011), it should be taken into account that the included studies exclusively examined extremely short-term interventions, which comprised between 1 and 13 sessions. Kleinstäuber et al. (2011) were able to identify the number of therapy sessions as a predictor of therapy success. In light of the fact that the study samples included patients with a symptom duration of 13 years, it is suggested by the authors that a longer duration of therapy could produce higher effects. At the same time, however, the authors discuss that in order to improve effectiveness in the future, not only should the number of sessions be increased, but the quality of therapy should be optimized.

Three randomized controlled trials of exposure-based pain management are available to date, demonstrating superiority of the intervention over a wait-list control group in terms of changes in functional level (Linton et al., 2008), pain intensity, depressive symptoms, symptom-related cognitive variables, and emotional variables (e.g., kinesiophobic symptoms, fear-avoidance thoughts, and catastrophizing thoughts) (Woods & Asmundson, 2008). In particular, with respect to cognitive variables (e.g., anxiety-avoidance thoughts, catastrophizing), exposure-based therapy was shown to be superior to increased physical activity at the conclusion of therapy and 6 months later (Leeuw et al., 2008). However, the results must be interpreted with caution as there were high dropout rates of up to 58% (Woods & Asmundson, 2008).

▪ Effectiveness of Depth Psychology-Oriented Therapy Approaches

There is currently no evidence of effectiveness at the highest level of evidence for depth psychology-oriented therapy for persistent somatic symptoms. The meta-analysis by Kleinstäuber et al. (2011) includes only one uncontrolled German-language paper (Tschuschke et al., 2007). In this study, patients with somatization disorder, undifferentiated somatoform disorder, and somatoform autonomic dysfunction were treated with psychodynamic and interpersonal elements in 20 weekly therapy sessions. What is problematic about this study is that primarily global rather than symptom-specific outcome measures were used at the self-report level. The authors report a significant reduction in psychological and symptomatic burden that was stable over the 6- and 12-month catamneses.

In addition to this work, there is another uncontrolled pre-post study (Melson et al., 1982) of psychodynamic group therapy, but this was not included in the meta-analysis by Kleinstäuber et al. (2011) due to the mixed sample (only 5% of patients suffer from a somatoform disorder and the remaining patients primarily have anxiety disorders, mood disorders or personality disorders). Group therapy took place in a day hospital setting over 2–5 weeks. For this mixed sample, the authors demonstrated a significant decrease in somatic symptoms that proved stable at the 6-month catamnesis. In addition, there was a significant increase in functional level at follow-up. Furthermore, the patients' external control beliefs increased significantly until the end of treatment. In summary, it must be emphasized that there is insufficient evidence for depth psychology-oriented therapy for patients with multiple persistent somatic symptoms.

▪ Effectiveness of Psychodynamic-Interpersonal Therapy Approaches

Two randomized controlled trials are currently available on psychodynamic-interpersonal therapy approaches for patients with persistent somatic symptoms, which were also included in the meta-analysis by van Dessel et al. (2014). For various outcome measures, psychodynamic-interpersonal therapy resulted in small or null effects at the end of therapy ($-0.11 \leq g \leq 0.39$) as well as at a 9- and 12-month follow-up after the end of treatment ($-0.02 \leq g \leq 0.35$; van Dessel et al., 2014).

▪ Effectiveness of Sports and Exercise Therapy

As described in ► Sect. 3.1.6, there has been one randomized controlled trial of exercise therapy for persistent somatic symptoms (Peters et al., 2002). In this study, 220 patients were randomly assigned to a group with aerobic exercises or a control group with stretching exercises. On self-report scales of somatization, depression, and anxiety, treated patients in both groups showed comparable symptom reduction. Improvement in general psychopathology showed stability at 6 months after training completion. In the different facets evaluated regarding social functioning impairments, patients in both groups showed a positive trend. On average, patients attended 11 of the 20 sessions. It should be particularly emphasized that in both groups healthcare utilization with regard to consultations with the primary care provider and prescriptions of medications, among other outcomes, could be reduced in a comparably significant and stable manner.

3.3.2 Effectiveness of Psychopharmacological Therapy

A meta-analysis is currently available on the psychopharmacological treatment of multiple, chronic somatoform symptoms (Kleinstäuber et al., 2014). This work comprises 26 randomized controlled trials in which a total of almost 2200 patients were treated. Pharmacotherapy in the individual studies lasted from 2 to 12 weeks. None of the included studies had a long-term follow-up, but patients were only interviewed immediately after treatment completion. Most of the included papers examined the efficacy of antidepressants, such as tricyclic antidepressants (e.g., amitriptyline) or various forms of new-generation antidepressant agents. The latter include:

- Selective serotonin reuptake inhibitors (SSRIs; e.g., fluoxetine),
- Norepinephrine reuptake inhibitors (NRIs; e.g., reboxetine),
- Serotonin-norepinephrine reuptake inhibitors (SNRIs; e.g., venlafaxine),
- Noradrenergic and specific serotonergic antidepressants (NaSSA; e.g. mirtazapine),
- Serotonin antagonists and reuptake inhibitors (SARIs; e.g., trazodone),
- Tetracyclic antidepressants (e.g., maprotiline).

Three of the studies were devoted to the efficacy of natural products, such as hypericum perforatum (St. John's wort). Another study assessed the efficacy of an antipsychotic and three studies investigated the efficacy of a combination treatment of an antidepressant and an antipsychotic. Although the total number of included studies was relatively high, only a small number of studies could be included in the individual comparisons per drug group. In addition, the quality of the studies was rated low to very low, limiting the interpretation of the results. For the tricyclic antidepressants, there was insufficient empirical evidence to evaluate their efficacy. In contrast, the new-generation antidepressants predominantly moderately reduced the expression of somatic symptoms, depression, and functional impairment compared with placebo ($0.26 \leq g \leq 0.91$). Likewise, herbal products showed good to high efficacy regarding physical and depressive symptoms ($0.64 \leq g \leq 0.83$). Studies comparing different types of antidepressants did not find any essential differences between tricyclic antidepressants or new generation antidepressants. A combined treatment of an antidepressant and an antipsychotic was found to be more effective than administration of an antidepressant alone ($0.26 \leq g \leq 0.95$) on several outcome measures. Discontinuation rates as a result of side effects were high in the antidepressant trials (0–32%) and low in the natural product trials (0–1.7%).

Furthermore, meta-analyses are available on specific functional syndromes such as irritable bowel syndrome (Ford et al., 2009), fibromyalgia (Häuser et al., 2009), premenstrual syndrome (Marjoribanks et al., 2013), or functional dyspepsia (Hojo et al., 2005) (■ Fig. 3.2). In these papers, mainly the effectiveness of antidepressants was investigated. Tricyclic antidepressants, selective serotonin reuptake inhibitors, and serotonin-norepinephrine reuptake inhibitors were found to be the most effective. Overall, however, only small to sometimes moderate effects were found for these groups of drugs with respect to both physical and psychological outcome measures. A decisive problem of these studies is that there is a lack of longitudinal studies including longterm follow-ups, so that no statements can be made about long-term effects.

3.4 Evidence-Based Guidelines for the Treatment of Persistent Somatic Symptoms

The existing empirical evidence on the treatment of persistent somatic symptoms and associated phenomena has been summarized in a total of two comprehensive guidelines of the Association of the Scientific Medical Societies in Germany (AWMF, 2012) and the German Society for Psychology (DGPs; Martin et al., 2013). Guidelines serve the purpose of quality assurance and have the task of systematically processing the existing knowledge and, in particular, empirical evidence on diagnostics and treatment in order to enable therapists and physicians as well as patients to make an informed selection of the best procedures with regard to diagnostics and therapy. Since the AWMF S3 guideline (Arbeitsgemeinschaft der Wissenschaftlichen Medizinischen Fachgesellschaften, 2012) focuses more on the medical care of patients in the context of primary care providers and specialists, the following will primarily address the contents of the DGPs guideline on diagnostics and psychotherapy in patients with persistent somatic symptoms.

As a necessary prerequisite for adequate treatment, both of the aforementioned guidelines cite careful diagnostics in both the somatic and psychopathological areas. With regard to medical diagnostics, a reasonable scope according to the principle "as much as necessary and as little as possible" seems advisable in order to counteract the danger of overdiagnosis in addition to overlooking possible somatic disease factors. The AWMF guideline also points out that in the area of appointment scheduling for patients with persistent somatic symptoms, a time-contingent approach is to be preferred over a symptom- or affect-contingent approach, since otherwise a perpetuation and amplification of symptoms and anxiety (in the sense of iatrogenicly caused symptoms) is possible via operant learning theory mechanisms. In addition to a thorough medical examination, which should be documented in the context of an outpatient psychological treatment, a careful classification and diagnosis of the patient's condition appears to be necessary in order to be able to create and implement an appropriate treatment plan. Prior to the use of extensive and time-consuming diagnostic interviews, the use of screening questionnaires (e.g. PHQ-15 and SOMS-2, ► Sect. 1.3.4) is recommended, particularly in primary and secondary medical settings, in order to obtain possible indications of the presence of a somatoform disorder. Since such screening instruments have a high degree of sensitivity with comparatively low specificity, the final diagnosis must be made on the basis of an appropriate clinical interview (e.g., SCID). In addition to the level of somatic symptoms and the associated impairment, cognitive (e.g., selective attention to bodily processes), affective (e.g., health anxiety), behavioral (e.g. avoidance and healthcare utilization behavior) and social contextual factors should also be carefully recorded. On the one hand, these are diagnostically relevant positive criteria of somatic symptom disorder according to DSM-5. On the other hand, according to current cognitive-behavioral disorder models, these factors function as essential factors in the perpetuation of persistent somatic symptoms with direct relevance for therapy planning.

With regard to the indication for psychological treatment, the DGPs guideline states, with reference to the AWMF guideline, that due to the high prevalence and the presentation of many patients in the primary and secondary medical setting, psychological treatment of all patients with somatoform disorder or functional somatic syndromes appears utopian. Psychotherapy is particularly indicated in the presence of diffuse polysymptomatic and long-standing symptomatology, as well as in the presence of comorbid mental disorders and a high degree of physical and psychological impairment (Martin et al., 2013). Other indications for psychotherapy include, but are not limited to, severe despair and suicidality, severe illness anxiety, and marked avoidance behaviors (Martin et al., 2013). In the case of acute suicidal tendencies and the patient's inability to dissociate, inpatient treatment must be considered (Arbeitsgemeinschaft der Wissenschaftlichen Medizinischen Fachgesellschaften, 2012).

▪ Symptom-Related Polysymptomatic Somatoform Disorders

For the treatment of symptom-related polysymptomatic somatoform disorders (somatization disorder and undifferentiated somatoform disorder), the DGPs guideline names cognitive behavior therapy (in individual and group settings and as short-term therapy) as the only psychological intervention with the highest level of evidence (evidence level I). Other therapy methods such as biofeedback-oriented therapy, psychodynamic-interpersonal psychotherapy (in individual settings) as well as GP-oriented brief interventions and psychiatric letters of recommendation only achieve evidence level II ("possibly effective").

▪ Health Anxiety

In the case of serious health anxiety, the guideline also recommends cognitive behavior therapy as the treatment method of choice (evidence level I). Inpatient psychoeducation in a group setting and internet-based cognitive behavior therapy are mentioned as possibly effective (evidence level II), although the coverage of internet-based psychotherapy by the funding agencies has not yet been clarified.

▪ Chronic Back Pain

Cognitive behavior therapy, self-regulatory therapies (biofeedback and relaxation techniques), exposure therapy to treat fear avoidance and multidisciplinary therapy are considered to be the methods of choice for chronic back pain symptoms (evidence level I). Behavior therapy, based on principles of operant learning, are only considered "possibly" effective (evidence level II).

▪ Chronic Fatigue Syndrome

With regard to chronic fatigue syndrome (or the ICD-10 disorder neurasthenia), the guideline recommends cognitive behavior therapy in an outpatient setting (individual and group therapy) for adults as well as for children and adolescents as an effective treatment method (evidence level I).

▪ Irritable Bowel Syndrome

One of the most common functional syndromes is irritable bowel syndrome, with an estimated population-wide prevalence of approximately 10%. For this functional syndrome with a focus on gastrointestinal symptoms, the guideline recommends, in addition to cognitive behavior therapy (individual and group setting), psychodynamic-interpersonal individual therapy, hypnotherapy, stress management therapy, and relaxation techniques as effective interventions with the highest level of evidence (Level I).

▪ Fibromyalgia

Fibromyalgia as a common chronic primary pain syndrome should be treated according to the guideline with the help of outpatient cognitive behavior therapy in a group setting, EMG biofeedback or hypnotherapy (evidence level I). Mindfulness-based approaches, behavior therapy and neurofeedback are currently only considered "possibly" effective (evidence level II).

▪ Noncardiac Chest Pain

For the disorder of non-cardiac chest pain, the guideline names cognitive behavior therapy in outpatient individual and group settings as the treatment method of choice (evidence level I).

▪ Environment-Related Persistent Somatic Symptoms and Somatoform Vertigo

In the area of environment-related persistent somatic symptoms (such as idiopathic environment-related intolerance, formerly "multiple chemical sensitivity") and in the area of somatoform vertigo, there is currently not enough evidence to be able to describe a treatment method as "effective" for these phenomena. For both areas, cognitive behavior therapy is currently considered "possibly" effective (evidence level II).

3.5 Conclusions for Future Cognitive Behavior Therapy for Persistent Somatic Symptoms

From the effectiveness findings on therapeutic approaches for persistent somatic symptoms, it can be concluded that cognitive behavior therapy is one of the best-studied therapeutic approaches. However, the evidence for cognitive behavior therapy developed to date does not yet show satisfactory effects. Evidence is emerging that the therapies examined in the studies are too brief for this chronically distressed patient population. In addition, a lack of high-quality therapeutic approaches investigated to date may also be responsible for the small effect sizes. With this in mind, the present manual offers a treatment approach that includes more sessions than has been the case in the studies examined to date. The present treatment manual also allows a flexible approach in the sense that the therapy modules can be put together according to the patient's individual needs. This represents a significant qualitative change in contrast to the strictly manualized ultra-short-term therapies investigated in previous studies.

3.6 Literature References of the Meta-Analyses of ◘ Fig. 3.1

Irritable Bowel Syndrome: Psychotherapy

- Altayar, O., Sharma, V., Prokop, L. J., Sood, A., & Murad, M. H. (2015). Psychological therapies in patients with irritable bowel syndrome: A systematic review and meta-analysis of randomized controlled trials. *Gastroenterology Research and Practice*. ▶ https://doi.org/10.1155/2015/549308
- Henrich, J. F., Knittle, K., De Gucht, V., Warren, S., Dombrowski, S. U., & Maes, S. (2015). Identifying effective techniques within psychological treatments for irritable bowel syndrome: A meta-analysis. *Journal of Psychosomatic Research, 78*(3), 205–222. ▶ https://doi.org/10.1016/j.jpsychores.2014.12.009
- Lackner, J. M., Mesmer, C., Morley, S., Dowzer, C., & Hamilton, S. (2004). Psychological treatments for irritable bowel syndrome: A systematic review and meta-analysis. *Journal of Consulting and Clinical Psychology, 72*(6), 1100–1113. ▶ https://doi.org/10.1037/0022-006X.72.6.1100
- Laird, K. T., Tanner-Smith, E. E., Russell, A. C., Hollon, S. D., & Walker, L. S. (2016). Short-term and long-term efficacy of psychological therapies for irritable bowel syndrome: A systematic review and meta-analysis. *Clinical* Gastroenterology *and Hepatology, 14*(7), 937–947.e4. ▶ https://doi.org/10.1016/j.cgh.2015.11.020
- Lee, H. H., Choi, Y. Y., & Choi, M. G. (2014). The efficacy of hypnotherapy in the treatment of irritable bowel syndrome: A systematic review and meta-analysis. *Journal of Neurogastroenterology and Motility, 20*(2), 152–162. ▶ https://doi.org/10.5056/jnm.2014.20.2.152
- Li, L., Xiong, L. S., Zhang, S. H., Yu, Q., & Chen, M. H. (2014). Cognitive-behavioral therapy for irritable bowel syndrome: A meta-analysis. *Journal of Psychosomatic Research, 77*(1), 1–12. ▶ https://doi.org/10.1016/j.jpsychores.2014.03.006
- Liegl, G., Plessen, C. Y., Leitner, A., Boeckle, M., & Pieh, C. (2015). Guided self-help interventions for irritable bowel syndrome: A systematic review and meta-analysis. *European Journal of Gastroenterology & Hepatology, 27*(10), 1209–1221. ▶ https://doi.org/10.1097/Meg.0000000000000428
- Pajak, R., Lackner, J., & Kamboj, S. K. (2013). A systematic review of minimal-contact psychological treatments for symptom management in irritable bowel syndrome. *Journal of Psychosomatic Research, 75*(2), 103–112. ▶ https://doi.org/10.1016/j.jpsychores.2013.05.007
- Park, S. H., Han, K. S., & Kang, C. B. (2014). Relaxation therapy for irritable bowel syndrome: A systematic review. *Asian Nursing Research, 8*(3), 182–192. ▶ https://doi.org/10.1016/j.anr.2014.07.001
- Schaefert, R., Klose, P., Moser, G., & Hauser, W. (2014). Efficacy, tolerability, and safety of hypnosis in adult irritable bowel syndrome: Systematic review and meta-analysis. *Psychosomatic Medicine, 76*(5), 389–398. ▶ https://doi.org/10.1097/Psy.0000000000000039
- Webb, A. N., Kukuruzovic, R. H., Catto-Smith, A. G., & Sawyer, S. M. (2007). Hypnotherapy for treatment of irritable bowel syndrome. *Cochrane Database of Systematic Reviews*, (4), Art. No.: CD005110. ▶ https://doi.org/10.1002/14651858.CD005110.pub2

- Zijdenbos, I. L., de Wit, N. J., van der Heijden, G. J., Rubin, G., & Quartero, A. O. (2009). Psychological treatments for the management of irritable bowel syndrome. *Cochrane Database of Systematic Reviews*, (1), Art. No.: CD006442. ▶ https://doi.org/10.1002/14651858.CD006442.pub2

Irritable Bowel Syndrome: Psychopharmacotherapy

- Andresen, V., Montori, V. M., Keller, J., West, C. P., Layer, P., & Camilleri, M. (2008). Effects of 5-hydroxytryptamine (serotonin) type 3 antagonists on symptom relief and constipation in nonconstipated irritable bowel syndrome: A systematic review and meta-analysis of randomized controlled trials. *Clinical Gastroenterology and Hepatology, 6*(5), 545–555. ▶ https://doi.org/10.1016/j.cgh.2007.12.015
- Chao, G. Q., & Zhang, S. (2013). A meta-analysis of the therapeutic effects of amitriptyline for treating irritable bowel syndrome. *Internal Medicine, 52*(4), 419–424. ▶ https://doi.org/10.2169/internalmedicine.52.9147
- Cremonini, F., Delgado-Aros, S., & Camilleri, M. (2003). Efficacy of alosetron in irritable bowel syndrome: A meta-analysis of randomized controlled trials. *Neurogastroenterology and motility, 15*(1), 79–86. ▶ https://doi.org/10.1046/j.1365-2982.2003.00389.x
- Ford, A. C., Brandt, L. J., Young, C., Chey, W. D., Foxx-Orenstein, A. E., & Moayyedi, P. (2009). Efficacy of 5-HT3 antagonists and 5-HT4 agonists in irritable bowel syndrome: Systematic review and meta-analysis. *American Journal of Gastroenterology, 104*(7), 1831–1843. ▶ https://doi.org/10.1038/ajg.2009.223
- Jackson, J. L., O'Malley, P. G., Tomkins, G., Balden, E., Santoro, J., & Kroenke, K. (2000). Treatment of functional gastrointestinal disorders with antidepressant medications: A meta-analysis. *American Journal of Medicine, 108*(1), 65–72. ▶ https://doi.org/10.1016/S0002-9343(99)00299-5
- Lesbros-Pantoflickova, D., Michetti, P., Fried, M., Beglinger, C., & Blum, A. L. (2004). Meta-analysis: The treatment of irritable bowel syndrome. *Alimentary Pharmacology and Therapeutics, 20*(11–12), 1253–1269.
- Rahimi, R., Nikfar, S., & Abdollahi, M. (2008a). Efficacy and tolerability of alosetron for the treatment of irritable bowel syndrome in women and men: A meta-analysis of eight randomized, placebo-controlled, 12-week trials. *Clinical Therapeutics, 30*(5), 884–901. ▶ https://doi.org/10.1016/j.clinthera.2008.05.002
- Rahimi, R., Nikfar, S., & Abdollahi, M. (2008b). Selective serotonin reuptake inhibitors for the management of irritable bowel syndrome: A meta-anlysis of randomized controlled trials. *Archives of Medical Sciences, 4*(1), 71–76.
- Rahimi, R., Nikfar, S., Rezaie, A., & Abdollahi, M. (2009). Efficacy of tricyclic antidepressants in irritable bowel syndrome: A meta-analysis. *World Journal of Gastroenterology, 15*(13), 1548–1553. ▶ https://doi.org/10.3748/wjg.15.1548
- Xie, C., Tang, Y. R., Wang, Y. F., Yu, T., Wang, Y., Jiang, L. Q., & Lin, L. (2015). Efficacy and safety of antidepressants for the treatment of irritable bowel syndrome: A meta-analysis. *Plos One, 10*(8). ▶ https://doi.org/10.1371/journal.pone.0127815

Irritable Bowel Syndrome: Combination or Comparison Psycho- and Psychopharmacotherapy

- Ford, A. C., Quigley, E. M. M., Lacy, B. E., Lembo, A. J., Saito, Y. A., Schiller, L. R., Soffer, E. E., Spiegel, B. M. R., & Moayyedi, P. (2014). Effect of antidepressants and psychological therapies, including hypnotherapy, in irritable bowel syndrome: Systematic review and meta-analysis. *American Journal of Gastroenterology, 109*(9), 1350–1365. ▶ https://doi.org/10.1038/ajg.2014.148
- Ford, A. C., Talley, N. J., Schoenfeld, P. S., Quigley, E. M., & Moayyedi, P. (2009). Efficacy of antidepressants and psychological therapies in irritable bowel syndrome: Systematic review and meta-analysis. *Gut, 58*(3), 367–378. ▶ https://doi.org/10.1136/gut.2008.163162

Chronic Fatigue Syndrome: Psychotherapy

- Castell, B. D., Kazantzis, N., & Moss-Morris, R. E. (2011). Cognitive behavioral therapy and graded exercise for chronic fatigue syndrome: A meta-analysis. *Clinical Psychology-Science and Practice, 18*(4),311–324. ▶ https://doi.org/10.1111/j.1468-2850.2011.01262.x
- Malouff, J. M., Thorsteinsson, E. B., Rooke, S. E., Bhullar, N., & Schutte, N. S. (2008). Efficacy of cognitive behavioral therapy for chronic fatigue syndrome: A meta-analysis. *Clinical Psychology Review, 28*(5), 736–745. ▶ https://doi.org/10.1016/j.cpr.2007.10.004. S0272-7358(07)00183-3.
- Marques, M. M., De Gucht, V., Gouveia, M. J., Leal, I., & Maes, S. (2015). Differential effects of behavioral interventions with a graded physical activity component in patients suffering from Chronic Fatigue (Syndrome): An updated systematic review and meta-analysis. *Clinical Psychology Review, 40*, 123–137. ▶ https://doi.org/10.1016/j.cpr.2015.05.009
- Price, J. R., Mitchell, E., Tidy, E., & Hunot, V. (2008). Cognitive behaviour therapy for chronic fatigue syndrome in adults. *Cochrane Database of Systematic Reviews*, (3), Art. No.: CD001027. ▶ https://doi.org/10.1002/14651858.CD001027.pub2.

Fibromyalgia: Psychotherapy

- Bernardy, K., Füber, N., Klose, P., & Häuser, W. (2011). Efficacy of hypnosis/guided imagery in fibromyalgia syndrome – A systematic review and meta-analysis of controlled trials. *Bmc Musculoskeletal Disorders, 12*. ▶ https://doi.org/10.1186/1471-2474-12-133
- Bernardy, K., Füber, N., Köllner, V., & Häuser, W. (2010). Efficacy of cognitive-behavioral therapies in fibromyalgia syndrome – A systematic review and metaanalysis of randomized controlled trials. *Journal of Rheumatology, 37*(10), 1991–2005. ▶ https://doi.org/10.3899/jrheum.100104
- Bernardy, K., Klose, P., Busch, A. J., Choy, E. H. S., & Hauser, W. (2013). Cognitive behavioural therapies for fibromyalgia. *Cochrane Database of Systematic Reviews*, (9), Art. No.: CD009796. ▶ https://doi.org/10.1002/14651858.Cd009796.Pub2
- Glombiewski, J. A., Bernardy, K., & Häuser, W. (2013). Efficacy of EMG and EEG biofeedback in fibromyalgia syndrome: A meta-analysis and a systematic review of randomized controlled trials. *Evidence-Based Complementary and Alternative Medicine*. ▶ https://doi.org/10.1155/2013/962741
- Glombiewski, J. A., Sawyer, A. T., Gutermann, J., Koenig, K., Rief, W., & Hofmann, S. G. (2010). Psychological treatments for fibromyalgia: A meta-analysis. *Pain, 151*(2), 280–295. ▶ https://doi.org/10.1016/j.pain.2010.06.011
- Lauche, R., Cramer, H., Dobos, G., Langhorst, J., & Schmidt, S. (2013). A systematic review and meta-analysis of mindfulness-based stress reduction for the fibromyalgia syndrome. *Journal of Psychosomatic Research, 75*(6), 500–510. ▶ https://doi.org/10.1016/j.jpsychores.2013.10.010
- Martinez, M. P., Miro, E., & Sanchez, A. I. (2016). Global clinical benefits of the cognitive-behavioural therapy for insomnia and of the mindfulness-based therapy applied to fibromyalgia: Systematic review and meta analysis. *Behavioral Psychology-Psicologia Conductual, 24*(3), 459–480.
- Theadom, A., Cropley, M., Smith, H. E., Feigin, V. L., & McPherson, K. (2015). Mind and body therapy for fibromyalgia. *Cochrane Database of Systematic Reviews*, (6), Art. No.: CD011735. ▶ https://doi.org/10.1002/14651858.Cd001980.Pub3

Fibromyalgia: Psychopharmacotherapy

- Arnold, L. M., Keck, P. E., & Welge, J. A. (2000). Antidepressant treatment of fibromyalgia. A meta-analysis and review. *Psychosomatics, 41*(2), 104–113. ▶ https://doi.org/10.1176/appi.psy.41.2.104
- Birse, F., Derry, S., & Moore, R. A. (2012). Phenytoin for neuropathic pain and fibromyalgia in adults. *Cochrane Database of Systematic Reviews*, (5), Art. No.: CD009485. ▶ https://doi.org/10.1002/14651858.Cd009485.Pub2

- Cooper, T. E., Derry, S., Wiffen, P. J., & Moore, R. A. (2017). Gabapentin for fibromyalgia pain in adults. *Cochrane Database of Systematic Reviews*, (1), Art. No.: CD012188. ► https://doi.org/10.1002/14651858.CD012188.pub2
- Cording, M., Derry, S., Phillips, T., Moore, R. A., & Wiffen, P. J. (2015). Milnacipran for pain in fibromyalgia in adults. *Cochrane Database of Systematic Reviews*, (10), Art. No.: CD008244. ► https://doi.org/10.1002/14651858.CD008244.pub3
- Corrigan, R., Derry, S., Wiffen, P. J., & Moore, R. A. (2012). Clonazepam for neuropathic pain and fibromyalgia in adults. *Cochrane Database of Systematic Reviews*, (5), Art. No.: CD009486. ► https://doi.org/10.1002/14651858.Cd009486.Pub2
- Derry, S., Cording, M., Wiffen, P. J., Law, S., Phillips, T., & Moore, R. A. (2016). Pregabalin for pain in fibromyalgia in adults. *Cochrane Database of Systematic Reviews*, (9), Art. No.: CD011790. ► https://doi.org/10.1002/14651858.CD011790.pub2
- Gaskell, H., Moore, R. A., Derry, S., & Stannard, C. (2016). Oxycodone for pain in fibromyalgia in adults. *Cochrane Database of Systematic Reviews*, (9), Art. No.: CD012329. ► https://doi.org/10.1002/14651858.Cd012329
- Gill, D., Derry, S., Wiffen, P. J., & Moore, R. A. (2011). Valproic acid and sodium valproate for neuropathic pain and fibromyalgia in adults. *Cochrane Database of Systematic Reviews*, (10), Art. No.: CD009183. ► https://doi.org/10.1002/14651858.CD009183.pub2
- Häuser, W., Bernardy, K., Üceyler, N., & Sommer, C. (2009a). Treatment of fibromyalgia syndrome with antidepressants: A meta-analysis. *JAMA Journal of the American Medical Association, 301*(2), 198–209.
- Häuser, W., Bernardy, K., Üceyler, N., & Sommer, C. (2009b). Treatment of fibromyalgia syndrome with gabapentin and pregabalin – A meta-analysis of randomized controlled trials. *Pain, 145*(1–2), 69–81. ► https://doi.org/10.1016/j.pain.2009.05.014
- Häuser, W., Petzke, F., Üceyler, N., & Sommer, C. (2011). Comparative efficacy and acceptability of amitriptyline, duloxetine and milnacipran in fibromyalgia syndrome: A systematic review with meta-analysis. *Rheumatology, 50*(3), 532–543. ► https://doi.org/10.1093/rheumatology/keq354
- Häuser, W., Urrutia, G., Tort, S., Üceyler, N., & Walitt, B. (2013). Serotonin and noradrenaline reuptake inhibitors (SNRIs) for fibromyalgia syndrome (Review). *Cochrane Database of Systematic Reviews*, (1), Art. No.: CD010292. ► https://doi.org/10.1002/14651858.Cd010292
- Hearn, L., Derry, S., & Moore, R. A. (2012). Lacosamide for neuropathic pain and fibromyalgia in adults. *Cochrane Database of Systematic Reviews*, (2), Art. No.: CD009318. ► https://doi.org/10.1002/14651858.Cd009318.Pub2
- Lee, Y. H., & Song, G. G. (2016). Comparative efficacy and tolerability of duloxetine, pregabalin, and milnacipran for the treatment of fibromyalgia: A Bayesian network meta-analysis of randomized controlled trials. *Rheumatology International, 36*(5), 663–672. ► https://doi.org/10.1007/s00296-016-3468-5
- Lunn, M. P. T., Hughes, R. A. C., & Wiffen, P. J. (2014). Duloxetine for treating painful neuropathy, chronic pain or fibromyalgia. *Cochrane Database of Systematic Reviews*, (1), Art. No.: CD007115. ► https://doi.org/10.1002/14651858.CD007115.pub3
- Moore, R. A., Derry, S., Aldington, D., Cole, P., & Wiffen, P. J. (2015). Amitriptyline for fibromyalgia in adults. *Cochrane Database of Systematic Reviews*, (7), Art. No.: CD011824. ► https://doi.org/10.1002/14651858.Cd011824
- Moore, R. A., Wiffen, P. J., Derry, S., Toelle, T., & Rice, A. S. C. (2014). Gabapentin for chronic neuropathic pain and fibromyalgia in adults. *Cochrane Database of Systematic Reviews*, (4), Art. No.: CD007938. ► https://doi.org/10.1002/14651858.Cd007938.Pub3
- O'Malley, P. G., Balden, E., Tomkins, G., Santoro, J., Kroenke, K., & Jackson, J. L. (2000). Treatment of fibromyalgia with antidepressants: A meta-analysis. *Journal of General Internal Medicine, 15*(9), 659–666. ► https://doi.org/10.1046/j.1525-1497.2000.06279.x
- Roskell, N. S., Beard, S. M., Zhao, Y., & Le, T. K. (2011). A meta-analysis of pain response in the treatment of fibromyalgia. *Pain Practice, 11*(6), 516–527. ► https://doi.org/10.1111/j.1533-2500.2010.00441.x
- Straube, S., Derry, S., Moore, R. A., & McQuay, H. J. (2010). Pregabalin in fibromyalgia: Meta-analysis of efficacy and safety from company clinical trial reports. *Rheumatology, 49*(4), 706–715. ► https://doi.org/10.1093/rheumatology/kep432
- Sultan, A., Gaskell, H., Derry, S., & Moore, R. A. (2008). Duloxetine for painful diabetic neuropathy and fibromyalgia pain: Systematic review of randomised trials. *BMC neurology, 8*. ► https://doi.org/10.1186/1471-2377-8-29
- Tofferi, J. K., Jackson, J. L., & O'Malley, P. G. (2004). Treatment of fibromyalgia with cyclobenzaprine: A meta-analysis. *Arthritis & Rheumatism-Arthritis Care & Research, 51*(1), 9–13. ► https://doi.org/10.1002/art.20076
- Tort, S., Urrutia, G., Nishishinya, M. B., & Walitt, B. (2012). Monoamine oxidase inhibitors (MAOIs) for fibromyalgia syndrome. *Cochrane Database of Systematic Reviews*, (4), Art. No.: CD009807. ► https://doi.org/10.1002/14651858.Cd009807
- Tzellos, T. G., Toulis, K. A., Goulis, D. G., Papazisis, G., Zampeli, V. A., Vakfari, A., & Kouvelas, D. (2010). Gabapentin and pregabalin in the treatment of fibromyalgia: A systematic review and a meta-analysis. *Journal of Clinical Pharmacy and Therapeutics, 35*(6), 639–656. ► https://doi.org/10.1111/j.1365-2710.2009.01144.x
- Üceyler, N., Sommer, C., Walitt, B., & Hauser, W. (2013). Anticonvulsants for fibromyalgia. *Cochrane Database of Systematic Reviews*, (10), Art. No.: CD010782. ► https://doi.org/10.1002/14651858.CD010782
- Walitt, B., Klose, P., Fitzcharles, M. A., Philipps, T., & Häuser, W. (2016). Cannabinoids for fibromyalgia. *Cochrane Database of Systematic Reviews*, (7), Art. No.: CD011694. ► https://doi.org/10.1002/14651858.CD011694.pub2
- Walitt, B., Klose, P., Ueceyler, N., Phillips, T., & Hauser, W. (2016). Antipsychotics for fibromyalgia in adults. *Cochrane Database of Systematic Reviews*, (6), Art. No.: CD011804. ► https://doi.org/10.1002/14651858.CD011804.pub2
- Walitt, B., Urrutia, G., Nishishinya, M. B., Cantrell, S. E., & Häuser, W. (2015). Selective serotonin reuptake inhibitors for fibromyalgia syndrome. *Cochrane Database of Systematic Reviews*, (6), Art. No.: CD011735. ► https://doi.org/10.1002/14651858.Cd011735
- Wiffen, P. J., Derry, S., Lunn, M. P. T., & Moore, R. A. (2013). Topiramate for neuropathic pain and fibromyalgia in adults. *Cochrane Database of Systematic Reviews*, (8), Art. No.: CD008314. ► https://doi.org/10.1002/14651858.Cd008314.Pub3
- Wiffen, P. J., Derry, S., & Moore, R. A. (2013). Lamotrigine for chronic neuropathic pain and fibromyalgia in adults. *Cochrane Database of Systematic Reviews*, (12), Art. No.: CD006044. ► https://doi.org/10.1002/14651858.Cd006044.Pub4
- Wiffen, P. J., Derry, S., Moore, R. A., & Kalso, E. A. (2014). Carbamazepine for chronic neuropathic pain and fibromyalgia in adults. *Cochrane Database of Systematic Reviews*, (4), Art. No.: CD005451. ► https://doi.org/10.1002/14651858.Cd005451.Pub3

Fibromyalgia: Combination or Comparison of Psycho- and Psychopharmacotherapy

- Garcia-Campayo, J., Magdalena, J., Magallon, R., Fernandez-Garcia, E., Salas, M., & Andres, E. (2008). A meta-analysis of the efficacy of fibromyalgia treatment according to level of care. *Arthritis Research & Therapy, 10*(4). ► https://doi.org/10.1186/Ar2455
- Häuser, W., Bernardy, K., Arnold, B., Offenbacher, M., & Schiltenwolf, M. (2009). Efficacy of multicomponent treatment in

fibromyalgia syndrome: A meta-analysis of randomized controlled clinical trials. *Arthritis & Rheumatism-Arthritis Care & Research, 61*(2), 216–224. ▶ https://doi.org/10.1002/art.24276

- Nüesch, E., Häuser, W., Bernardy, K., Barth, J., & Juni, P. (2013). Comparative efficacy of pharmacological and non-pharmacological interventions in fibromyalgia syndrome: Network meta-analysis. *Annals of the Rheumatic Diseases, 72*(6), 955–962. ▶ https://doi.org/10.1136/annrheumdis-2011-201249
- Papadopoulou, D., Fassoulaki, A., Tsoulas, C., Siafaka, I., & Vadalouca, A. (2016). A meta-analysis to determine the effect of pharmacological and non-pharmacological treatments on fibromyalgia symptoms comprising OMERACT-10 response criteria. *Clinical Rheumatology, 35*(3), 573–586. ▶ https://doi.org/10.1007/s10067-015-3144-2
- Rossy, L. A., Buckelew, S. P., Dorr, N., Hagglund, K. J., Thayer, J. F., McIntosh, M. J., Hewett, J. E., & Johnson, J. C. (1999). A meta-analysis of fibromyalgia treatment interventions. *Annals of Behavioral Medicine, 21*(2), 180–191. ▶ https://doi.org/10.1007/Bf02908299

Premenstrual Disorder: Psychotherapy

- Busse, J. W., Montori, V. M., Krasnik, C., Patelis-Siotis, I., & Guyatt, G. H. (2009). Psychological intervention for premenstrual syndrome: A meta-analysis of randomized controlled trials. *Psychotherapy and Psychosomatics, 78*(1), 6–15. ▶ https://doi.org/10.1159/000162296

Premenstrual Disorder: Psychopharmacotherapy

- Dimmock, P. W., Wyatt, K. M., Jones, P. W., & O'Brien, P. M. S. (2000). Efficacy of selective serotonin-reuptake inhibitors in premenstrual syndrome: A systematic review. *Lancet, 356*(9236), 1131–1136
- Marjoribanks, J., Brown, J. P. W., O'Brien, P. M. S., & Wyatt, K. M. (2013). Selective serotonin reuptake inhibitors for premenstrual syndrome. *Cochrane Database of Systematic Reviews*, Art. No.: CD001396. ▶ https://doi.org/10.1002/14651858.CD001396.pub3
- Shah, N. R., Jones, J. B., Aperi, J., Shemtov, R., Karne, A., & Borenstein, J. (2008). Selective serotonin reuptake inhibitors for premenstrual syndrome and premenstrual dysphoric disorder: A meta-analysis. *Obstetrics and Gynecology, 111*(5), 1175–1182. ▶ https://doi.org/10.1097/AOG.0b013e31816fd73b

Premenstrual Disorder: Combination or Comparison Psycho- and Psychopharmacotherapy

- Kleinstäuber, M., Witthöft, M., & Hiller, W. (2012). Cognitive-behavioral and pharmacological interventions for premenstrual syndrome or premenstrual dysphoric disorder: A meta-analysis. *Journal of Clinical Psychology in Medical Settings, 19*(3), 308–319. ▶ https://doi.org/10.1007/s10880-012-9299-y

Non-Cardiac Chest Pain: Psychotherapy

- Kisely, S. R., Campbell, L. A., Yelland, M. J., & Paydar, A. (2015). Psychological interventions for symptomatic management of non-specific chest pain in patients with normal coronary anatomy. *Cochrane Database of Systematic Reviews*, (6), Art. No.: CD004101. ▶ https://doi.org/10.1002/14651858.Cd004101.Pub5

Non-Cardiac Chest Pain: Psychopharmacotherapy

- Atluri, D. K., Chandar, A. K., Fass, R., & Falck-Ytter, Y. (2015). Systematic review with meta-analysis: Selective serotonin reuptake inhibitors for noncardiac chest pain. *Alimentary Pharmacology & Therapeutics, 41*(2), 167–176. ▶ https://doi.org/10.1111/apt.13015

Functional Dyspepsia: Psychotherapy

- Soo, S., Moayyedi, P., Deeks, J., Delaney, B., Lewis, M., & Forman, D. (2005). Psychological interventions for non-ulcer dyspepsia. *Cochrane Database of Systematic Reviews*, (2), Art. No.: CD002301. ▶ https://doi.org/10.1002/14651858.CD002301.pub4

Functional Dyspepsia: Psychopharmacotherapy

- Hiyama, T., Yoshihara, M., Matsuo, K., Kusunoki, H., Kamada, T., Ito, M., Tanaka, S., Chayama, K., & Haruma, K. (2007). Treatment of functional dyspepsia with serotonin agonists: A meta-analysis of randomized controlled trials. *Journal of Gastroenterology and Hepatology, 22*(10), 1566–1570. ▶ https://doi.org/10.1111/j.1440-1746.2006.04723.x
- Hojo, M., Miwa, H., Yokoyama, T., Ohkusa, T., Nagahara, A., Kawabe, M., Asaoka, D., Izumi, Y., & Sato, N. (2005). Treatment of functional dyspepsia with antianxiety or antidepressant agents: Systematic review. *Journal of Gastroenterology, 40*(11), 1036–1042. ▶ https://doi.org/10.1007/s00535-005-1687-8
- Lu, Y. Y., Chen, M., Huang, Z. Y., & Tang, C. W. (2016). Antidepressants in the treatment of functional dyspepsia: A systematic review and meta-analysis. *Plos One, 11*(6). ▶ https://doi.org/10.1371/journal.pone.0157798

Persistent Somatic Symptoms: Psychotherapy

- Kleinstäuber, M., Witthöft, M., & Hiller, W. (2011). Efficacy of short-term psychotherapy for multiple medically unexplained physical symptoms: A meta-analysis. *Clinical Psychology Review, 31*(1), 146–160. ▶ https://doi.org/10.1016/j.cpr.2010.09.001
- van Dessel, N., Den Boeft, M., van der Wouden, J. C., Kleinstäuber, M., Leone, S. S., Terluin, B., Numans, M. E., van der Horst, H. E., & van Marwijk, H. (2014). Non-pharmacological interventions for somatoform disorders and medically unexplained physical symptoms (MUPS) in adults. *Cochrane Database of Systematic Reviews*, (11), Art. No.: CD011142. ▶ https://doi.org/10.1002/14651858.CD011142.pub2

Persistent Somatic Symptoms: Psychopharmacotherapy

- Kleinstäuber, M., Witthöft, M., Steffanowski, A., van Marwijk, H., Hiller, W., & Lambert, M. J. (2014). Pharmacological interventions for somatoform disorders in adults. *Cochrane Database of Systematic Reviews*, (11), Art. No.: CD010628. ▶ https://doi.org/10.1002/14651858.CD010628.pub2

References

Aiarzaguena, J. M., Grandes, G., & Gaminde, I. (2007). A randomized controlled clinical trial of a psychosocial and communication intervention carried out by GPs for patients with medically unexplained symptoms. *Psychological Medicine, 37*(2), 283–294. https://doi.org/10.1017/S0033291706009536

Allen, L. A., Escobar, J. I., Lehrer, P. M., Gara, M. A., & Woolfolk, R. L. (2002). Psychosocial treatments for multiple unexplained physical symptoms: A review of literature. *Psychosomatic Medicine, 64*(6), 939–950. https://doi.org/10.1097/01.PSY.0000024231.11538.8F

Allen, L. A., Woolfolk, R. L., Escobar, J. I., Gara, M. A., & Hamer, R. M. (2006). Cognitive-behavioral therapy for somatization disorder: A randomized controlled trial. *Archives of Internal Medicine, 166*(14), 1512–1518. https://doi.org/10.1001/archinte.166.14.1512

Arbeitsgemeinschaft der Wissenschaftlichen Medizinischen Fachgesellschaften. (2012). S3 Leitlinie. Umgang mit Patienten mit nicht-spezifischen, funktionellen und somatoformen Körperbeschwerden (Registernr.: 051-00).

Arbeitskreis PISO. (2012). *Somatoforme Störungen: Psychodynamisch-Interpersonelle Therapie (PISO)*. Hogrefe.

Blankenstein, A. H., van der Horst, H. E., Schilte, A. F., de Vries, D., Zaat, J. O. M., Knottnerus, J. A., et al. (2002). Development and feasibility of a modified reattribution model for somatising patients, applied by their own general practitioners. *Patient Education and Counseling, 47*(3), 229–235. https://doi.org/10.1016/S0738-3991(01)00199-9

Bleichhardt, G., Timmer, B., & Rief, W. (2004). Cognitive-behavioural therapy for patients with multiple somatoform symptoms – A randomised controlled trial in tertiary care. *Journal of Psychosomatic Research, 56*(4), 449–454. https://doi.org/10.1016/S0022-3999(03)00630-5

Bowlby, J. (1969). *Attachment*. Basic Books.

Busch, A. J., Barber, K. A. R., Overend, T. J., Peloso, P. M. J., & Schachter, C. L. (2007). Exercise for treating fibromyalgia syndrome. *Cochrane Database of Systematic Reviews*, (4), Art. No.: CD003786. https://doi.org/10.1002/14651858.CD003786.pub2

Cohen, J. (1977). *Statistical power analysis for the behavioral sciences*. Academic.

Cooper, T. E., Derry, S., Wiffen, P. J., & Moore, R. A. (2017). Gabapentin for fibromyalgia pain in adults. *Cochrane Database of Systematic Reviews*, (1), Art. No.: CD012188. https://doi.org/10.1002/14651858.CD012188.pub2

Derry, S., Cording, M., Wiffen, P. J., Law, S., Phillips, T., & Moore, R. A. (2016). Pregabalin for pain in fibromyalgia in adults. *Cochrane Database of Systematic Reviews*, (9), Art. No.: CD011790. https://doi.org/10.1002/14651858.CD011790.pub2

Edmonds, M., McGuire, H., & Price, J. (2004). Exercise therapy for chronic fatigue syndrome. *Cochrane Database of Systematic Reviews*, (3), Art. No.: CD003200. https://doi.org/10.1002/14651858.CD003200.pub2

Escobar, J. I., Gara, M. A., Diaz-Martinez, A. M., Interian, A., Warman, M., Allen, L. A., et al. (2007). Effectiveness of a time-limited cognitive behavior therapy type intervention among primary care patients with medically unexplained symptoms. *Annals of Family Medicine, 5*(4), 328–335. https://doi.org/10.1370/afm.702

Fink, P., Rosendal, M., & Toft, T. (2002). Assessment and treatment of functional disorders in general practice: The extended reattribution and management model. *Psychosomatics, 43*(2), 93–131. https://doi.org/10.1176/appi.psy.43.2.93

Fjorback, L. O., Arendt, M., Ornbøl, E., Walach, H., Rehfeld, E., & Schröder, A. (2013). Mindfulness therapy for somatization disorder and functional somatic syndromes – Randomized trial with one-year follow-up. *Journal of Psychosomatic Research, 74*(1), 31–40. https://doi.org/10.1016/j.jpsychores.2012.09.006

Ford, A. C., Talley, N. J., Schoenfeld, P. S., Quigley, E. M., & Moayyedi, P. (2009). Efficacy of antidepressants and psychological therapies in irritable bowel syndrome: Systematic review and meta-analysis. *Gut, 58*(3), 367–378. https://doi.org/10.1136/gut.2008.163162

Freidl, M., Spitzl, S. P., Prause, W., Zimprich, F., Lehner-Baumgartner, E., Baumgartner, C., et al. (2007). The stigma of mental illness: Anticipation and attitudes among patients with epileptic, dissociative or somatoform pain disorder. *International Review of Psychiatry, 19*(2), 123–129. https://doi.org/10.1080/09540260701278879

Goldberg, D., Gask, L., & O'Dowd, T. (1989). The treatment of somatization: Teaching techniques of reattribution. *Journal of Psychosomatic Research, 33*(6), 689–695. https://doi.org/10.1016/0022-3999(89)90084-6

Guthrie, E. (1996). Psychotherapy for somatisation disorders. *Current Opinion in Psychiatry, 9*(3), 182–187.

Hahn, S. R., Kroenke, K., Spitzer, R. L., Brody, D., Williams, J. B., Linzer, M., et al. (1996). The difficult patient: Prevalence, psychopathology, and functional impairment. *Journal of General Internal Medicine, 11*(1), 1–8. https://doi.org/10.1007/BF02603477

Harber, V. J., & Sutton, J. R. (1984). Endorphins and exercise. *Sports Medicine, 1*(2), 154–171. https://doi.org/10.2165/00007256--198401020-00004

Häuser, W., Bernardy, K., Üceyler, N., & Sommer, C. (2009). Treatment of fibromyalgia syndrome with antidepressants: A meta-analysis. *JAMA-Journal of the American Medical Association, 301*(2), 198–209. https://doi.org/10.1001/jama.2008.944

Hiller, W., Fichter, M. M., & Rief, W. (2003). A controlled treatment study of somatoform disorders including analysis of healthcare utilization and cost-effectiveness. *Journal of Psychosomatic Research, 54*(4), 369–380. https://doi.org/10.1016/S0022--3999(02)00397-5

Hojo, M., Miwa, H., Yokoyama, T., Ohkusa, T., Nagahara, A., Kawabe, M., et al. (2005). Treatment of functional dyspepsia with antianxiety or antidepressive agents: Systematic review. *Journal of Gastroenterology, 40*(11), 1036–1042. https://doi.org/10.1007/s00535-005-1687-8

Jackson, J. L., O'Malley, P. G., & Kroenke, K. (2006). Antidepressants and cognitive-behavioral therapy for symptom syndromes. *CNS Spectrums, 11*(3), 212–222. https://doi.org/10.1017/S1092852900014383

Kanwischer, H. (2006). Somatoforme Störungen. In F. Leichsenring (Hrsg.), *Lehrbuch der Psychotherapie für die Ausbildung zur/zum PsychologischenPsychotherapeutIn und für die ärztliche Weiterbildung* (3. Aufl., Bd. 2, S. 173–182). CIP-Medien.

Kashner, T. M., Rost, K., Cohen, B., Anderson, M., & Smith, G. R. J. (1995). Enhancing the health of somatization disorder patients. Effectiveness of short-term group therapy. *Psychosomatics, 36*(5), 462–470. https://doi.org/10.1016/S0033-3182(95)71627-9

Kleinstäuber, M., Witthöft, M., & Hiller, W. (2011). Efficacy of short-term psychotherapy for multiple medically unexplained physical symptoms: A meta-analysis. *Clinical Psychology Review, 31*(1), 146–160. https://doi.org/10.1016/j.cpr.2010.09.001

Kleinstäuber, M., Witthöft, M., Steffanowski, A., van Marwijk, H., Hiller, W., & Lambert, M. J. (2014). Pharmacological interventions for somatoform disorders in adults. *Cochrane Database of Systematic Reviews*, (11), Art. No.: CD010628. https://doi.org/10.1002/14651858.CD010628.pub2

Kleinstäuber, M., Gottschalk, J., Weiß, F., Schwarz, J., & Rief, W. (2016). Cognitive Behavior Therapy Enriched with Emotion Regulation Training (ENCERT) for patients with multiple medically unexplained symptoms: Preliminary results. *International Journal of Behavioral Medicine, 23*(Suppl. 1), S183–S184. https://doi.org/10.1007/s12529-016-9586-3

Kroenke, K. (2007). Efficacy of treatment for somatoform disorders: A review of randomized controlled trials. *Psychosomatic Medicine, 69*(9), 881–888. https://doi.org/10.1097/PSY.0b013e31815b00c4

Kroenke, K., & Swindle, R. (2000). Cognitive-behavioral therapy for somatization and symptom syndromes: A critical review of controlled clinical trials. *Psychotherapy and Psychosomatics, 69*(4), 205–215. https://doi.org/10.1159/000012395

Larisch, A., Schweickhardt, A., Wirsching, M., & Fritzsche, K. (2004). Psychosocial interventions for somatizing patients by the general practitioner. A randomized controlled trial. *Journal of Psychosomatic Research, 57*(6), 507–514. https://doi.org/10.1016/j.jpsychores.2004.04.372

Leeuw, M., Goossens, M. E. J. B., van Breukelen, G. J. P., de Jong, J. R., Heuts, P. H. T. G., Smeets, R. J. E. M., et al. (2008). Exposure in vivo versus operant graded activity in chronic low back pain patients: Results of a randomized controlled trial. *Pain, 138*(1), 192–207. https://doi.org/10.1016/j.pain.2007.12.009

Leibbrand, B. (1997). *Therapieeffekte bei somatoformen Störungen in Abhängigkeit vom zusätzlichen Vorliegen von Persönlichkeitsstörungen* (Bd. 15). Empirische Pädagogik.

Linton, S. J., Boersma, K., Jansson, M., Overmeer, T., Lindblom, K., & Vlaeyen, J. W. S. (2008). A randomized controlled trial of exposure in vivo for patients with spinal pain reporting fear of work-related activities. *European Journal of Pain, 12*(6), 722–730. https://doi.org/10.1016/j.ejpain.2007.11.001

Looper, K. J., & Kirmayer, L. J. (2002). Behavioral medicine approaches to somatoform disorders. *Journal of Consulting and Clinical Psychology, 70*(3), 810–827. https://doi.org/10.1037/0022-006X.70.3.810

Margraf, J., & Schneider, S. (1990). *Panik: Angstanfälle und ihre Behandlung* (2. Aufl.). Springer.

Marjoribanks, J., Brown, J. P. W., O'Brien, P. M. S., & Wyatt, K. M. (2013). Selective serotonin reuptake inhibitors for premenstrual syndrome. *Cochrane Database of Systematic Reviews*, Art. No.: CD001396. https://doi.org/10.1002/14651858.CD001396.pub3

Martin, A., Rauh, E., Fichter, M., & Rief, W. (2007). A one-session treatment for patients suffering from medically unexplained symptoms in primary care: A randomized clinical trial. *Psychosomatics, 48*(4), 294–303. https://doi.org/10.1176/appi.psy.48.4.294

Martin, A., Härter, M., Henningsen, P., Hiller, W., Kröner-Herwig, B., & Rief, W. (2013). *Evidenzbasierte Leitlinie zur Psychotherapie somatoformer Störungen* (Bd. 4, Evidenzbasierte Leitlinien Psychotherapie). Hogrefe.

Melson, S. J., Clark, R. D., Rynearson, E. K., Snyder, A. I., & Dorizbach, J. (1982). Short-term intensive group psychotherapy for patients with 'functional' complaints. *Psychosomatics, 23*(7), 689–695. https://doi.org/10.1016/S0033-3182(82)73343-2

Minor, M. A. (1991). Physical activity and management of arthritis. *Annals of Behavioral Medicine, 13*(3), 117–124.

Moore, R. A., Straube, S., Wiffen, P. J., Derry, S., & McQuay, H. J. (2009). Pregabalin for acute and chronic pain in adults. *Cochrane Database of Systematic Reviews*, (3), Art. No.: CD007076. https://doi.org/10.1002/14651858.CD007076.pub2

Morriss, R., Dowrick, C., Salmon, P., Peters, S., Dunn, G., Rogers, A., et al. (2007). Cluster randomised controlled trial of training practices in reattribution for medically unexplained symptoms. *British Journal of Psychiatry, 191*(6), 536–542. https://doi.org/10.1192/bjp.bp.107.040683

Murray, A. M., Toussaint, A., Althaus, A., & Löwe, B. (2016). The challenge of diagnosing non-specific, functional, and somatoform disorders: A systematic review of barriers to diagnosis in primary care. *Journal of Psychosomatic Research, 80*, 1–10. https://doi.org/10.1016/j.jpsychores.2015.11.002

Nanke, A., & Rief, W. (2003). Biofeedback-based interventions in somatoform disorders: A randomized controlled trial. *Acta Neuropsychiatrica, 15*(4), 249–256. https://doi.org/10.1034/j.1601-5215.2003.00028.x

Nezu, A. M., Nezu, C. M., & Lombardo, E. R. (2001). Cognitive behavioural therapy for medically unexplained symptoms: A critical review of the treatment. *Behavior Therapy, 32*(3), 537–583. https://doi.org/10.1016/S0005-7894(01)80035-6

Nickel, M., Cangoez, B., Bachler, E., Muehlbacher, M., Lojewski, N., Mueller-Rabe, N., et al. (2006). Bioenergetic exercises in inpatient treatment of Turkish immigrants with chronic somatoform disorders: A randomized, controlled study. *Journal of Psychosomatic Research, 61*(4), 507–513. https://doi.org/10.1016/j.jpsychores.2006.01.004

Peters, S., Stanley, I., Rose, M., Kaney, S., & Salmon, P. (2002). A randomized controlled trial of group aerobic exercise in primary care patients with persistent, unexplained physical symptoms. *Family Practice, 19*(6), 665–674. https://doi.org/10.1093/fampra/19.6.665

Rief, W., & Birbaumer, N. (2006). *Biofeedback. Grundlagen, Indikationen, Kommunikation, praktisches Vorgehen in der Therapie*. Schattauer.

Rief, W., & Hiller, W. (2011). *Somatisierungsstörung* (Bd. 1, Fortschritte der Psychotherapie). Hogrefe.

Rief, W., Hiller, W., Geissner, E., & Fichter, M. M. (1995). A two-year follow-up study of patients with somatoform disorders. *Psychosomatics, 36*(4), 376–386. https://doi.org/10.1016/S0033--3182(95)71647-4

Rief, W., Shaw, R., & Fichter, M. M. (1998). Elevated levels of psychophysiological arousal and cortisol in patients with somatization syndrome. *Psychosomatic Medicine, 60*(2), 198–203. https://doi.org/10.1097/00006842-199803000-00016

Rost, K., Kashner, T. M., & Smith, R. G., Jr. (1994). Effectiveness of psychiatric intervention with somatization disorders. *General Hospital Psychiatry, 16*(6), 381–387. https://doi.org/10.1016/0163--8343(94)90113-9

Schilte, A. F., Portegijs, P. J. M., Blankenstein, A. H., van der Horst, H. E., Latour, M. B. F., van Eijk, J. T. M., et al. (2001). Randomised controlled trial of disclosure of emotionally important events in somatisation in primary care. *British Medical Journal, 323*(7304), 86. https://doi.org/10.1136/bmj.323.7304.86

Speckens, A. E. M., van Hemert, A. M., Spinhoven, P., Hawton, K. E., Bolk, J. H., & Rooijmans, H. G. (1995). Cognitive behavioural therapy for medically unexplained physical symptoms: A randomised controlled clinical trial. *British Medical Journal, 311*(7016), 1328–1332. https://doi.org/10.1136/bmj.311.7016.1328

Stuart, S., & Noyes, R. (1999). Attachment and interpersonal communication in somatization. *Psychosomatics, 40*(1), 34–43. https://doi.org/10.1016/S0033-3182(99)71269-7

Stuart, S., & Noyes, R., Jr. (2006). Interpersonal psychotherapy for somatizing patients. *Psychotherapy and Psychosomatics, 75*(4), 209–219. https://doi.org/10.1159/000092891

Sullivan, H. S. (1953). *The interpersonal theory of psychiatry*. Norton.

Sumathipala, A. (2007). What is the evidence for the efficacy of treatments for somatoform disorders? A critical review of previous intervention studies. *Psychosomatic Medicine, 69*(9), 889–900. https://doi.org/10.1097/PSY.0b013e31815b5cf6

Sumathipala, A., Siribaddana, S., Abeysingha, M. R. N., Silva, P., Dewey, M., Prince, M., et al. (2008). Cognitive-behavioural therapy v. structured care for medically unexplained symptoms: Randomised controlled trial. *British Journal of Psychiatry, 193*(1), 51–59. https://doi.org/10.1192/bjp.bp.107.043190

Taerk, G., & Gnam, W. (1994). A psychodynamic view of the chronic fatigue syndrome. The role of object relations in etiology and treatment. *General Hospital Psychiatry, 16*(5), 319–325. https://doi.org/10.1016/0163-8343(94)90018-3

Taylor, G. J. (1992). Psychoanalysis and psychosomatics: A new synthesis. *Journal of the American Academy of Psychoanalysis, 20*(2), 251–275.

Tschuschke, V., Weber, R., Horn, E., Kiencke, P., & Tress, W. (2007). Ambulante psychodynamische Kurzgruppenpsychotherapie bei Patienten mit somatoformen Störungen [Psychodynamic short-term outpatient group therapy with patients suffering from somatoform disorders]. *Zeitschrift für Psychiatrie, Psychologie und Psychotherapie, 55*(2), 87–95.

United States Department of Health and Human Services. Agency for Health Care Policy and Research. (1993). *Acute pain management: Operative or medical procedures and trauma*. AHCPR.

van Dessel, N., Den Boeft, M., van der Wouden, J. C., Kleinstäuber, M., Leone, S. S., Terluin, B., et al. (2014). Non-pharmacological interventions for somatoform disorders and medically unexplained physical symptoms (MUPS) in adults. *Cochrane Database of Systematic Reviews*, (11), Art. No.: CD011142. https://doi.org/10.1002/14651858.CD011142.pub2

van Ravesteijn, H., Lucassen, P., Bor, H., van Weel, C., & Speckens, A. (2013). Mindfulness-based cognitive therapy for patients with medically unexplained symptoms: A randomized controlled

trial. *Psychotherapy and Psychosomatics, 82*(5), 299–310. https://doi.org/10.1159/000348588
Veehof, M. M., Oskam, M. J., Schreurs, K. M. G., & Bohlmeijer, E. T. (2011). Acceptance-based interventions for the treatment of chronic pain: A systematic review and meta-analysis. *Pain, 152*(3), 533–542. https://doi.org/10.1016/j.pain.2010.11.002
Vlaeyen, J. W. S., Kolesnijders, A. M. J., Boeren, R. G. B., & Vaneek, H. (1995). Fear of movement (re)injury in chronic low-back-pain and its relation to behavioral performance. *Pain, 62*(3), 363–372. https://doi.org/10.1016/0304-3959(94)00279-N
Vlaeyen, J. W. S., De Jong, J., Geilen, M., Heuts, P. H. T. G., & van Breukelen, G. (2001). Graded exposure in vivo in the treatment of pain-related fear: A replicated single-case experimental design in four patients with chronic low back pain. *Behaviour Research and Therapy, 39*(2), 151–166. https://doi.org/10.1016/S0005--7967(99)00174-6
Von Uexküll, T., & Köhle, K. (1996). *Psychosomatische Medizin: Modelle ärztlichen Denkens und Handelns* (6. Aufl.). Urban & Schwarzenberger.
Wambach, S., Rohr, P., & Häuser, W. (2001). Abuse of opioid therapy in somatoform pain disorder. A contribution from a psychosomatic/pain therapist point of view to the discussion of the indication of opioids in nonmalignant pain based on 8 cases. *Schmerz, 15*(4), 254–264. https://doi.org/10.1007/s004820000035
Westin, V. Z., Schulin, M., Hesser, H., Karlsson, M., Noe, R. Z., Olofsson, U., et al. (2011). Acceptance and Commitment Therapy versus Tinnitus Retraining Therapy in the treatment of tinnitus: A randomised controlled trial. *Behaviour Research and Therapy, 49*(11), 737–747. https://doi.org/10.1016/j.brat.2011.08.001
Weyerer, S., & Kupfer, B. (1994). Physical exercise and psychological health. *Sports Medicine, 17*(2), 108–116. https://doi.org/10.2165/00007256-199417020-00003
Wilkinson, P., & Mynors-Wallis, L. (1994). Problem-solving therapy in the treatment of unexplained physical symptoms in primary care: A preliminary study. *Journal of Psychosomatic Research, 38*(6), 591–598. https://doi.org/10.1016/0022-3999(94)90056-6
Woods, M. P., & Asmundson, G. J. G. (2008). Evaluating the efficacy of graded in vivo exposure for the treatment of fear in patients with chronic back pain: A randomized controlled clinical trial. *Pain, 136*(3), 271–280. https://doi.org/10.1016/j.pain.2007.06.037

Practice: The Manual: Basics and Initial Phase

Contents

Cognitive-Behavioral Individual Therapy for Patients with Persistent Somatic Symptoms, Somatoform Disorders, and Somatic Symptom Disorders: Basics and Initial Phase

Contents

M. Kleinstäuber et al., *Cognitive Behavior Therapy for Persistent Somatic Symptoms and Somatic Symptom Disorder*, https://doi.org/10.1007/978-3-662-69726-9_4

4.1 Introduction to the Structure of the Manual

This therapy manual is structured in modules. Since the effectiveness of the therapy concept could be proven by adhering to the module sequence or the structured procedure (▶ Chap. 14), we recommend that you follow the suggested sequence of therapy modules as far as possible. The manual comprises a total of 7 modules (◘ Table 4.1), which are divided into 20 individual therapy sessions, and one excursus module. The treatment is introduced with exercises designed to help build up **motivation for therapy or change**. The topic of **stress and stress management** is divided into 2 modules. The first stress module directly

◘ **Table 4.1** Modules of the therapy manual

Module	Therapy session(s)	Therapy goals	Therapy Techniques
Module 1: Treatment motivation	1	Clarification of the therapy goals Building motivation for change	Guided imagery for goal clarification
Module 2: Stress and stress management (Part 1)	2–3	Building knowledge of the human stress and relaxation response Improvement of the ability to relax	Psychoeducation on functions of human stress response, on the structure of the autonomic nervous system, on the physical stress and relaxation response Progressive muscle relaxation
Module 3: Attention refocusing	4–6	Experience of the effect of attention on the perception of bodily changes Learning to refocus attention Enhancement of enjoyment	Demonstration exercises/behavioral experiments to teach the role of attention in the perception of physical discomfort Spotlight metaphor Attention refocusing strategies Mindfulness practice
Module 4: Cognitive reappraisal	7–11	Recognition of connections between feelings, thoughts, behavior and somatic symptoms	ABC model and its transfer to somatic symptoms Cognitive reappraisal techniques in combination with behavioral experiments to induce somatic symptoms Concept of health
Module 5: Illness Behavior	12–15	Reduction of avoidance behavior Reduction of sick-role behaviors Reduction of excessive use of healthcare services	Short- and long-term consequences of illness behaviors Vicious circle model of illness behavior Integrating physical activity and exercise in everyday life Techniques for identifying symptom-related, less helpful thoughts and cognitive reappraisal Behavioral experiments Techniques for building self-care Strategies for reducing reassurance behavior
Module 6: Stress and stress management (Part 2)	16–19	Building stress management skills	Psychoeducation on the transactional stress model according to Lazarus Stress management strategies Time management strategies Strategies for building social support Identification of stress-inducing cognitions Mindfulness practices
Module 7: The explanatory symptom and treatment model	20	Summary of experiences on correlations between psychosocial aspects and somatic symptoms Relapse prevention	Conveying a comprehensive, psychosocial explanatory model of somatic symptoms Relapse prevention plan with future coping strategies
Excursus module: Communication about symptoms in everyday life and with the physician	Flexible number of therapy sessions depending on the problem area	Improving communication about the somatic symptoms and related needs with the social environment	Role plays to switch perspectives Role plays to practice assertive patient-doctor interactions or to practice interactions of different people in the social environment

follows the section on therapy motivation, while the second stress module should be done just before the end of therapy. In addition, the patient is repeatedly taught stress management techniques as practice of the week in the other modules. Two further modules of the manual deal with **attention** and dysfunctional **cognitive appraisals**. The manual also contains a module on **changing dysfunctional behaviors**. These typically include protective behaviors, sick role behaviors, and medical service utilization behaviors. Numerous practical exercises as well as practice of the week assignments distributed throughout the manual enable patients to gradually experience and understand the connections between psychosocial aspects and their somatic symptoms through "guided discovery". These crucial findings are then summarized in the final module, and based on this, an individual **explanatory symptom model** can be derived together with the patient. Compared to the cognitive behavior therapy of other mental disorders, it may at first seem unusual that the symptom model is only taken up at the end of therapy. The advantages and disadvantages of this approach, as well as possible deviations from it that may be necessary under certain circumstances, are explained in ► Sect. 4.1.1. In addition, for patients who have difficulties in **communicating with their psychologist and physicians, relatives or friends**, an excursus module is presented from which content can be used to supplement the manual, which was originally designed with 20 sessions. The individual therapy modules are presented in more detail in ◘ Table 4.1.

The individual therapy sessions predominantly have a fixed structure:

- They are first introduced with **the discussion of practice of the week**. This section should not be underestimated in its importance. Only continuous feedback from the therapist on the practice of the week helps the patient take this practice seriously and feeling motivated to deal intensively with the therapy content between sessions.
- A large proportion of the therapy modules include **practical demonstration exercises, behavioral experiments or guided discovery exercises**, which are designed to give patients new connections and perspectives on their symptoms through practical experience. These experiences are then often combined with a psychoeducational element on the corresponding module topic.
- Each therapy session is rounded off with the **planning a "practice of the week"**.

Instructional texts are provided for the exercise instructions. Numerous worksheets, whose contents are tailored to the respective sessions, have been prepared as therapy material for the patient.

Although it is advisable to follow the prescribed order of the therapy modules, modifications are of course possible. Suggestions regarding tailoring the manual according to patients' needes are described in ► Sects. 4.1.1 and 4.1.2.

4.1.1 Application of the Manualized-Structured Approach in Everyday Practice: Opportunities and Problems

The interested reader will quickly realize when reading the following treatment program that it is a very structured and manualized approach. A total of 20 individual therapeutic sessions (and, depending on the problem area, a flexible number of excursion sessions) were worked out in detail on the basis of therapist instructions and worksheets for the patients as well as suggestions for concrete practices of the week. Such a "strict" standardized procedure may seem strange to some readers who work in a more individualized way. We would therefore like to briefly reflect on the "chances" and "problems" of such a standardized procedure, which have arisen from our therapeutic and supervisory work with the present manual.

▪ High Degree of Structuring

In the exchange with therapists who have already worked with the present treatment concept, the most frequent fear that emerged was that the therapist would not be able to pay sufficient attention to possible current and individual concerns and problems of individual patients due to the high information density per session. Consequently, significant problems, especially with regard to the therapeutic relationship, were anticipated. Interestingly, these fears proved to be largely unfounded. The vast majority of patients reacted extremely positively to the high degree of structuring, experienced the program as professional and were also committed to working with the planned therapy content between sessions. From the therapist's side, too, the structured procedure was mostly experienced as helpful in keeping a "common thread" across the individual sessions and not getting too caught up in current problems. This structured approach can be particularly helpful for patients who tend to get lost in trivialities or who use a digressive discussion of trivial problems in order to avoid having to deal with their actual problems. However, it should be kept in mind at this point that the procedure outlined has been conceptualized primarily for patients for whom persistent somatic symptoms and associated emotional distress and disability are currently the main focus (► Sect. 4.2.2, "For whom is this treatment approach indicated?"). In cases such as a comorbid major depression or a severe personality disorder (e.g. borderline personality disorder), an alternative treatment plan is undoubtedly preferable. In this case, individual modules of our treatment concept can also be incorporated into the therapy of the primary disorder. Overall, we encourage you to use the individual treatment modules and materials as an suggested potential approach, knowing that in any treatment there will be events in the patient's life that necessitate a temporary deviation from the planned course of action (e.g., death of close relatives or separation). In addition, you may feel that some treatment sessions are a bit too "packed" (e.g., introducing progressive muscle relaxation). At this point, feel free to shorten content or spread the material over two sessions if necessary. The question of how quickly certain content can be conveyed always depends on certain patient-related characteristics (e.g., reflective or insightful ability).

▪ Sequence of the Modules

Furthermore, according to previous experience, the strict adherence to the module sequence has been critically questioned. In this context, we would like to share with you some considerations that we associate with this sequence of therapy modules. We consider the division of the topic "stress and stress management" into two parts to be particularly important. This has the advantage that the handling of the physical stress reaction is updated and supplemented again and again in the course of the therapy. The patient does not have to learn several stress management techniques at once, but can acquire them step by step during the course of therapy. In addition, we have deliberately filled the first section of the manual with concrete stress management techniques, such as progressive muscle relaxation, and attention control techniques. Both can usually be taught and implemented relatively quickly. Moreover, they often lead to initial successes in a short time. This also helps to maintain the patient's motivation for therapy.

Another special feature—in comparison with the usual sequence of therapeutic techniques in manuals for other mental disorders—is that the reflection of a biopsychosocial explanatory model of the development and maintenance of somatoform symptoms is only provided for at the end of the manual. This is done against the background that patients with a biomedical symptom attributions should not be overtaxed at the beginning of treatment and should not lose themselves too early in theoretical debates about the causes of their symptoms (and thereby possibly waste valuable therapeutic working time). By means of the strategy of guided discovery, patients can repeatedly gather new experiences throughout the entire course of therapy, which expands their initially often rather biomedical view of their symptoms. These experiences can finally be summarized in the biopsychosocial explanatory model, which patients can then usually accept and internalize much better.

From our point of view, however, it also seems possible to change the order of certain therapeutic interventions. For individual patients, for example, who show a very strong need for transparency of the treatment rationale or who already accept a biopsychosocial model, the discussion of such an overall model can rather be placed at the beginning of the therapy. In addition, it must be taken into account that the group of patients with somatoform symptoms is an extremely heterogeneous patient sample. Accordingly, the problems that are in the foreground of each affected person are individually very different. In one patient, dysfunctional attention focusing and associated somatosensory amplification processes are paramount, whereas in another patient, dysfunctional appraisal processes are more predominant. ► Section 4.1.2 explains in more detail how the manual can be used, particularly for patients with more monosymptomatic functional syndromes, and which focal points are recommended.

▪ Application of the Manual to Patients with Perfectionistic Personality Traits

Another certain "risk" of the strongly manualized procedure has arisen from our previous experience with persons with clearly pronounced perfectionist personality traits or an obsessive-compulsive personality disorder. It is precisely these persons who show a high level of commitment to the implementation of the individual therapy's content and the practices of the week. In the case of these supposedly "ideal patients" it seems important from our therapeutic experience not to reinforce the pattern of "rigid fulfilment of duty" (e.g., in the form of perfectly done practice of the week) too much. Instead, new experiences should be made possible, in the sense of a caring approach to oneself as well as the consideration of one's own needs, independent of supposed external expectations. With this group of patients, it has also frequently been shown that, with regard to dysfunctional behavior, instead of avoidance behavior, there may rather be a very excessive, boom and bust behavior. According to their very high standards, the patients try to master their everyday life in a perfectionist way despite their symptoms and the accompanying impairments. In doing so, they often disregard the signals of their body, which make it clear to them that they are exceeding their limits. In this case, we have had good experience with addressing this dysfunctional-excessive behavior in the corresponding sessions dealing with the topic of "avoidance behavior". As with the avoidance behavior, positive and negative consequences of the dysfunctional behaviors can be inferred and the techniques described can be used to modify behavior-related cognitions. Exercises to increase physical fitness should rather be discussed under consideration of "I do something good for myself, I take care of myself". The psychologist is on a tightrope walk in which, on the one hand, they should value the patient's ambition as a resource and strength. On the other hand, it should be worked out that too much pressure to perform particularly well can have a negative effect on the successful implementation of the exercises.

In general, we see the manualization as an opportunity to treat somatoform symptoms in a targeted and effective way. Towards the end of this book, we will discuss the first study results (► Chap. 14), which can be interpreted as indications of the effectiveness of the treatment manual.

▪ Linking the Contents of the Manual with Procedures of the "Third Wave" of Cognitive Behavior Therapy

Depending on the patient's individual treatment assignment, this manual can be very well combined with strategies of more modern approaches of cognitive behavior therapy, such as acceptance-commitment therapy, dialectical-behavioral therapy, or mindfulness-based therapy. In the following we give examples for possible ways of connecting the approach promoted in this manual and "third wave" approaches of cognitive behavior therapy.

A common primary emotion that may occur with persistent somatic symptoms is anger. Patients may, for example, develop strong anger toward the symptomatology that prevents them from functioning as they once did, or toward their own bodies, whose functioning they can no longer trust. A common reaction to this anger emotion is to "fight" the discomfort, which manifests itself in patients desperately and very persistently seizing every opportunity to eliminate their somatic symptoms. This fighting against the symptom usually leads to frustration and draws even more attention to the discomfort. Here, for example, strategies of Acceptance Commitment Therapy (for more in-depth information, see e.g. Eifert, 2011) can be helpful, which can help the patient to let go of their fight-against-the-symptom and to develop an accepting attitude towards their symptoms. For example, the concept of "creative hopelessness" helps the patient to clarify that it is not they themselves who are hopeless, but their previous attempts to find solutions and to cope, such as consulting new specialists over and over again. On the one hand, the patient should develop an understanding of which aspects of their symptomatology can be controlled and for what the more solution-oriented strategies in this manual can be used. On the other hand, patients should learn to recognize what about their somatic symptoms is less controllable and for what acceptance-based strategies are important. This creates room for new possibilities of action for the patient. In this context, it is important to consider that many patients with somatoform symptoms, although they often experience strong negative emotions, have limited access to their emotional world. In this context, it would be useful, for example, to supplement the manual modules with a stronger focus on the emotions associated with somatic symptoms. Psychoeducational elements on the perception and handling of feelings from dialectical-behavioral therapy could be used for this purpose (for more detailed information, see e.g. Bohus & Wolf, 2009). In addition to the more change-oriented strategies taught in this manual, complementary mindfulness-based strategies for learning acceptance can be taught (Michalak et al., 2012). These help patients to initially accept and observe their symptoms and associated feelings instead of fighting them.

4.1.2 Recommendations for Therapeutic Priorities in the Treatment of Monosymptomatic Functional Syndromes

The treatment manual is primarily aimed at patients with multiple somatic symptoms. In practice, special constellations of somatoform symptoms sometimes occur, which are also referred to as "functional (somatic) syndromes" in the relevant literature (e.g. Wessely et al., 1999; ► Sects. 1.2.2 and 1.3.1). So far, it is unclear whether these functional syndromes are ultimately the same type of disorder (in the sense of a superordinate somatoform disorder) merely with a different name (Wessely et al., 1999) or whether the various functional syndromes really represent distinct disorder entities. Possibly both views have their justification. For example, there is at least a high degree of comorbidity between individual functional syndromes, and certain medical specialties prefer individual functional syndromes as a label for persistent somatic symptoms (Wessely et al., 1999). The most common functional syndromes include:
- Irritable Bowel Syndrome (IBS),
- Chronic fatigue syndrome,
- Idiopathic environmental intolerance (formerly also called multiple chemical sensitivity),
- Fibromyalgia syndrome,
- Premenstrual syndrome and
- Noncardiac chest pain.

4

Table 4.2 Functional syndromes and central treatment topics and goals

Functional syndrome	Treatment topics/goals
Irritable bowel syndrome	Normalization of nutrition Reduction of diet-related avoidance behavior Reduction of social withdrawal If necessary, reduction of medication abuse (e.g. laxative medication)
Chronic fatigue syndrome	Slow and gradual build-up of physical activity and increase in physical fitness (see Gaab & Ehlert, 2005)
Idiopathic environmental intolerance (formerly: multiple chemical sensitivity)	Reduction of social withdrawal If necessary, systematic desensitisation with the aid of fragrances that trigger symptoms
Fibromyalgia syndrome	Reduction of pain-reinforcing boom and bust behavior Build healthy activity levels (e.g., positive activities, relaxation) If necessary, reduction of pain-promoting avoidance behavior Reduction of operant, pain-reinforcing mechanisms
Premenstrual syndrome	Psychoeducation on the functioning of the menstrual cycle Nutrition management Building positive and sporting activities Promotion of positive communication in partnership
Noncardiac chest pain	Reduction of checking behavior (e.g., regularly checking heart rate and blood pressure) Reduction of excessive healthcare utilization behavior (especially with regard to diagnostic cardiological examinations) Questioning/reappraising catastrophizing interpretations of pain symptoms Reduction of avoidance behavior

The present treatment manual appears to be largely suitable for successfully treating these functional syndromes as well, although a certain emphasis may be necessary in individual cases. For example, IBS is one of the most common functional syndromes in the population, with a prevalence of approximately 10%. Patients with IBS often show marked agoraphobia-like avoidance behavior regarding places and situations where a toilet is not available. In addition, certain foods are often avoided out of fear and concern that they could lead to increased gastrointestinal upset. The result here is a progressive sensitization of the gastrointestinal tract due to an increasingly restricted food palette. As a consequence, the gastrointestinal tract reacts more and more sensitively to deviations from the norm, e.g. new foods. It is not uncommon for medications to be used prophylactically before important events (e.g., against diarrhoea). The problems described make it clear that additional treatment goals and elements are required in the treatment of IBS. In particular, it is important to reduce social and food-related avoidance behavior with the help of in vivo exposure (e.g., longer train journeys in regional trains without a toilet, eating in unfamiliar restaurants).

A separate treatment plan for each individual functional syndrome would go beyond the scope of this manual. In some cases, excellent manuals are already available for specific functional syndromes such as chronic fatigue syndrome (e.g. Gaab & Ehlert, 2005). Table 4.2 provides a brief overview of which treatment topics and goals are of central importance for certain functional syndromes. These are intended to serve as a suggestion for specific treatment targets in the application of the present therapy manual to functional syndromes.

4.2 Initial Phase of Therapy

Before the patient and psychologist can begin with the therapy modules, the initial conditions for the start of therapy must first be created in an initial phase. According to the 7-stage process model of psychotherapy according to Kanfer et al. (2006), before planning, selecting and implementing specific therapeutic methods, several phases first follow with the goals of establishing a cooperative patient-psychologist relationship, clarifying the patient's expectations of the therapy, defining the patient's problem precisely or weighing up which therapeutic interventions appear to be indicated for the patient. When working with patients with persistent somatic symptoms, this initial phase can be characterized by various peculiarities, which will be discussed in the following two sections.

4.2.1 Initial Contact and the Patient's Expectations of Therapy

A special feature of the initial contact with patients with somatoform symptoms compared to other disorders is that the patient's symptoms are primarily of somatic nature. The psychologist is therefore usually not the first contact person in a treatment. Patients often have a history of many consultations with physicians before they see a therapist for the first time. Therefore, in the first contact it is of particular importance to carefully explore the patient's motivation and concerns for the therapy. It is helpful to adopt an interested, open, respectful or "naive" attitude. In this way, you support the patient from the initial interview onwards to concretize facts and contexts. Based on Kanfer et al. (2006), the following initial questions can be helpful:

Helpful Questions to Start the Initial Interview

- Can you tell me your concern or reasons for seeking psychotherapy?
- What was the trigger for you to seek psychotherapy at this point in time?
- From whom did you receive the referral or who referred you? How did you become aware of our institution?

With the help of these initial questions, initial information can be obtained about where the patient stands with regard to his or her understanding of the illness and motivation for therapy. Patients can seek psychotherapy with a very different awareness of the problem. While some go to a therapist primarily on the advice of their family physician, without knowing specifically why psychotherapy should be helpful for their symptoms, other patients come to the initial contact with already biopsychosocially shaped ideas about their symptoms. Accordingly, there can be substantial interindividual differences in the motivation to change one's own behavior. Even though the transtheoretical model of behavioral change ("Stages of Change Model") according to Prochaska and DiClemente (1982; ◘ Fig. 4.1) actually originates from the therapy of addictive disorders, it can provide valuable information regarding the motivation to change in the treatment of persistent somatic symptoms. For example, patients may still be in the first phase (precontemplation), in which they have no knowledge of the biopsychosocial connections of their symptoms or do not want to acknowledge them and accordingly are not motivated to change anything about themselves. On the other hand, they may already be in the next phase—contemplation—in which they become aware of the connections between their symptoms and biopsychosocial factors and consider changes in their behavior.

> The key message is that the therapist should understand patients' motivation to change their own behavior.

This understanding of patients' motivation is often most difficult with patients who have sought psychotherapy primarily on the advice of their family physician, but who at the same time signal ambivalence towards psychological interventions. Such patients often have primarily biomedical theories of their symptoms and a strong need for transparency in the therapeutic process. In the following, some important hints and strategies are explained that can facilitate the handling of this special group of patients.

◘ **Fig. 4.1** The six stages of behavior change of the transtheoretical model of behavior change. (Based on Prochaska and DiClemente (1982))

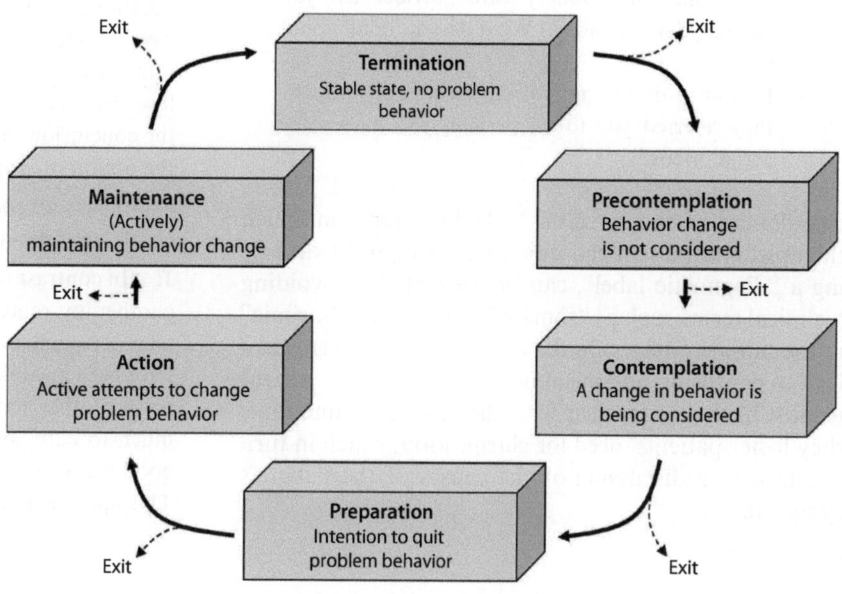

4

Dealing with Patients' Biomedical Explanatory Models in the Initial Contact

Due to the primarily somatic nature of the symptoms, it is not surprising that those affected often have biomedical ideas about the origin of their symptoms at the beginning. They usually cannot explain why they were referred to a therapist. In some cases, this referral can also have a negative effect on the doctor-patient relationship, as the patient feels stigmatized as "mentally ill" or as a "malingerer". In this case, the patient can be expected to have a pronounced sceptical or negative attitude towards psychotherapy. In order to pave the way to therapy in this case, it is important to explore patients' ideas about their symptoms in an interested and appreciative manner. Too early an emphasis on the fact that, in addition to biological causes, psychosocial aspects also play an important role in symptom development and maintenance should be avoided in the initial interview. Affected persons are usually not yet able to accept a biopsychosocial models of their symptoms at this stage and regard the therapist's behavior as an "attempt to persuade" them. In addition, the patient may feel misunderstood or labelled as a "malingerer". The risk of an unfruitful discussion of the causes of the disorder developing during the initial contact can therefore be counteracted with the help of an interested and appreciative exploration of patients' personal theories to explain their own symptoms. The patient should feel taken seriously and understood. The following questions can be helpful for this:

Helpful Questions for Exploring the Patient's Personal Theories to Explain their Symptoms

- Perhaps you have already thought about what caused your symptoms? Do you have any ideas or suspicions?
- What did your primary care provider tell you caused your symptoms? What do you think about it?
- If your primary care provider hasn't told you why they referred you to us, perhaps you have some assumptions?

The danger of the so-called "labelling trap", in which therapist and patient can quickly get caught by attaching a "diagnostic label", can be prevented by avoiding technical terms such as "somatoform" or "psychogenic" in the initial contact. On the one hand, these terms can lead to confusion and misunderstandings, as the patient is most likely not familiar with them. At the same time, they foster patients' need for clarification, which in turn can lead to a discussion of the causes of the patient's symptoms.

Transparency from the Start of Therapy

Particularly for those affected, for whom it is unclear why psychotherapy should be helpful with their symptoms, transparency in therapy is very important from the first contact. But now the problem arises how to create transparency concerning the contents and goals of therapy without getting caught up in a discussion of the causes of the symptoms. Instead of confronting the patient directly with the fact that psychotherapy can be helpful because there are psychosocial factors associated with somatic symptoms in addition to biomedical ones, psychotherapy can be conveyed as an "additional treatment offer". This should enable new perspectives regarding the symptoms. New approaches to the symptoms can possibly open up new ways in which patients can improve their well-being independently of the somatic symptoms. It should be made transparent from the first contact that, in contrast to medical therapies, the actual goal of psychological interventions is to improve management of the symptoms and not a cure in the sense of complete elimination of all symptoms. At the same time, it should be made clear to patients that they have nothing to lose by embarking on a completely different path in addition to the previous cure-oriented treatment attempts. Of course, care should be taken to ensure that the patient does not pursue any counterproductive alternative therapies. The concrete implementation of the procedure becomes clear in the following example dialogue between patient (P) and therapist (T).

▶ Example

P: – I'm actually not really clear yet how psychotherapy can help me with my symptoms. I have pain and no problem in my head. I rather think that I am out of place here.

T: – You have already told me a lot about the many examinations as well as treatment offers you have taken up because of your symptoms. Perhaps it will help you to see psychotherapy for your symptoms as another treatment offer or an "experiment" in which you have nothing to lose. You try it out and if, as you go along, you come to the conclusion that it is not helping you, you always have the option of stopping it.

P: – That's all good, but it's still not clear to me why psychotherapy should be helpful.

T: – In contrast to your previous treatment attempts, psychotherapy represents a different path. It can give you new perspectives on your symptoms that you may not have been aware of before. In this way, it can help you to try out other ways of getting better. The goal is not so much to cure your symptoms, but to help you regain a good measure of quality of life, regardless of your pain. This approach has had success with many other patients with symptoms similar to those you are experiencing. In some cases, a changed, more helpful way of dealing with the discomfort can then even lead to a reduction in pain in the long term.

P: – I can't imagine regaining quality of life without my pain finally stopping.

T: – I can understand that very well. After all, psychotherapy does not necessarily mean that you have to say goodbye to the hope that at some point a way will be found to reduce your pain, or at best even cure it. Unfortunately, such an approach is currently not available. Nevertheless, you should get better. Accordingly, it is perhaps all the more worthwhile to take a "multi-path" approach, and to try out a completely new approach in addition to the treatment paths you have used so far. You do not have to give up the other way because of that.

P: – That sounds plausible. Actually, I can't lose anything. It's at least worth a try.

T: – You can think it over and we can talk about it again in the next session. ◀

It is important to grant the patient autonomy at all times with regard to his decision for or against this treatment offer. However, in order to indirectly increase the patient's motivation for the treatment, the positive consequences of cognitive behavior therapy can be made clear to the patient. At the same time, these can be contrasted with the discomfort and distress that the patient is currently experiencing. It is important that the therapist shows patience and does not put pressure on the patient. As was made clear in ► Sect. 1.4.4, persistent somatic symptoms have an increased risk of developing a chronic manifestation. Many patients who seek psychotherapy have already been suffering from their symptoms for many years and can hardly imagine a life in which somatic symptoms are not the primary concern. Accordingly, it seems understandable that the decision to engage into a psychological intervention is not easy to make for many patients.

▪ Clarification of the Basic Principles of Cognitive Behavior Therapy

In addition to unrealistic ideas of the patient regarding the treatment results, the patient may also come to the initial contact with "myths" about the therapeutic procedure. Ideas such as, for example, that the symptoms and stresses of everyday life are exclusively talked about or that therapy consists of "conversations about childhood problems and experiences" are not uncommon. Thus, in the initial contact with patients, their expectations and ideas about the mode of action and effectiveness of psychotherapy should also be explored. In accordance with the concept of transparency, it should be made clear from the beginning of the therapy that, in addition to the support of the therapist, the therapy requires a great deal of personal commitment on the part of the patient. In contrast to the idea of only having conversations together and remaining "passive", patients should be aware that they must actively practice and experiment with the strategies they are provided with. Only in this way they can find a good way for themselves to make use of what they have learned. In this sense, the division of roles between therapist and patient should be made transparent from the beginning of therapy. The idea that psychotherapy is primarily based on childhood history should be put into perspective by pointing out that cognitive behavior therapy is primarily based on the patient's currently existing problems. Although childhood experiences or all experiences in the past play an important role in deriving an individual explanatory model of patients' symptoms, they do not represent the main target of psychological interventions. The following example of formulation can be an aid in conveying the principles of cognitive behavior therapy.

► Sample Formulation to Convey the Approach of Cognitive Behavior Therapy

In our institution we provide the so-called cognitive behavior therapy. A fundamental characteristic of this form of therapy is that it starts with patients' current problems and tries to develop possible solutions. Since psychotherapy cannot directly change or cure your somatic symptoms, the primary goal is to restore your quality of life and well-being in the present, regardless of the somatic symptoms. You should be able to concentrate on the important things in your life again, and the somatic symptoms should no longer dominate your life as before. An associated positive effect may be that your somatic symptoms are reduced or no longer affect you as much. To achieve this, it will be necessary for you to try to apply the techniques you learn during therapy on your own and experiment with them beyond the therapy sessions. Since there is no "recipe" that is equally effective for everyone, you will have to figure out for yourself how to integrate what you learn into your daily life. The therapist's function is to give you "the tools" and to support you in the implementation or in the difficulties that arise. So it becomes clear that the role of the patient in cognitive behavior therapy is a very active one. Only in this way does the treatment have a chance of being effective. Talks about your past or childhood are not the main focus of cognitive behavior therapy. However, they are an important part of the therapy section, in which we will try together to develop a model for the development and maintenance of your symptoms. ◀

▪ **Basic Medical Knowledge**

In order to treat patients with persistent somatic symptoms, it is not necessary to be an expert on medical issues related to the corresponding somatic symptoms. However, in the initial interview as well as in the further course of therapy (e.g., in psychoeducational treatment sections) it can be helpful to be able to fall back on a basic medical knowledge of the patient's symptoms. This supports the professionalism and credibility of the therapist. Particularly in the case of patients who have pronounced hypochondriacal fears along with somatic symptoms, a certain basic medical knowledge helps to better assess the patient's fears. In addition, it can be better assessed to what extent certain behaviors of the patients can be classified as functional or dysfunctional (Bleichhardt & Weck, 2011). It is important, however, that the therapist at the same time emphasizes his or her professional boundaries and continues to respect the physician as well as the patient as experts on the somatic symptoms. Appropriate basic knowledge can be obtained from medical literature (e.g., a detailed introduction to various pain-related disorders can be found in Kröner-Herwig et al., 2007). It may also be interesting to take a look at Internet portals that are frequently visited by patients (e.g. ▶ http://www.netdoktor.de).

▪ **Basic Strategies for the Beginning**

For the communication with the patient in the initial contact, but also in the further course of therapy, the consideration of some basic techniques from motivational interviewing approach ("motivational interviewing"; Miller & Rollnick, 2004) can be helpful. They are particularly valuable for patient groups in which a certain ambivalence towards psychotherapy and the associated changes in their own behavior can be found.

▪ **Ask Open Questions**

For patients with persistent somatic symptoms, who have often had the previous experience of not being taken seriously, it is particularly important to experience understanding in the initial consultation. To achieve this, openly asked questions about the patient's symptoms and expectations can be helpful. They convey an interested, understanding therapist attitude.

▪ **Active Listening**

According to Thomas Gordon (cited in Miller & Rollnick, 2004), there are 12 different types of so-called communication barriers. These include lecturing, moralising, or criticizing. They can have a blocking or distracting effect after an (open-ended) question has been asked. Once an (open-ended) question has been asked, the next step is active listening. It is crucial that the therapist assesses the importance of what the patient has said. Therapists should try to paraphrase in their own words what they understood to ensure that they correctly understood the meaning of what has been said. In this way, therapists offer patients a statement that includes what they have understood, without this feedback becoming a communication block.

▪ **"Check in" with the patient**

To promote open exploration and build the patient's trust in the therapist, it can be helpful for therapists to frequently check in whether they understand correctly of what patients have been said. This can take the form of acknowledgement or statements conveying understanding. Using summarizing ensures mutual understanding of the discussion so far.

▶ Examples of Confirmatory Statements

- I can well imagine that you are severely impaired in your everyday life due to your symptoms.
- It is a sign of strength that you have agreed to talk to me today, even though you have absolutely no idea what to expect in therapy.
- Thank you for being so open with me today about your discomfort. ◀

▪ **Paraphrazing**

Paraphrazing in one's own words have several positive effects on therapist-patient communication. On the one hand, they reinforce what has been said. Furthermore, they demonstrate that you as a therapist have listened attentively and at the same time motivate the patient to continue. They can also connect topics of conversation and create structure in the conversation.

▪ **Change Talk**

The communication techniques explained so far create an important basis for the resolution of the patient's ambivalence. However, this alone does not lead to a reduction of ambivalence. For this, a communication technique such as Change Talk is important. In contrast to a confrontational approach, patients should be enabled to collect and express arguments speaking in favor of a therapy and a change themselves. In a confrontational approach, the patient would be forced to defend the position that speaks against a change or new view. For example, if patients with biomedical assumptions about their persistent somatic symptoms are confronted right from the first contact with the fact that their symptoms may also have psychosocial causes and that psychotherapy is therefore necessary, they will automatically put themselves in the defensive position. Of course, Change Talk is not only an important communication strategy in the initial contact, but throughout the entire course of therapy. Change Talk comprises the following **four components**:

- Recognize the disadvantages of the status quo (e.g., "Because of my pain, I am severely limited in both my personal and professional life."),
- Recognizing the benefits of change or a new perspective (e.g., "If I could manage to let my pain fade more into the background, I could at least partially regain my old quality of life."),
- Developing confidence about change (e.g., "If I do my exercises regularly, I can do it.") and
- Developing an intention to change (e.g., "I believe it is time not to hope for a magic pill alone, but to change something in my life or in myself.").

While the last two components tend to play an important role in the later course of therapy, the first two principles can also be significant in the initial contact or in the introductory phase of therapy, e.g., when the therapist explores patients' current symptoms and functional impairment and communicates the content and goals of therapy to them.

Taking into account the special features of initial contact with patients with persistent somatic symptoms, the basic questions listed in the following overview should be clarified in the initial interview (based on Wendisch & Neher, 2003).

Important Questions That Should Be Clarified in the Initial Interview

- **Questions about the current reason for seeking psychotherapy**
  - Current reason for treatment request?
  - Clarification of the assignment context?
- **Symptoms and previous treatments**
  - What somatic symptoms does the patient have?
  - Is it a single specific symptom, a monosymptomatic syndrome or a polysymptomatic syndrome?
  - Are there any findings of medical examinations concerning these symptoms?
  - How long have the symptoms already existed?
  - Did the symptoms occur continuously since their onset or were there also symptom-free periods?
  - How do the symptoms behave during the course of the day? Are there fluctuations in intensity?
  - How to the symptoms interfere with patients' everyday life functioning (in professional as well as private life)?
  - How does the social environment deal with the patient's symptoms?
  - Are the symptoms associated with certain behaviors (avoidance behavior, use of medical services, body checking)?
  - What attempts at change or treatment has the patient already made? What success did these have?
  - Is the patient currently taking medication? If yes, which ones and in which dosage? Are the medications prescribed by a physician?
  - Does the patient have underlying physical illnesses (independent of the somatoform symptoms)?
  - What explanation does the patient have for his or her symptoms?
  - Are there any indications of comorbid disorders?
- **Biography**
  - What is the patient's current life situation (professional situation, partnership, family, hobbies, social network, resources)?
  - Is there a history of particular stressful events that may be related to the symptoms?
- **Expectations**
  - Initial clarification of expectations of psychotherapy
- **Closing situation**
  - Questions from the patient about the course of therapy
  - Clarification of the basic principles of cognitive behavior therapy
  - Does the patient would like to add something to what has been said so far?
  - Discussion of the further procedure
  - If applicable, gain consent to contact the patient's primary care physician and other healthcare providers who are involved in the treatment of the somatic symptoms

4.2.2 Important Issues of the Further Course of Therapy

▪ **For whom is this treatment indicated?**

As already mentioned in ► Sect. 1.4.3, patients with persistent somatic symptoms are at increased risk of developing comorbid mental disorders. These include anxiety and mood disorders in particular, but personality disorders also seem to be increasingly associated with somatoform symptoms. For the therapy process, it plays a decisive role to clarify diagnostically to what extent it is primarily a matter of somatoform symptoms or whether, from a differential diagnostic point of view, the symptoms are secondary to another primary psychiatric condition. In addition, it must be clarified to what extent it is a polysymptomatic or monosymptomatic phenomenon. A good diagnosis and the therapeutic indication derived from it are the decisive basis for the development of a successful therapy plan at the end of the initial therapy phase. Information on the steps and tools of the diagnostic procedure have already been described in detail in ▶ Sect. 1.3. It must be emphasized at this point that the structured, manualized procedure described in ▶ Chaps. 5, 6, 7, 8, 9, 10, 11 and 12 is intended for patients who have persistent somatic symptoms as their primary problem. If additional comorbid disorders are present, the therapy plan should implement more flexibility for the therapist. Modules of the present manual can be combined with therapy components recommended for the corresponding comorbid disorders. If the somatic symptoms are only symptoms of another primary mental health condition, the primary disorder should be treated first. Of course, suitable modules of this manual can be integrated into the therapy. The presence of monosymptomatic functional syndromes (e.g. fibromyalgia, chronic fatigue syndrome, irritable bowel syndrome) may require a specific focus in therapy planning, as described in ▶ Sect. 4.1.2.

Furthermore, the initial phase of therapy should be used to inform the patient in detail about the basic principles of the cognitive behavior therapy approach (▶ Sect. 4.2.1).

> It is important that patients decide for themselves to engage in this form of therapy and that they are sufficiently motivated to actively participate in the therapy and to change something about themselves.

If it becomes clear that the patient is unable to engage in this therapeutic approach despite various attempts to build up motivation for change, it should be seriously questioned whether another therapeutic approach might not seem more suitable for this individual case. The same is the case if the patient attaches great importance to working through childhood experiences in therapy, which may be related to the somatic symptoms. Here the patient could be recommended a depth psychology-oriented therapy. It is crucial for the last two cases mentioned that the patient is sufficiently informed about the therapeutic procedure and is given enough leeway to make a decision for or against a cognitive behavior therapy.

▪ Cooperation with the Patient's Physicians

In the therapy of persistent somatic symptoms, there are several reasons why close cooperation between physician and therapist is particularly important. As already mentioned several times, primary care physicians or other physicians seem to be the first point of contact for patients. It is common that patients with persistent somatic symptoms have gone through a long history of medical examinations, thus it can be assumed that the treating physician already knows the patient and their symptoms over a long period of time. Furthermore, in the context of the therapy of persistent somatic symptoms, the medical examination of the symptoms plays a pivotal role. Therefore, a medical report from the patient's primary care physician which is supposed to provide information about possible medical causes of the somatic symptom should be requested. Another important reason to request the patient's medical report is related to a central goal of the therapy—extending patient's primarily biomedical perspective on their symptoms by psychosocial aspects—it is important that therapist and physician "work together". If statements of the therapist and the physician contradict each other, this can lead to strong uncertainty of the patient or, in the long run, force the patient to take sides for the "medical" or "psychological" perspective. A cooperative physician-therapist relationship, including regular exchanges, can prevent this. The reasons explained for establishing good cooperation with the patient's primary care physician suggest contacting the primary care physician after the initial consultation. After obtaining informed consent from the patient, should send a letter that summarizes the psychological assessment and treatment plan to the primary care physician or other healthcare providers who are involved in the patient's treatment.

▪ Behavior Analysis

In order to prepare the actual therapeutic interventions, a detailed behavioral analysis is necessary in the initial therapy phase. This is an important component of any cognitive behavior therapy. As a rule, it forms the basis for the derivation of a biopsychosocial explanatory model of the patient's symptoms as well as the therapy goals. In addition to this general function, however, in the therapy of patients with persistent somatic symptoms it also has the task of laying a foundation for extending the patient's often biomedical explanations by psychosocial components. It enables patients to experience the connections between their symptoms and psychosocial aspects through guided discovery based on everyday experiences. In the case of persistent somatic symptoms, its focus is usually on the problematic emotional as well as behavioral reactions to the somatic symptoms. The following is an example of a behavioral analysis of a patient with somatoform symptoms. It is based on the classical SORCK scheme according to Kanfer and Saslow (1965), which distinguishes between situation (S), organism variables (O), (problematic) reactions on emotional, physiological, cognitive and behavioral levels (R), contingency (C) as well as consequences (K).

▶ Behavior Analysis of a Patient with Persistent Somatic Symptoms

This is a patient with persistent pain in the left shoulder as well as in the left chest.

- **Situation**
  - The patient is sitting at home and reading. He perceives an intensification of his pain in the left shoulder radiating into the left chest.
- **Organism Variables**
  - Increased general anxiety since childhood, a principle the patient had been taught by his mother: "Somatic symptoms can be dangerous and threatening, they must be taken very seriously."
  - Death of mother from a heart attack two years ago, since then the patient experiences increased sensitivity to perceived physical changes in his body.
  - Passivity and lack of self-efficacy with regard to a proactive self-management of his symptoms.
- **Reactions**
  - Emotional: fear, helplessness, despair, anger.
  - Physiological: inner tension, further amplification of pain.
  - Cognitive: "Now this is getting worse again? What am I going to do? What do I do if it doesn't get better? Maybe there is something wrong with the heart after all? Should I call 911?"
  - "I'm going to take a painkiller and rest for now."
  - "That's so annoying that it's starting again. Then I'll have to cancel my meeting with Bernd later. It just won't do any good for me to meet with him under these circumstances, it'll only make things worse."—"I'll go to the family doctor right away on Monday."
  - Motor-behavioral: Patient stops reading and gets a painkiller prescribed by his family physician for cases of need. Before he lies down, he calls his friend Bernd and cancels the planned meeting.
- **Consequences**
  - C^+: In the short term, the patient experiences a calming effect through his behavior.
  - C^-: The painkillers cause the discomfort to subside promptly.
  - C^+: He forgoes meeting his friend, missing an opportunity to experience positive distraction.
  - C^-: While resting, attention to the somatic symptoms and negative ruminations about the symptoms get amplified. The mood deteriorates further. In the long term, the patient's behavior leads him to withdraw more and more from his social network. In the long run, the avoidance behavior implies that the patient's physical condition deteriorates. His self-confidence in being able to cope with his symptoms decreases significantly. ◀

Taking into account the special issues listed in this chapter, the therapy modules can be started after completion of the initial phase. These are introduced with the derivation of the therapy goals and the preparation of the therapy plan. The formulation of therapy goals is dealt with in more detail in ▶ Sect. 5.1—the first module of this individual therapy manual. The basis for the preparation of the therapy plan is the complete manual (▶ Chaps. 5, 6, 7, 8, 9, 10, 11 and 12) as well as additional instructions for the application of the manual in ▶ Sect. 4.1.

▪ Things to Consider in an Inpatient Setting

Especially in inpatient psychiatric and psychotherapeutic settings, disturbance patterns with severe, persistent somatic symptoms are among the most frequent problem areas. Therefore, the question arises whether and, if so, how exactly the present treatment program can also be implemented in inpatient settings. Since inpatient stays are usually only 4–6 weeks, the complete implementation of the program seems unrealistic due to the limited time available. Moreover, many facilities rely on a multimodal and interdisciplinary treatment program, in which psychotherapy embodies only one approach among many. Therefore, it seems advisable to use the limited time of an inpatient treatment primarily for a detailed and conscientious diagnosis as well as for a first motivation building towards a longer-term outpatient psychological treatment. Accordingly, we suggest that Module 1 (treatment motivation) and Module 2 (stress and stress management - part 1) be tackled first during a stay in hospital. Depending on time resources, modules 3 (attention refocusing) and 4 (cognitive reappraisal) can also be addressed. In our opinion, however, the following Module 5 on the subject of illness-related behavior should, if possible, only be addressed in an outpatient treatment setting. Module 5 involves the modification of old and the development of new behavioral habits, which may be strongly linked to the patient's private environment. Modifying behavioral habits in an inpatient setting will be probably challenging for patients to maintain in their home environment. In addition, the inpatient treatment setting is not very well suited for implementing changes in patients' healthcare utilization behavior, which, however, is a central and important component of treatment in many cases (e.g., in the case of severe health anxiety). Overall, we consider the sometimes high pressure to change resulting from the comparatively short duration of inpatient treatments is not necessarily a facilitating factor for therapy. Based on clinical experience and meta-analytical findings, according to which changes in the area of persistent somatic symptoms require a longer-term treatment framework, we advise the development of realistic goals during an inpatient stay and the planning and preparation of follow-up outpatient psychological treatment.

▪ Dealing with Invalidity Retirement Claims

A further complication of treatment in both the inpatient and outpatient setting can be when patients submit claims for invalidity retirement. A dilemma can arise for therapists and physicians as well as patients from the fact that a significant improvement in symptomatology is accompanied by a loss of pension entitlements and thus the patient's coverage of living expenses. It should be noted that simulation of symptoms is not a frequently observed phenomenon in this context. The problem is usually rather that many affected persons can hardly imagine a life without persistent somatic symptoms and are therefore understandably very afraid of losing financial support to cover living expenses if pension support is discontinued. We generally do not see an existing pension claim as a contraindication for inpatient or outpatient psychological treatment and suggest that this problem be openly addressed and, at the same time, solutions to the supposed dilemma be sought together with the patient and positive future scenarios be carefully developed.

4.3 Special Features of Therapy with Patients with Migration Background

The patient's cultural background can have a strong influence on how somatic symptoms are experienced and expressed (Kohrt et al., 2014). Although persistent somatic symptoms are a phenomenon that exists worldwide (▶ Sect. 1.4.2), the nature and frequency of somatic symptoms and how they are understood and expressed by those affected can vary greatly. In ▶ Sect. 1.4.2, various culturally linked concepts of suffering were presented in this regard. These cultural differences require, on the one hand, that the cultural background of patients, especially patients with a migration background, be taken into account from the first contact. On the other hand, the therapist should be aware of the risk of stigmatizing patients with persistent somatic symptoms based on cultural stereotypes.

According to the fifth revision of the Diagnostic and Statistical Manual of Mental Disorders (DSM-5; Falkai et al., 2015), the aspects of **cultural formulation** mentioned below should be asked about in the early phase of therapy and taken into account throughout the course of therapy. The concept of cultural formulation provides "a frame of reference for assessing information about culturally bound features of a person's mental health problems and how these relate to social, cultural, and historical context" (Falkai et al., 2015). It includes, but is not limited to.

- The cultural identity of a person,
- Culturally bound concepts of distress (▶ Sect. 1.4.2),
- Psychosocial stressors,
- Cultural specificities of vulnerabilities and resilience as well as the
- Cultural characteristics of the relationship between the patient and the therapist or physician.

With regard to **cultural identity**, patients with a migration background should, for example, be explored separately in terms of how they are integrated into the culture of their region of origin on the one hand and how they are integrated into the culture of the country they now live in, on the other hand. Knowledge about cultural reference groups that influence the person's relationship behavior and about their use of resources should be taken into account. In this context, e.g., language barriers play an important role, as they can make access to treatment services more difficult and may require interpreters. In addition to the **culturally linked concepts of distress** (▶ Sect. 1.4.2), it is important to ask about **cultural characteristics relating to psychosocial stressors and resources** in the patient's social environment. The role of religion, along with the family environment and other social networks, as a source of social support should not be underestimated. Finally, **cultural characteristics of the relationship between the patient and the therapist or physician** play an important role in treatment **and** diagnosis. Differences in culture, language and perception of social status between therapist or physician and patient can lead to misunderstandings in communication and thus result in difficulties in establishing and maintaining a therapeutic relationship.

As a tool for a targeted exploration of a patient's cultural background, the DSM-5 introduces the so-called **Cultural Formulation Interview (CFI)**, which is also accessible online (▶ www.psychiatry.org/dsm5). The CFI is a semi-structured interview with 16 questions covering the following four areas:

- Cultural definition of the concerns with which the patient visits the therapist or physician,
- Cultural specificities in the perception of causes and in the context of reported problems as well as in the handling and support from the patient's social environment,
- Cultural factors influencing self-help and past help-seeking behavior,
- Cultural factors that influence current help-seeking behavior.

References

Bleichhardt, G., & Weck, F. (2011). *Kognitive Verhaltenstherapie bei Hypochondrie und Krankheitsangst* (2. akt. Aufl.). Springer.

Bohus, M., & Wolf, M. (2009). *Interaktives SkillsTraining für Borderline-Patienten. Manual zur CD-ROM für die therapeutische Arbeit*. Schattauer.

Eifert, G. H. (2011). *Akzeptanz- und Commitment-Therapie (ACT). Fortschritte der Psychotherapie* (Band 45). Hogrefe.

Falkai, P., Wittchen, H.-U., Döpfner, M., Gaebel, W., Maier, W., Rief, W., et al. (2015). *Diagnostisches und Statistisches Manual Psychischer Störungen. DSM-5*. Hogrefe.

Gaab, J., & Ehlert, U. (2005). *Chronische Erschöpfung und Chronisches Erschöpfungssyndrom (Fortschritte der Psychotherapie Band 26)*. Hogrefe.

Kanfer, F. H., & Saslow, G. (1965). Behavioral analysis: An alternative to diagnostic classification. *Archives of General Psychiatry, 12*(6), 529–538. https://doi.org/10.1001/archpsyc.1965.01720360001001

Kanfer, F. H., Reinecker, H., & Schmelzer, D. (2006). *Selbstmanagement-Therapie. Ein Lehrbuch für die klinische Praxis* (4. Aufl.). Springer.

Kohrt, B. A., Rasmussen, A., Kaiser, B. N., Haroz, E. E., Maharjan, S. M., Mutamba, B. B., et al. (2014). Cultural concepts of distress and psychiatric disorders: Literature review and research recommendations for global mental health epidemiology. *International Journal of Epidemiology, 43*(2), 365–406. https://doi.org/10.1093/ije/dyt227

Kröner-Herwig, B., Frettlöh, J., Klinger, R., & Nilges, P. (2007). *Schmerzpsychotherapie* (6. Aufl.). Springer.

Michalak, J., Heidenreich, T., & Williams, J. M. G. (2012). *Achtsamkeit (Fortschritte der Psychotherapie)*. Hogrefe.

Miller, W. R., & Rollnick, S. (2004). *Motivierende Gesprächsführung*. Lambertus.

Prochaska, J. O., & DiClemente, C. C. (1982). Transtheoretical therapy: Toward a more integrative model of therapy. *Psychotherapy: Theory, Research, and Practice, 19*(3), 267–288. https://doi.org/10.1037/h0088437

Wendisch, M., & Neher, M. (2003). The initital session of behaviour therapy – A guide. *Verhaltenstherapie, 13*(2), 122–129.

Wessely, S., Nimnuan, C., & Sharpe, M. (1999). Functional somatic syndromes: One or many? *Lancet, 354*(9182), 936–939. https://doi.org/10.1016/S0140-6736(98)08320-2

Practice: The Manual: Therapeutic Phase

Contents

Module 1: Treatment Motivation

Contents

M. Kleinstäuber et al., *Cognitive Behavior Therapy for Persistent Somatic Symptoms and Somatic Symptom Disorder*, https://doi.org/10.1007/978-3-662-69726-9_5

5.1 Session 1

Contents and Materials of the 1st Session

- **Contents**
  - Summary of the therapy's content
  - What are the patient's symptom attributions?
  - Clarifying therapy goals: Guided imagery
  - Formulation of therapy goals
  - The purpose of the practice of the week
  - Practice of the week: Elaboration of Worksheet 5.2 (My personal therapy goals)
- **Materials**
  - Worksheet 5.1: Therapy's content
  - Worksheet 5.2: My personal therapy goals
  - Quick file for the patient

5.1.1 Summary of the Therapy's Content

At the beginning of this session it is recommended to provide patients with a folder for their therapy documents. Afterwards, a summary of the therapy's content and the course of the therapy is given. The patient receives Worksheet 5.1 (Therapy's content). The therapist briefly explains the bulletpoints.

5.1.2 What Are the Patient's Symptom Attributions?

Together with the therapist, patients should record their personal explanatory model of their symptoms or their ideas about the origin of their symptoms on a blank sheet of paper and then file it away. The following questions can be helpful:

- What explanations do you have for your symptoms?
- Which aspects play an important role in the development, deterioration, and perpetuation of your symptoms?
- Do you think your symptoms are caused by one or multiple factors?

The therapist emphasizes that there is usually more than one explanation for the symptoms. Now the therapist collects factors that accompany or exacerbate the patient's somatic symptoms.

- What factors can contribute to physical discomfort?
- What factors can exacerbate your somatic symptoms?

Patient and therapist collect and complete together different possible explanations (e.g., bad sleep, muscle tension, inactivity, hyperventilation). In the following overview you will find a list of possible factors that can contribute to the development of somatoform symptoms as a suggestion.

Possible Factors Facilitating the Development of Somatoform Symptoms

- Minimal organic dysfunctions: e.g., constipation, minor illnesses (such as the common cold)
- Harmless swellings/skin irregularities: e.g., oedema, premenstrual water retention, moles, warts
- Autonomic or hormonally induced arousal: e.g., physical emotional reactions
- Muscle tension: e.g., neck or back pain
- Hyperventilation: e.g., dizziness, lightheadedness, heart sensations, tingling sensations
- Inactivity: e.g., "sore muscles", low physical resilience, palpitations
- Poor sleep: e.g., tiredness, drowsiness, concentration problems
- Physiological effects of foods or drink: e.g., digestive problems after eating bad food, flatulence, effects of alcohol including withdrawal symptoms or "hangover".
- Side effects of medication: e.g., dry mouth, restlessness, tiredness, tremor

Your draft of an explanatory model of the patient's symptoms should look something like ◘ Fig. 5.1 and is best drawn by hand in the session and expanded in the next session.

5.1.3 Clarifying the Therapy Goals: Guided Imagery

Now a guided imagery can be conducted to clarify therapy goals. The following instructional example can serve as a basis for this exercise.

▪ Instruction: Guided Imagery to Generate Therapy Goals

In the following, I would like to take you on a little guided imagery that can make it a little more tangible to you what a life with less burden from the somatic symptoms could look like. The aim of this guided imagery is to develop positive perspectives for the future, even if these may seem unrealistic at the moment, perhaps even represent a utopia. Nevertheless, try to engage with this exercise!

I now ask you to make yourself comfortable in your chair. Sit down in a relaxed position. Try to breathe in and

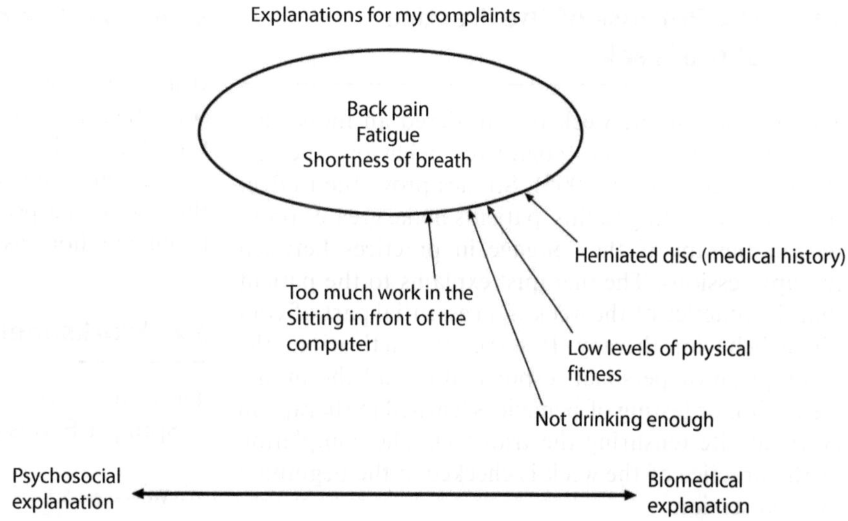

Fig. 5.1 Explanatory model of somatic symptoms

out calmly and deeply. If you like, close your eyes. Slowly come to rest. Now imagine that you are sitting in a room in which you feel very comfortable …

In front of you is a large suitcase, which is open … Now try to put into this suitcase all that you feel as a burden and restriction due to your somatic symptoms. Pack everything that constricts your joy of life into it. When you feel that you have put everything that is a burden into the suitcase, then close it.

Now the door opens and a porter comes in. Silently he takes the suitcase and carries it out. Now that the suitcase is gone, you feel free and unencumbered. Enjoy the feeling of being liberated. And it seems to you as if a heavy burden has fallen from you….

Now stand up in thought and walk around the room lightly and carefree. After you have wandered around a little, open the door and leave the room.

Now go in your thoughts to a person who is close to you. Go to one of your family members, to your partner, to your children, or even to one of your friends. Pick out someone who is personally close to you. Now, what if you stand in front of this person without any limitation due to your somatic symptoms? How will this person behave towards you? What will have changed in your relationship with this person? What will this person notice about you? Will this person say something to you?

Free and light-hearted, you now leave this person and next visit your workplace (if you don't have a job, then imagine your normal everyday life). What will be different when you no longer feel limited by pain or other physical discomfort? What jobs will you be able to do again? What will change?

Now leave your workplace in your mind and imagine your leisure time. What will you be able to do? What activities will you be involved in? How will you spend your weekends? Is there perhaps something you have wanted to do for a long time? Think about vacation destinations as well. Is there perhaps a place you have always wanted to visit?

Now let all the images, thoughts and feelings that came up during your little journey sink in again … Try to memorize the mood so that you can remember this state better later.

Now slowly return to this room in your mind, count from 5 to 1, and when you reach 1, open your eyes again!

After carrying out the exercise, it is particularly important to discuss and evaluate it together with the patient. The following questions can be helpful:

- How well was the patient able to engage with the guided imagery?
- Any problems?
- With what impressions did the patient return?

To make it easier for the patient to remember, the therapist can mention again the areas mentioned in the guided imagery (social relationships, work, leisure time).

5.1.4 Formulation of Therapy Goals

The therapist hands out Worksheet 5.2 (My personal therapy goals) and supports the patient in formulating goals. When defining goals, the therapist should first and foremost make sure that the goals are realistic. In addition, vague ideas for goals should be made concrete, the patient's capacities should be assessed, existing resources and inhibiting factors in the environment should be taken into account, and ethical and moral aspects should be considered. If time is short, the worksheet can also be given as additional practice of the week.

5.1.5 The Purpose of the Practice of the Week

The practice of the week is considered an indispensable element in any cognitive behavior therapy (Wunschel & Linden, 2005). Studies prove their effectiveness. According to this, patients make greater progress in therapy if they engage in practices between therapy sessions. The therapist explains to the patient that the practice of the week is an essential part of cognitive behavior therapy. It serves the activation, the assumption of personal responsibility and the implementation or testing of behaviors learned in therapy in everyday life (ensuring the transfer). The completion of the practice of the week is checked at the beginning of each session.

5.1.6 Practice of the Week

If it was not possible to work on Worksheet 5.2 (My personal therapy goals) during the session due to a lack of time, this can be handed out as practice of the week to be worked on. The patient should be motivated to consider the discussed aspects of therapy goal formulation and to formulate short- as well as long-term therapy goals.

5.2 Worksheets

These worksheets are also available for download online at Springer Extras (► extras.springer.com).

Worksheet 5.1	Therapy's content	◘ Figure 5.2
Worksheet 5.2	My personal therapy goals	◘ Figure 5.3

◘ **Fig. 5.2** Worksheet 5.1: Therapy's content

Worksheet 5.1: Therapy's content?

During treatment, we will deal with somatic symptoms whose causes can be more or less sufficiently explained by an illness or medical condition. The aim will be to work out various possible explanations for your symptoms and to get to know and practice strategies that will help you managing your symptoms and can also lead to a reduction in your symptoms.

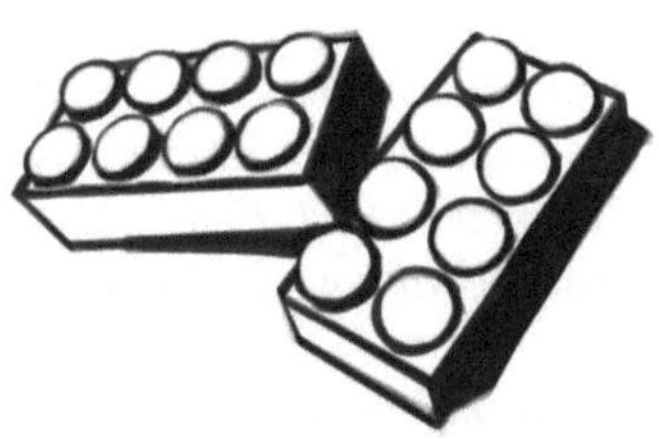

In detail, we will deal with the following topics in the course of the therapy:

- Stress, and its connection with persistent somatic symptoms
- Components and functions of the autonomic nervous system and how it regulates the body's stress response
- Relaxation, introduction to progressive muscle relaxation
- How our attention works and how it is connected to your somatic symptoms, strategies of refocusing attention
- The role of thoughts and their connection with somatic symptoms; checking and challenging thoughts that are related to somatic symptoms; developing alternative thoughts about somatic symptoms
- Avoidance or, the opposite, "boom and bust" behavior and its effects on somatic symptoms; strategies to increase resilience of your body
- Strategies to deal successfully with illness
- Strategies to deal with chronic distress caused by somatic symptoms
- Coping strategies to manage your persistent symptoms

Fig. 5.3 Worksheet 5.2: My personal therapy goals

Worksheet 5.2: My personal therapy goals

Please enter which goals you would like to achieve with the help of the therapy in the medium term (at the end of treatment) and in the long term (1-3 years after the end of therapy)! You are welcome to add further target areas! Tip for creating your goals: Be as specific as possible so that the achievement of the respective goal can be verified! You may also be able to create short-term goals (positive changes within the next few weeks, i.e., small progress)?

	(short term)	medium-term	long-term
somatic symptoms			
work			
recreation			

Reference

Wunschel, I., & Linden, M. (2005). Hausaufgaben. In M. Linden, & M. Hautzinger (Hrsg.), *Verhaltenstherapiemanual* (5. Aufl., S. 176–179). Springer.

Module 2: Stress and Stress Management (Part 1)

Contents

M. Kleinstäuber et al., *Cognitive Behavior Therapy for Persistent Somatic Symptoms and Somatic Symptom Disorder*, https://doi.org/10.1007/978-3-662-69726-9_6

6.1 Session 2

Contents and Materials of the 2nd Session

- **Contents**
  - Discussion of the practice of the week
  - Extension of the patient's explanatory model
  - Functions of stress
  - Structure of the nervous system
  - Physical stress reaction and signs of inner tension
  - Practice of the week: Fill in Worksheet 6.4 (Journal of well-being: How have I been today?)
- **Materials**
  - Patient's notes on the explanatory model from session 1
  - Worksheet 6.1: What you should know about stress?
  - Worksheet 6.2: Structure of the nervous system
  - Worksheet 6.3: Effects of sympathetic and parasympathetic nervous system
  - Worksheet 6.4: Journal: How have I been today? (7 copies)

6.1.1 Discussion of the Practice of the Week

Assuming that Worksheet 5.2 (My personal therapy goals) was given as practice of the week in the first session, this should be discussed first. The therapist should make sure that the goals drafted by the patient are realistic and verifiable. If this is not the case, concrete suggestions to rephrase the goals can be made to the patient.

6.1.2 Extension of the Patient's Explanatory Model

By means of "guided discovery", it should be worked out with patients on the basis of their explanatory model of their symptoms, which was created in the previous session, that the explanations for the symptoms cannot always be clearly classified into the categories "psychological" and "somatic":

?
- What did you notice as you "sorted" the explanations?
- When "sorting" the explanations according to "purely psychological" vs. "purely somatic", did you possibly notice that there are hardly any explanations that are 100% somatic or 100% psychological (e.g., a previous illness is a learning experience and learning is something psychological; muscle tension shows especially in stressful situations or with negative emotions)?

Furthermore, it is explored whether the patient can think of other explanations that also have a psychological component:

?
- Has anyone ever said to you, "This is something psychological or psychosomatic?" Do you have any idea what they meant?

Here it is important to consider that every psychological factor also has a physical component (at the latest on the level of neurotransmitters etc.). At this point the example of phantom limb pain can be explained if necessary: Phantom limb pain occurs when a limb has been removed and yet it continues to hurt. The pain is real even though the corresponding body part is missing. This is because the experience originates in the brain. Exploration for other factors can continue as follows:

?
- What other factors can you think of that have an impact on your symptoms?
- For example, when are your symptoms worse? When are they better?

The information collected is written down together and then, if necessary, supplemented by the therapist in the following areas

- Stress,
- Perception and appraisals,
- Behaviors,
- Emotions.

The patient can be informed at this point that we know from scientific research that these areas have an influence on the extent of somatic symptoms. It is important to emphasize here that the experience of stress can very often be accompanied by physical changes and somatic symptoms. Therefore, in the following, it is first important to look more deeply into the role of stress in relation to somatic symptoms.

6.1.3 Functions of Stress

With the help of guided discovery, some general questions about stress should first be explored with the patient. The therapist should be careful to acknowledge and respond to the patient's thoughts on each question. Should this be necessary, the information below can be conveyed to the patient.

❓ What actually is stress?

Originally, the term comes from the technical field, more precisely from materials science, and is to be understood as follows: Stress on a material leads to strain on it. This model can also be applied to humans. **Stress** is always neutral (neither good nor bad) and can be measured objectively. **Stress**, on the other hand, is experienced individually differently and can only be measured subjectively. The degree of stress is influenced by the individual's **abilities**, **skills** and **coping strategies**. A distinction is made between positively experienced stress, so-called **eustress**, and negatively experienced stress, so-called **distress**. Eustress is associated with feelings of challenge and satisfaction, whereas distress is associated with feelings of being overwhelmed. From a medical or biological point of view, stress is a natural reaction of the human body to stress of all kinds (dangerous situations, problematic situations, internal and external demands). Stress triggers the "alarm behavior" program that is anchored in every human being.

❓ How long has there been stress?

Stress has been around since time immemorial. The physical stress reaction is a (Stone Age) old behavior pattern. It is not acquired or learned, but is innate and therefore a normal phenomenon.

❓ What kind of stress did humans suffer from at the beginning of evolution?

Humans suffered from the threat of predators, hostile tribes, interpersonal conflicts, extreme weather conditions, search for food, and disease.

❓ What would a person do in a typical dangerous situation (e.g., attack by a wild animal)?

The person would **fight** or **escape** ("fight or flight"). The third behavioral response is the so-called **"freezing" reflex**. This is a kind of psychological shock that sets in when all previous coping mechanisms have failed. It is associated with a feeling of being overwhelmed and activates a kind of paralysis ("rigid with fear"). In order to be able to fight or escape, the body needs a lot of energy. This is made available to it by the automatically triggered stress reaction. The body is prepared for action within a very short time. Seen in this way, the physical stress reaction represents a **natural adaptation mechanism**, a protective reaction to threat. Accordingly, this alarm behavior makes biological sense; physical performance is increased. However, the physical stress reaction loses its biological sense if it is triggered in objectively harmless situations (e.g., phobias or specific anxiety disorders), if it lasts for a long time or if it occurs too frequently. At the end of this information, the patient receives Worksheet 6.1 (What you should know about stress?).

6.1.4 Structure of the Autonomic Nervous System

In the following you will find suggestions for knowledge transfer on the topic "autonomic nervous system and physical stress reaction". Here, too, we recommend using the principle of guided discovery with the help of questions.

❓ Do you know who or what is responsible for triggering and controlling the physical stress response?

The **autonomic nervous system** (ANS) is responsible for this. It is called ANS because it is largely removed from voluntary control. The ANS regulates the internal balance of the body's systems and ensures that the organism is constantly adapting to a changing environment. The ANS monitors and regulates blood circulation, cardiac activity, blood pressure, respiration, body temperature, and digestion. Simplified, the ANS consists of the two subsystems **sympathetic** and **parasympathetic**. The effects of the two systems on the organs are often opposing, which allows for precise control of organ function. Most organs are innervated by both the sympathetic and the parasympathetic nervous system, but some are not (e.g., the sweat glands; these are innervated exclusively by the sympathetic nervous system). In simple terms, the sympathetic nervous system induces activation of the body during work or in situations requiring a rapid response (threat, stress/strain). It serves to mobilize the organism. The parasympathetic nervous system, on the other hand, serves to build up energy resources during periods of rest and mainly supports functions such as digestion and reproduction. It is important to emphasize that the two systems do not compete with each other, but rather work "hand in hand" to enable optimal interaction of the body organs in each case in adaptation to the respective requirements (Ehlert, 2003). The patient then receives Worksheet 6.2 (Structure of the nervous system).

In case the patient is knowledgeable regarding the human body and/or keenly interested, the following information about the **influence of hormones** in regulating the body's stress response can be given as an option.

Hormones in the Regulation of the Physical Stress Response

Stress hormones are released when the sympathetic nervous system is activated or under strong internal or external stress. These are primarily **adrenaline** (and **noradrenaline**) from the adrenal medulla and **cortisol** from the adrenal cortex. Both adrenaline and cortisol initiate processes that quickly make more energy available to the organism (e.g., increase in blood sugar levels, release of fatty acids from fat depots). In addition, they increase blood pressure and the stroke volume of the heart and can lead to vasoconstriction in certain vascular areas (Faller, 1995).

The hormones of the adrenal cortex, which include cortisol, enable the organism to respond to internal and external stress. **Glucocorticoids** are indispensable for coping with severe stress situations. In this context, cortisol is the physiologically most important glucocorticoid (Mutschler & Schäfer-Korting, 1996). Cortisol (also hydrocortisone) is a vital hormone. The complete absence of cortisol as a result of illness or after adrenalectomy leads to certain death in a few days (Kuschinsky et al., 1993).

The **adrenal glands** are two small, yellowish-looking glands that sit cap-like on the upper pole of the kidneys. Each weighs about 4 grams and consists of two morphologically and functionally completely different organs, namely the adrenal cortex and the adrenal medulla. The adrenal cortex is divided into three layers. The innermost layer (zona reticularis) produces predominantly androgens (male sex hormones). The outermost layer (zona glomerulosa) produces mainly mineralocorticoids. The middle layer, the zona fasciculata, produces the group of glucocorticoids, the most important of which is cortisol. The glucocorticoids support processes that ensure that sufficient glucose ("fuel" or "energy") is made available to the cells of the body. In addition, glucocorticoids have a number of other roles, most notably in metabolism, behavior, and the immune system. Cortisol release is controlled by one of the four glandotropic hormones of the anterior pituitary lobe (HVL), ACTH, which in turn is under the control of the pituitary releasing hormone CRH. Cortisol circulating in the blood has an inhibitory effect on the further release of CRH and ACTH in the hypothalamus and the HVL, respectively, via a negative feedback mechanism. Many stressors lead to an increased release of CRH, which in turn induces an increased release of ACTH. Severe stress situations can be so intense that excess ACTH is found in the blood, as more ACTH is produced than is necessary for maximal cortisol secretion (Birbaumer & Schmidt, 2010).

High cortisol levels cause amino acids to be converted to glucose in the liver. This process is called **gluconeogenesis**. This process, to which glucocorticoids owe their name, is activated especially during fasting and starvation, so that after depletion of glycogen stores, blood glucose levels are maintained as constant as possible. The amino acids required for gluconeogenesis are obtained by breaking down body protein (→ protein catabolic effect). The catabolic effect is mainly seen in the muscles, skin and skeleton. Under the conditions mentioned, cortisol also activates the release of glycerol and fatty acids from the body's fat stores (→ lipolysis) to provide further cellular fuel (Birbaumer & Schmidt, 2010).

Adrenaline and noradrenaline, together with dopamine, form the group of **catecholamines**. Catecholamines are formed from the amino acid phenylalanine by the following enzymatic steps: Phenylalanine → p-tyrosine → dopa → dopamine → norepinephrine → epinephrine. Adrenaline, like noradrenaline, is secreted from the adrenal medulla by activation of the sympathetic nervous system (80% adrenaline, 20% noradrenaline) and serves primarily to provide energy rapidly (→ metabolic action). Thus, adrenaline and noradrenaline are primarily considered **metabolic hormones**. Adrenaline mobilizes free fatty acids from adipose tissue and glucose and lactate from glycogen. In emergency situations (e.g., blood loss, hypothermia, burns or extreme physical stress) and during intense emotional stress, the release of adrenaline and noradrenaline from the adrenal medulla increases. Oxygen and nutrients or fuels (glucose and free fatty acids) are increasingly transported to the brain, heart and skeletal muscles. The release is in turn controlled by the hypothalamus and the limbic system (Birbaumer & Schmidt, 2010).

Adrenaline acts primarily on the heart by increasing its frequency and beating force. Norepinephrine causes an increase in blood pressure, primarily through vasoconstriction of the arterioles and internal organs, so that blood is directed towards the muscles and brain. Catecholamines also cause an increase in attention and alertness via stimulation of the central nervous system (CNS) (Kapit et al., 1992).

6.1.5 Physical Stress Reaction and Signs of Inner Tension

Individual physical stress reactions and signs of tension can be explored with the following question:

? When you are tensed or under great stress, what physical changes do you notice?

The patient's answers are collected on the flip chart. It is helpful to go through the individual organ systems if the patient has difficulty answering the question. A helpful question from the therapist to the patient might be:

? For example, do you notice a change in your heartbeat or breathing?

Changes that might be related to the patient's physical complaints should be highlighted. The patient is given Worksheet 6.3 (Effects of sympathetic and parasympathetic nervous system).

6.1.6 Practice of the Week

The patient is asked to keep a diary of his or her state of mind until the next session (Worksheet 6.4). The therapist introduces the task with the following words: "In order to change the impairment caused by the symptoms in the long term, it is first important to monitor your symptoms and the circumstances in which they occur. For this reason, I would like to ask you to keep this so-called diary of well-being during the next week. From this you can see whether the symptoms always remain the same or whether they change, whether there are influencing conditions and how much you are affected by the symptoms in your life."

The therapist hands out seven copies of Worksheet 6.4 (Journal of well-being: How have I been today?) (assuming that the next session will take place in exactly 1 week). The individual questions are gone through with the patient and, if necessary, explained with examples. The patient is instructed to complete the diary daily. It is important to point out to patients that they are not keeping the diary for the therapist, but for themselves, i.e., in their own interest.

6.2 Session 3

Contents and Materials of the 3rd Session

- **Contents**
  - Discussion of the practice of the week
  - Relaxation response
  - Background information on progressive muscle relaxation (PMR)
  - PMR practice (long form, duration approx. 30 minutes)
  - Typical difficulties in performing PMR in the context of persistent somatic symptoms
  - Practice of the week: Keeping a relaxation log (Worksheet 6.8)
- **Materials**
  - Worksheet 6.5: Relaxation response
  - Worksheet 6.6: Progressive muscle relaxation (PMR)
  - Worksheet 6.7: Instructions for progressive muscle relaxation
  - Worksheet 6.8: Relaxation log
  - PMR CD

6.2.1 Discussion of the Practice of the Week

Session 3 begins with the evaluation of the journal of well-being (Worksheet 6.4). Helpful questions in this regard can be:

- Were there any difficulties in processing?
- Has the patient discovered any connections?
- Were there any particular triggers for the symptoms or changes in the symptoms (see point 8 on Worksheet 6.4)?
- How frequent, how intense were the symptoms, or what was the extent of the distress?

6.2.2 Relaxation Response

One way to have a positive effect on the physical stress reaction is to activate the parasympathetic nervous system. This is possible by regularly practicing a relaxation technique.

In the following, the therapist explains the typical physical and psychological changes that characterize the physical relaxation response and hands out Worksheet 6.5: (relaxation response) to the patient. In addition, Worksheet 6.3 (Effects of sympathetic and parasympathetic nervous system) can be used again to explain the effects of the parasympathetic nervous system. The relaxation response, like the stress response discussed earlier, is a biologically anchored, and therefore innate, behavioral program.

Regularly performed relaxation exercises lead to a reduction of the sympathetic nervous system's readiness to respond, i.e. to a decrease in the general level of arousal. It should be noted that the stimulation and stabilization of a relaxation reaction requires continuous practice. With longer, regular practice, an increasing serenity can develop, which helps to better cope with stress and the burdens of everyday life. Performing a relaxation procedure provides an opportunity to better cope with stress that you cannot, or cannot yet, change. In the long run, relaxation exercises can lead to the fact that one looks at things with more serenity and calmness, that one is no longer so easily "driven up the wall", that one acquires a thicker skin for stressful situations and that one does not react to small annoyances or an accumulation of these in the same way as the famous "HB male" named Bruno.

6.2.3 Background Information on Progressive Muscle Relaxation

Progressive muscle relaxation (PMR) was developed by the American physician and physiologist Edmund Jacobson around 1930. The basic principle of PMR is to focus attention on a specific region of the body, tense the muscles, hold the tension for a short time and release the tension again when exhaling and relax. The procedure of PMR—achieving relaxation through targeted physical tension—seems paradoxical at first glance. But on closer examination, the supposed contradiction dissolves. The practitioner should pay close attention to the differences between tension and relaxation. The relaxation of the musculature can be perceived better if the opposite (tension of the musculature) took place before (contrast effect). This makes the seemingly paradoxical procedure understandable. The aims of PMR are to improve body awareness and to be able to recognise muscular tension at an early stage and to actively reduce it. The patient receives Worksheet 6.6 (Progressive muscle relaxation).

The therapist emphasizes that learning a relaxation technique involves commitment, effort and time. Concentration and regular practice over several weeks are important for the success of the training. This is no different for similar activities such as learning a new sport or musical instrument. In this respect, the saying "No master has ever fallen from the sky", "Practice makes perfect" and "No pain, no gain" is true. Transferred to the patient and the learning of a relaxation technique, this means that he must/should practice daily in order to be able to bring about the feeling of relaxation at some point in a targeted and rapid manner, that he must have patience with himself, that he cannot force relaxation and that he should not expect too much of himself at the beginning. Accordingly, "the gun" should not be "thrown in the basket" if the desired relaxation does not occur immediately after the first runs.

6.2.4 PMR Practice

The therapist performs the long form of PMR using the following instruction, which takes about 30 minutes. It is useful to discuss the exercises for the individual muscle groups with the patient before starting. It should also be discussed that unusual physical sensations (e.g., a feeling of warmth or tingling in the extremities) may occur during the exercise. These are completely harmless and can be explained by increased blood circulation.

- **Instruction: Progressive Muscle Relaxation (Long Form)**

Bring yourself in a posture, as comfortable as possible and be prepared to get in a relaxed state.—Make sure that you are sitting relaxed and upright.—You lean back to the back of your chair and your feet firmly touch the ground.—Arms and hands rest loosely in your lap.—Your head is in a comfortable position.—Closing your eyes can improve your focus on your body.—You can close your eyes now or later.—You may want to get a little more comfortable.—Go through your body in your mind and try to notice which muscles are tight and try to loosen them a little bit more.—Take a few deep breaths and then slowly exhale.—Observe how your abdominal wall rises slightly as you inhale and slowly lowers again as you exhale.—You may also be able to feel the air flowing in through your nose in a cool way and—warmed by your body—flowing out again warmed up.—We are about to begin the exercises.—Please pay close attention to your sensations as you tense and then relax your muscles.—It is not important to tense the muscles strongly, but only to notice clearly the differences between tension and relaxation.—Please increase the tension to the point where you can clearly feel the tension.—But only to the point that it does not hurt or cramp.—Continue to breathe calmly, in your rhythm, even while tensing the muscles.—Please always perform the tightening of the muscles only when I say "NOW!".

First, focus your attention on your right hand and forearm.—How do your right hand and forearm feel?—Clench your right hand into a fist—NOW!—Increase the tension until you feel it clearly, but not too tight.—And with your next exhale, release the tension in your hand and forearm and let your arm and hand be completely loose and comfortable.—Also try to let the fingers become completely loose.—Notice the difference between tension before and relaxation.—Allow some time for the muscles to release a little more.—Let go completely!—Now focus on your upper right arm and become aware of how it feels.—Bend your right arm towards your shoulder with your hand open—NOW!—Feel the tension.—With the next exhale, lower the arm and relax.—Again, notice the difference in sensation between tension before and relaxation.—Notice how, as the tension eases, the relaxation can come very slowly.

Now concentrate on your left hand and forearm.—Close your left hand into a fist—NOW!—Pay close attention to the tension that arises.—And with the next exhale, release again.—Notice how comfortable it is as the muscles transition from the tense to the relaxed state.—Again, pay attention to the relaxation in each finger.—Now focus on your upper left arm and become aware of how it feels.—With your hand open, bend your left arm toward your shoulder and tense your left upper arm muscle—NOW!—Feel the tension.—With your next exhale, lower your arm back down and relax.—Again, notice the difference in sensation between tension before and relaxation.—Notice how as the tension eases, the relaxation can come very slowly.—Clench both hands into a fist—NOW!—Again, pay attention to the tension that is created.—Release again with the next exhalation.—Again, notice the difference between tension before and the pleasant relaxation.—Let your forearms rest heavily and concentrate again on each finger.

Now concentrate again on your right arm.—Stretch it so far that you feel an intense tension at the back of your arm—NOW!—Pay attention to the tension again.—On your next exhale, release your arm again and rest it comfortably.—Focus your attention on your left arm.—Stretch your left arm so that you feel an intense tension at the back of the arm—NOW!—Again, pay attention to the tension.—With your next exhale, release the tension and let it become completely loose and relaxed.—Again, notice the difference between tension before and the pleasant relaxation.—Now try to tense both upper and lower arms and hands at the same time—NOW!—Feel the tension.—With the next exhale, lower both arms and hands again and relax.—Try to let the muscles in your arms become completely loose.—Let your arms become heavier and heavier.—Concentrate again on each individual finger.

Now concentrate on your forehead—pull your eyebrows upwards so that horizontal wrinkles appear on your forehead—NOW!—Hold the tension.—With the next exhale, release again.—Now let your forehead become smooth and released like a smooth, empty surface.—As you relax your forehead, try to let your whole head cover become loose.—Again, notice the difference between tension before and the feeling of relaxation.—Now draw your eyebrows together so that there are vertical wrinkles on your forehead—NOW!—Notice the tension again.—With the next exhale, release the tension again.—Notice the transition from tension to comfortable relaxation.—Let your forehead become more and more loosened and relaxed.—Try to form horizontal and vertical wrinkles on your forehead at the same time—NOW!—Your forehead is now completely tense.—With your next exhale, release the tension.—Let your forehead muscles become completely loose—looser and looser,—until your forehead feels like a smooth and empty surface.—Now concentrate on your eyes.—Squeeze your eyes tightly shut—NOW!—Notice the tension in your eye area.—With the next exhale, release again.—Now keep your eyes very slightly closed.—Again, notice the difference between the tension before and the feeling of relaxation.—Let your eyelids become heavy—heavier and heavier—and make sure that your forehead muscles are also completely loosened and relaxed.

Now concentrate on your nose.—Wrinkle your nose by pulling it upwards—NOW!—Feel the tension in the nose area.—With the next exhale, release again.—Allow your nostrils to relax and release completely.—Let your eyelids become heavier and heavier as well.—And pay attention to your forehead, which is smooth and loosened.

Now concentrate on your teeth.—Bite your molars firmly together—NOW!—Notice the tension in your jaw.—With your next exhale, release the tension and allow your jaw to loosen again.—Allow your lips and all facial muscles to become completely loose.—Try to relax your facial muscles more and more.—Pay attention to your forehead—your eyelids—and your nostrils.—Notice the feeling of calm that spreads as you relax your face more and more.—Now focus on your tongue—press your tongue firmly against the roof of your mouth—NOW!—Notice the tension.—With the next exhale, release the tension again and let your tongue fall back into a relaxed position.—Again, notice the difference between tension before and the feeling of relaxation.—Now focus on your mouth and lips.—Press your lips firmly together—NOW!—Notice the tension in your lips and mouth area.—With the next exhale, release again.—Notice again the contrast between the tension before and the pleasant relaxation that gradually spreads.

Now try to tense your entire face, i.e. your forehead, the top of your head, the eye area, your nose, your lips, your cheeks, your jaw and your chin—NOW!—Notice the tension.—With the next exhale, relax again.—Notice that your jaw becomes completely loose, your cheeks are relaxed, your forehead becomes smooth and detached, and your eyelids become heavy.—Notice the feeling of calm that gradually spreads as you relax your facial muscles more and more.

Now concentrate on your neck muscles.—Push your head forward as if you wanted to touch your chest with your chin and at the same time try to prevent this—NOW!—Hold this tension.—With your next exhale, release the tension.—Again, notice the difference between the tension before and the feeling of relaxation.—Now balance your head so that your neck muscles become completely loose and released.—Try to relax further and further.

Now concentrate on your shoulders.—Pull your shoulders up and hold the tension—NOW!—Notice the tension that is created.—With the next exhalation let your shoulders hang loosely down again.—Pay attention only to the pleasant feeling of relaxation.—Let your shoulder muscles become more and more relaxed.—Now let the relaxation radiate all the way down your back.—Let your neck, throat, jaw and whole face become completely relaxed as well.—Let the relaxation radiate out further and further—into your arms and hands—all the way to your fingertips.—Again, pay attention to each individual finger.—Try to relax further and further.

Now concentrate on your breath—notice how the air flows in and out again.—After inhaling, hold your breath for a short time—NOW!—Notice the tension in your chest—Now let the air flow out again.—As you exhale, notice how your chest relaxes comfortably and becomes loose again.—Hold your breath again after inhaling—NOW!—Notice the tension in your chest again—Now breathe out slowly.—Pay attention to the pleasant feeling of relaxation.—Now follow the inflow and outflow of your breath.—Talk inwardly as you breathe in and out again.—As you inhale and exhale.—As you do so, pay attention to the feeling of calm that gradually spreads through your body.

Now focus on your abdomen.—Tighten your abdominal muscles, make your abdomen hard, as if you wanted to absorb a blow—NOW!—Pay attention to the tension this creates.—With your next exhale, release again.—Allow your abdominal muscles to become completely loose and released.—Again, notice the difference between tension before and the feeling of relaxation.

Now concentrate on your back.—Arch your back by bending far forward—NOW!—Notice the tension along your spine.—With your next exhale, straighten back up and ease back into the chair.—Allow your back to relax and release.—Let the relaxation of the back muscles radiate forward—to the chest and abdominal muscles—to the shoulder area—to the arms and hands—and to the face.—Now, again, pay attention only to the inflow and outflow of your breath.—Talk inwardly as you breathe in and out again.—Let yourself fall deeper and deeper into relaxation.

Now try to tense your entire body—your arms—the shoulders—the face—the chest—and the belly—NOW!—Pay attention to the tension.—With the next exhale, release again.—Again, pay attention to the transition between tension and relaxation.—Try to relax further and further.—Again, pay attention only to the inflow and outflow of your breath.

Now focus on your legs—stretch your legs forward and tense your thighs and glutes—NOW!—Pay attention to the tension.—On the next exhale, lower your legs again and release.—Pay attention to the transition from tension to relaxation.—Now press your heels firmly to the floor and pull your toes up at the same time—NOW!—Notice the tension this creates in your feet and lower legs.—With your next exhale, release again.—Notice again the difference between tension before and relaxation.—Now press your toes into the floor and simultaneously pull your heels upwards—NOW!—Notice the tension in your calf muscles.—With your next exhale, lower your heels again and release the tension in your calves.—Again, notice the difference between tension before and relaxation.—Now press your entire foot firmly against the floor, as if you were trying to push the floor down or as if you were trying to stand up but preventing it at the same time—NOW!—Notice the tension in your lower legs, thighs and glutes.—With the next exhale, release the tension.—Allow your leg muscles to become completely loose and released.—Again, pay attention to the transition from tension to release.—Notice how the feeling of relaxation radiates down into your feet—all the way to the tips of your toes.—Let your legs become more and more relaxed and heavy.

Now let the feeling of relaxation flow up from the feet—through the legs to the back—into the chest—into the stomach area—into the shoulders—into the arms and hands—into the fingertips—into the neck—up to the face.—Let your entire body become loose and relaxed.—Your forehead resembles a smooth and empty surface—your eyelids are heavy—and your jaw is completely slack.—Let your body rest on the chair with its entire weight.—Now pay attention to your breathing once again.—Try not to influence it at all, just observe it.—Talk inwardly as you breathe in and out again.—Just register this inflow and outflow of your breath.—Try to relax more and more as you do this.—Enjoy this state of peace and relaxation for a while by yourself.—Now tell yourself that you are gradually ending the exercise.—Now slowly tense your body again—and return to this room in your mind.—And when you are ready, slowly open your eyes again.

Afterwards there is a short evaluation of the exercise, which can be done with the help of the following questions:

- What sensations occurred (e.g., heaviness, lightness, warmth, cold, tingling, changes of your body schema)?
- Were there any difficulties with individual exercises?
- How deep is the experienced relaxation rated on a scale of 0–100?

Finally, the patients receive a CD with instructions for PMR (e.g., available from health insurance companies) as well as written PMR instructions (Worksheet 6.7), so that they can practice independently at home.

6.2.5 Typical Difficulties in Performing PMR in the Context of Persistent Somatic Symptoms

In the following you will find a list of typical difficulties that the therapist may be confronted with in the application of PMR with patients with persistent somatic symptoms, as well as appropriate suggestions for solutions and handling. Individual problems in learning relaxation techniques can have very different causes. The following overview in ◘ Table 6.1 does not claim to be complete, but merely provides a selection of possible solutions.

◘ Table 6.1 Difficulties in the application of PMR in patients with persistent somatic symptoms and ways of dealing with them for therapists

Typical problems with the application of PMR	What causes can play a role and how can I behave as a therapist?
"It just doesn't work for me."	*Excessive expectations* Explain that learning a relaxation technique takes practice, just like other skills (e.g. driving a car) Reassure patients and, if necessary, challenge excessive expectations of PMR First, ask for the patient's patience to practice PMR for a certain period of time. If it becomes apparent that PMR is really not a suitable method for the patient, then alternative methods (e.g., imagination exercises) can be practiced
	Other causes Exploring the reasons for problems during performance in detail (if necessary, by observing behavior during PMR performance in session; relaxation protocol) and working out possible solutions with the patient (e.g., if the patient feels uncomfortable in a lying position, PMR should be practiced in other body positions at an early stage, aids such as pillows and blankets should be used or shorter exercise sequences should be carried out throughout the day) Emphasize small advances in the process and explain various goals of PMR (in addition to relaxation skills, improved body awareness alone is an important goal)

Table 6.1 (continued)

Typical problems with the application of PMR	What causes can play a role and how can I behave as a therapist?
"I don't have time."	*Problems with scheduling* See ► Sect. 10.2 (Time management)
	Problems doing something good for yourself Resource-oriented work: balancing stressors and stress resistance Exploring and questioning cognitions behind the problem Euthymic strategies and strategies to promote enjoyment skills Mindfulness-based strategies for building self-care
"My discomfort gets stronger during PMR."	*Excessive tension of certain muscle groups (possibly due to the patient's motive to perform the exercise "as well and as correctly as possible")* Emphasis on the fact that the relaxation and not the tension phase is the most important in PMR Muscles are only tensed to such an extent that there is a slight feeling of tension and a difference to the relaxation phase is noticeable If necessary combination with EMG biofeedback If necessary, questioning the patient's performance thinking when carrying out relaxation exercises Before conducting a PMR session, first test the optimal level of tension for individual PMR exercises with patients
"My discomfort gets stronger during PMR."	*Parts of the body where symptoms occur are very sensitive to muscle tension* Certain muscle groups that become too painful for patients under tension can be omitted at first, if necessary, and integrated later step by step Search for alternative muscle tightening exercises for certain parts of the body that cause less pain Imagination of muscle tension Emphasize the voluntary nature and autonomy of the patient, who can stop the exercise at any time if it is unbearable for him or her
	Attention Shifting Problem Normalization of the lack of a distraction effect: When the patient is in a resting situation, there is an increased risk that attention will be directed towards the body's symptoms (this problem should be anticipated with the patient before PMR is performed) In addition to the relaxation effect, PMR can be used as an exercise to practice shifting attention (patient can consciously practice attention-shifting between body perception and therapist's voice, see also ► Chap. 7) In the long term, the relaxation effect will increase and body symptoms will remain in the background (if necessary, exchange about positive experiences of other patients)
"My thoughts are rambling."	Normalization that rambling thoughts are normal, especially during the first attempt to practice PMR Mindfulness-based exercises (e.g., thoughts are imagined as clouds that are perceived without judgement and pass by)
"During the relaxation exercise, even more somatic symptoms come to the fore."	*Psychoeducation* Focusing attention on the body causes bodily perceptions to come to the fore that are otherwise not conscious Physical relaxation reaction (activation of the parasympathetic nervous system) is accompanied by physical changes (e.g., sensations of warmth in extremities)
"I might fall asleep and start snoring. Then I disturb other group members."	Explanation that falling asleep can be a normal reaction in the initial practice phase Positive reframing: falling asleep shows that the patient is engaged in the exercise In the long term, of course, a differentiation between relaxation and falling asleep should be learned In the context of group therapy, it can be agreed with the patients that they lie down/sit down near the therapist and a sign can be agreed with which the therapist may wake the patients when they fall asleep or snore Patients can be offered to do exercises sitting up instead of lying down, which reduces the risk of falling asleep

(continued)

6

Table 6.1 (continued)

Typical problems with the application of PMR	What causes can play a role and how can I behave as a therapist?
"I've done PMR so many times. It's not for me."	Exploration of the patient's previous experience and possible reasons why PMR has not been effective so far (e.g., lack of professional guidance) Suggest to the patient to perform PMR in long form at least once during the session under therapist instruction (→ give space for new experiences in a new setting) If it turns out that despite correct implementation the patient cannot experience relaxation through PMR, other relaxation methods can be tried (→ Emphasis that not every relaxation strategy is equally effective for everyone and that it is useful to have a repertoire of relaxation strategies)
	Dysfunctional behavioral pattern: "briefly touch on many strategies and drop them when there is no sense of achievement" Some patients tend to abandon coping strategies prematurely if they do not immediately show the desired effect. Therapist and patient should reflect on this behavior pattern and it should be questioned (especially if the behavior pattern is used to justify passive behavior: "I have already tried PMR. It does not work for me. So I can leave it alone.") Motivate patients to really engage in exercises for once
"I cannot relax during relaxation exercises. On the contrary, I feel strong inner restlessness."	First of all, a detailed analysis of the problem is recommended Respect that some patients are not good at using relaxation techniques to bring themselves into a state of relaxation and take seriously and validate patient difficulties in relaxing Individual exploration of which alternative positive activities relax the patient Have patient perform physical or mental activity before relaxation exercise
"When my discomfort is this severe, I have no chance of getting into a state of relaxation."	Validation and understanding to patients that relaxation exercises are difficult to perform under body symptomatology Building acceptance of expected symptom amplification during the first PMR sessions and emphasizing that in the long run the exercises will lead to success and symptom reduction
"I can't get into relaxation because I feel like I'm giving up too much control."	PMR in a different form: e.g., keep the eyes open during the exercise and fixate on a distant point (e.g., on a wall), do only short exercises Emphasize the "experimental character": Patients should experiment with the PMR exercises and find out what does them good
"I can't practice at home because I just don't have a quiet room."	Validation that relaxation is difficult without an appropriate setting At the same time, emphasis should be placed on increasing the ability to relax in the long term, especially in situations that are perceived as stressful (→ conscious practice in a less relaxing atmosphere can be helpful for this in the long term)

6.2.6 Practice of the Week

Patient should perform PMR daily and record their experiences using Worksheet 6.8 (Relaxation log).

6.3 Worksheets

These worksheets are also available for download online at Springer Extras (► extras.springer.com).

Worksheet 6.1	What you should know about stress?	Figure 6.1
Worksheet 6.2	Structure of the nervous system	Figure 6.2
Worksheet 6.3	Effects of sympathetic and parasympathetic nervous system	Figure 6.3
Worksheet 6.4	Journal of well-being: How have I been today?	Figure 6.4
Worksheet 6.5	Relaxation response	Figure 6.5
Worksheet 6.6	Progressive muscle relaxation (PMR)	Figure 6.6
Worksheet 6.7	Instructions for progressive muscle relaxation	Figure 6.7
Worksheet 6.8	Relaxation log	Figure 6.8

Fig. 6.1 Worksheet 6.1: What you should know about stress!

Worksheet 6.1: What should I know about stress?

- The physical stress response of our body is genetically determined and makes sense from a biological point of view!
- From a biological point of view, our physical stress response enables human beings to cope with a dangerous situation. Either through fight or flight. To do this, the body needs a lot of energy, which is made available by triggering the physical stress reaction!
- Under stress, the physical stress response is automatically initiated!

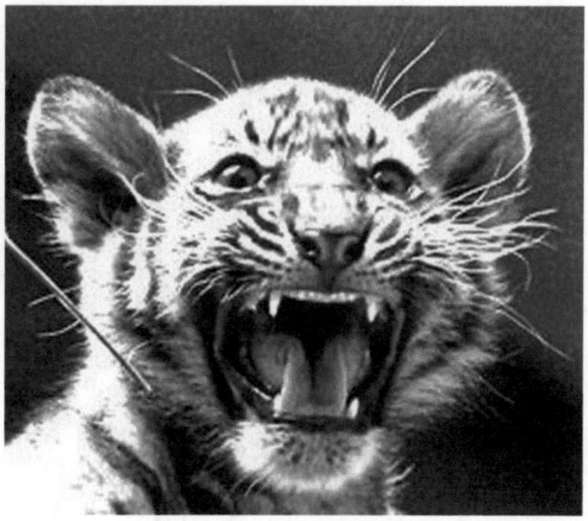

If we are in danger, we have to have to be responsive and act quickly. If we are exposed to a tiger, for example, we can either escape or fight.

Fig. 6.2 Worksheet 6.2: Structure of the nervous system

Worksheet 6.2: Structure of the nervous system

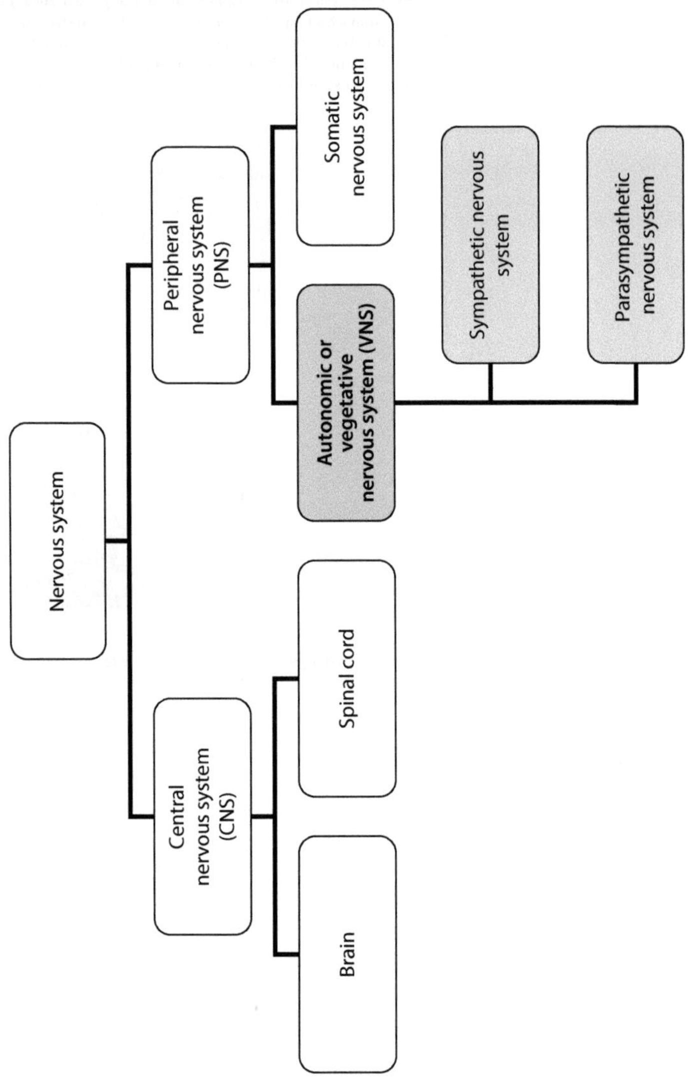

Fig. 6.3 Worksheet 6.3: Effects of sympathetic and parasympathetic nervous system

Worksheet 6.3: Effects of the sympathetic and parasympathetic nervous system

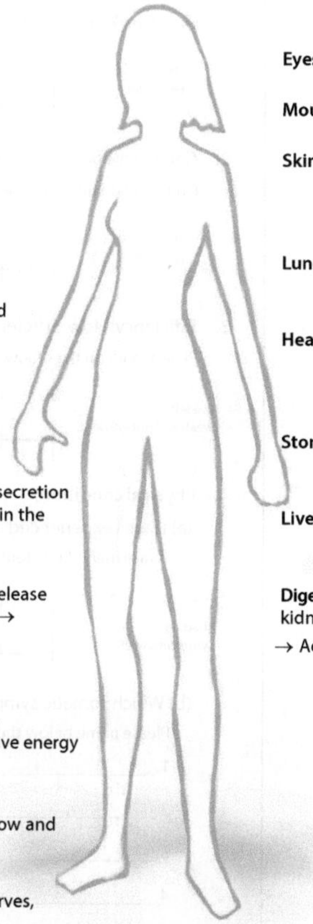

SYMPATHIC
→"Fight or flight"
Mobilization of the body's own energy reserves

CNS → Increased attention

Eyes → Pupil dilation

Mouth → Inhibition of salivation

Skin → Increased perspiration

Lungs → Dilatation of the airways, faster breathing, increased oxygen uptake

Heart → Acceleration of heart rate and increase of the blood pressure

Stomach → Inhibition of gastric juice secretion and the blood circulation in the stomach wall

Liver → Breakdown of glycogen, release of glucose into the blood → Energy!

Digestive organs (pancreas, kidneys, urinary bladder, intestine) → Inhibition of the digestive process to save energy

Skeletal muscles → Increased blood flow and increase in muscle tension

Adipose tissue → Depletion of fat reserves, Release of fatty acids into the blood → Energy!

Blood → Bleeding tendency decreases, the blood clots faster (in case of injury)

Hair → Erection of the body hair (goose bumps) which is a threatening gesture

PARASYMPATHETIC
→"Rest and digestion"
accumulation of energy reserves

Eyes → Pupil constriction

Mouth → Stimulation of salivation

Skin → No effect, sweat glands are only innervated by the sympathetic nervous system

Lungs → Narrowing of the airways, slower breathing

Heart → Slowing of the pulse rate and lowering of blood pressure

Stomach → Activation of gastric juice secretion

Liver → Storage of glucose as glycogen

Digestive organs (pancreas, kidneys, bladder, intestines)
→ Activation of the digestive process

Fig. 6.4 Worksheet 6.4: Journal of well-being: How have I been today?

Worksheet 6.4: Journal of well-being: How have I been today?

Name/Patienten code:______________________________ Date/time:________________

1. **Tension/stress:** How tense or under pressure or stress did you feel today?

   Please mark the amount of tension or inner pressure you have felt today:

   I felt very calm. 0 1 2 3 4 5 6 7 8 9 10 I felt very tense and under pressure.

2. **General mood:** How was your mood today in general?

   On the following scale, please mark how you felt in general today:

   My mood was very bad. 0 1 2 3 4 5 6 7 8 9 10 My mood was very good.

3. **Efficiency:** How efficient did you feel today?

   Please mark on the following scale how fit and efficient you felt today:

   I've felt weak and not efficient. 0 1 2 3 4 5 6 7 8 9 10 I've felt in good shape and efficient.

4. **Physical condition:**

   (a) Have I experienced any physical discomfort or symptoms today?

   Please mark the extent of your physical discomfort that you have experienced today, on the following scale:

   I had no symptoms at all. 0 1 2 3 4 5 6 7 8 9 10 I had very severe somatic symptoms.

   (b) Which somatic symptoms have I experienced today?

   Please name below the symptoms you experienced today:

   1.____________________ 6.____________________

   2.____________________ 7.____________________

   3.____________________ 8.____________________

   4.____________________ 9.____________________

   5.____________________ 10.____________________

5. **Fear of physical complaints:** Have you experienced fear today that your somatic symptoms could be a sign of a serious illness?

   On the following scale, mark the extent to which you fear that your somatic symptoms could be a sign of a serious illness:

   I have no fear of being critically ill. 0 1 2 3 4 5 6 7 8 9 10 I have very intense fear of being critically ill.

Fig. 6.4 (continued)

6. **Coping:**

   (a) Did you have the impression that you were able to cope with or manage your somatic symptoms today?

   Please indicate on the following scale how well you are coping with or managing your somatic symptoms today:

   I was not able to cope with my somatic symptoms at all. 0 — 1 — 2 — 3 — 4 — 5 — 6 — 7 — 8 — 9 — 10 I was able to cope with my somatic symptoms very well.

   (b) What have you done to manage your symptoms?

   Please list below all the things that you have done today to cope with your symptoms:

   1.__________ 4.__________

   2.__________ 5.__________

   3.__________ 6.__________

7. **Daily activities:** What did I do today?

   Please list below all the activities that you did today, regardless of your somatic symptoms. These include professional, social, private, physical, and any other other activities. Also, using the time scale, mark the times at which you want to carry out the activities by blackening cells in the following graph. In the last line you can record the course of your somatic symptoms. Blacken the cells according to the periods of time when your symptoms worsened, and enter a circle when your symptoms improved.

Activities \ Time	1	2	3	4	5	6	7	8	9	10	11	12	13	14	15	16	17	18	19	20	21	22	23
1.																							
2.																							
3.																							
4.																							
5.																							
6.																							
7.																							
8.																							
9.																							
10.																							
Somatic symptoms:																							

Fig. 6.5 Worksheet 6.5: Relaxation response

6

Worksheet 6.5: Relaxation response

- **Physiological changes in my body**
  - Muscle relaxation
  - Improved blood circulation in the limbs, resulting in a feeling of warmth and heaviness, sometimes tingling sensations in arms and legs
  - Slowing of heart rate and blood pressure
  - Slowing and deepening of breathing
  - Decrease in skin conductivity or sweat gland activity
  - Change in brain electrical activity, increase in low frequency brain waves

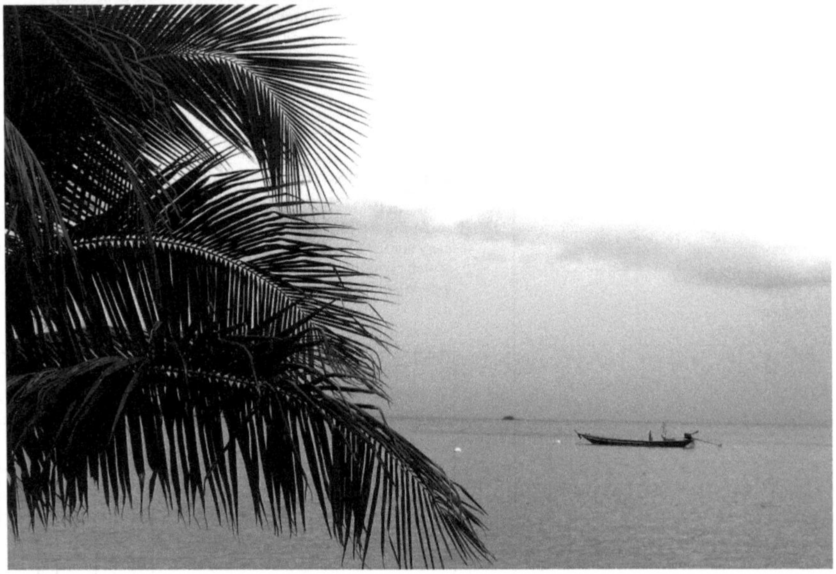

- **Psychological changes**
  - Sense of serenity
  - Increase in perceptional thresholds (external stimuli such as sounds, changes in lighting, or tactile stimulation or touch increasingly loses the ability to trigger a reaction)
  - Mental freshness, improvement of the ability to concentrate
  - Feeling of well-being and balance
  - Decrease in stressful thoughts ("switching off")

Fig. 6.6 Worksheet 6.6: Progressive muscle relaxation (PMR)

Worksheet 6.6: Progressive muscle relaxation (PMR)

- **How does PMR work?**
  Basic principle: Certain muscle groups are first tensed and then relaxed in a specific sequence, while at the same time you concentrate on the differences between tension and relaxation. The tension of the muscles creates a contrasting effect to the subsequent relaxation, so that the relaxation can be felt quickly and intensively.

- **What is the purpose of muscle relaxation?**
  PMR is a rather physiological relaxation technique. With the help of PMR, under consideration that it is practiced regularly, physical and mental tension and nervousness can be reduced and everyday stressful situations can be dealt with more easily. Regular relaxation training can lead to more peace, balance and well-being lead!

- **What you should pay attention to!**
  - Practice daily at the beginning and log your experiences
  - Be patient with yourself, because no one is born a master!
  - The tension of the muscles should be noticeable, but not exaggerated
  - Ideal practice environment is a quiet, darkened room
  - Remove constricting clothing or accessories beforehand (e.g. shoes, belts, glasses, wristwatch, rings).
  - Adopt a comfortable and relaxed sitting position, the feet should have good contact with the floor
  - Emerging bodily sounds or sensations (e.g., stomach growling, tingling sensations, muscle twitching, increased salivation) as well as letting distracting thoughts come and go – they are normal and not a cause for concern

Fig. 6.7 Worksheet 6.7: Instructions for progressive muscle relaxation

Worksheet 6.7: Instructions for progressive muscle relaxation

Preparation

Sit as comfortably as possible and try to keep your muscles as loose as possible! Start the exercise with the right hand. The tension should always be held for a few seconds before you relax your muscles again. Always pay attention to the tension and the subsequent transition into pleasant relaxation!

How to tense the individual muscles

1. Right hand and right forearm	→ Clench right hand into fist
2. Right upper arm	→ Bend elbow with open hand
3. Left hand and left forearm	→ Clench left hand into fist
4. Left upper arm	→ Bend elbow with open hand
5. Forehead	→ Raise *or* pull together eyebrows
6. Eyes	→ Squint eyes and wrinkle nose (after pull up)
7. Jaw and mouth	→ Clench teeth, press lips together, Press tongue upwards against the palate
8. Neck and nape	→ Pull the head in a little and press it backwards or pull head forward onto chest
9. Shoulders and upper back	→ Pull shoulders upwards *or* shoulder blades downwards
10. Chest	→ Take a deep breath and hold it briefly, tense chest muscles
11. Lower back	→ Make make a slight hollow back by tilting the pelvis forward *or* bending the torso forward
12. Abdomen	→ Make the abdominal wall "hard" or retract and tighten
13. Buttocks	→ Squeeze buttocks together
14. Thighs	→ Press heels on the floor and point toes up
15. Lower leg/calves	→ Lift heels slightly off the floor to tense the calves or pull your toes up
16. Feet	→ Press toes in ground or spread toes

Ending the relaxation practice

Finish your relaxation practice slowly by counting from 4 to 1!

- At **4**, move your arms and legs a little!
- At **3**, whole body stretch!
- On **2**, press your feet on the floor!
- And on the count of **1**, open your eyes, yawn if necessary, and say to yourself "I'm awake and feel refreshed, recovered and concentrated"!

Note: If you want to use the this practice to fall asleep, just leave out the instructions to finish the practice!

Fig. 6.8 Worksheet 6.8: Relaxation log

Worksheet 6.8: Relaxation log

Date	Time	Place where practice performed (e.g., sofa, bed, room, standing or lying)	Relaxation thermometer* (0 to 1000) see explanation below	Difficulties or pecularities while practicing

* Relaxation thermometer: After performing the exercise, estimate the degree of relaxation! For this purpose, enter a number between 0 (= maximum tension) and 100 (= maximum relaxation; absolutely calm and relaxed)!

References

Birbaumer, N., & Schmidt, R. F. (2010). *Biologische Psychologie* (7. Aufl.). Springer.Ehlert, U. (2003). *Verhaltensmedizin*. Springer.

Faller, A. (1995). *Der Körper des Menschen: Einführung in Bau und Funktion* (12. Aufl.). Thieme.

Kapit, W., Macey, R. I., & Meisami, E. (1992). *Physiologie-Malatlas*. Arcis.

Kuschinsky, G., Lüllmann, H., & Mohr, K. (1993). *Kurzes Lehrbuch der Pharmakologie und Toxikologie* (13. Aufl.). Thieme.

Mutschler, E., & Schäfer-Korting, M. (1996). *Arzneimittelwirkung: Lehrbuch der Pharmakologie und Toxikologie*. Wissenschaftliche Verlagsgesellschaft.

Module 3: Attention Refocusing

Contents

M. Kleinstäuber et al., *Cognitive Behavior Therapy for Persistent Somatic Symptoms and Somatic Symptom Disorder*, https://doi.org/10.1007/978-3-662-69726-9_7

7

7.1 Session 4

Contents and Materials of the 4th Session

- **Contents**
  - Discussion of the practice of the week
  - Body scan
  - Spotlight metaphor
  - The role of attention in the perception of somatic symptoms
  - What's important to us ...
  - Strategies for attention refocusing: The fakir
  - Practice of the week: Worksheet 7.3 (My strategies for refocusing attention)
- **Materials**
  - Worksheet 7.1: Characteristics of attention
  - Worksheet 7.2: Coping with physical discomfort through distraction
  - Worksheet 7.3: My strategies for refocusing attention

7.1.1 Discussion of the Practice of the Week

Session 4 begins with an evaluation of the progressive muscle relaxation (PMR; Worksheet 6.8) log. The following introductory questions may be helpful:

- What is the patient's experience with PMR?
- Has the patient been practicing regularly?
- Was there any trouble?
- Has there been any progress?

The patient is encouraged to continue practicing PMR on a daily basis. It should be emphasized again that regular training is important in order to learn and successfully apply PMR.

7.1.2 Body Scan

The following exercise, which takes about 20 minutes including debriefing, is based on an exercise by Bleichhardt and Weck (2011). The instruction was slightly modified. The pauses indicated in the text should be about 5 seconds each.

Instruction: Body Scan

I now ask you to sit down as comfortably and relaxed as possible.—Try to come to rest.—Place your hands on the backrest or on your thighs.—Close your eyes if you wish.—If this makes you feel uncomfortable, fixate on a point in the room as far away as possible.

I would now like to take you on a little mental journey through your body.—In the process, you may experience some physical sensations, but they are all harmless.—Some of them may be pleasant to you, some a little unpleasant, and some neither.—When we finish the exercise, the sensations will fade back into the background.—In between, I will ask you a question from time to time.—But you do not need to answer it aloud.—Your inner reaction already represents the answer to the question.—Now concentrate on your breathing.—Try to notice how the air flows in through your nose, enters your lungs and finally flows out again.—PAUSE—Try to pay close attention to your sensations at your nose.—You may notice that when you breathe in, there is a rather cool breeze in your nose.—PAUSE—And you may also notice that as you exhale, warmer air tends to leave your body.—PAUSE—In this accuracy, try to pay attention to all the sensations on and in your nose.—What do you feel on the right nostril, what on the left, and what on the partition between them?

Now continue with your body scan and move your attention to your back.—PAUSE—Pay close attention to where your back makes contact with the back of the chair.—Do you feel the pressure on your back?—Do you perhaps also feel warmth, cold or a slight tingling sensation?—Try to pay close attention to the sensations in your back.

Now move on in your mind to your buttocks and thighs.—PAUSE—Notice how your weight rests on the seat of the chair.—Can you feel the pressure?—PAUSE—You may also notice how your sitting bones are pressing on the chair?—PAUSE—Or perhaps you notice a feeling of cold or warmth?

Now try to shift your attention further down, along your legs, to your feet.—PAUSE—Notice where your feet make contact with the floor.—PAUSE—Do you feel any pressure?—PAUSE—Where on your feet is the feeling of pressure strongest?—PAUSE—What do you feel in your feet when you focus closely on them?—Do your feet feel warm or rather cold?—PAUSE—Are there any places where your feet tingle slightly?—PAUSE—You may also notice that your feet feel moist or dry?—PAUSE—Now pay attention to everything you can perceive in the area of your feet in terms of sensations.

Now take a big leap on the journey through your body from your feet up to your throat, more specifically to your larynx.—PAUSE—Now direct your complete attention to your larynx.—PAUSE—Try to feel the surface, the texture of your larynx.—PAUSE—Does it feel flat or rather a little rough or even scratchy?—PAUSE—If you have to swallow, pay close attention to how your larynx feels when you swallow and immediately after you swallow.—PAUSE—It may feel like it is in the way or even swollen when you swallow.—PAUSE—Pay as close atten-

tion as you can to any sensations you can feel in and around your larynx.

Now leave your larynx in your thoughts and let your attention wander once more to your nose, the starting point of your body scan.—PAUSE—Breathe calmly and evenly.—Notice again how cooler air flows into your nose and warmer air flows out again.—PAUSE—Try to pay attention once again to everything you can perceive about your nose in connection with your breathing.

Now gradually complete your body scan and return with your mind in this room.—PAUSE—Stretch a little and breathe deeply in and out a few times.—PAUSE—Count in your mind from 5 to 1 and open your eyes again at 1!

This is followed by a discussion or evaluation of the exercise. This can be done with the following questions:

- What bodily sensations did you notice?
- Were these sensations there before the exercise?
- How do you explain the appearance of these sensations now, after the exercise?
- How would you have explained the sensations that occurred if they had occurred outside of this exercise?
- Why do you think I did this exercise with you?

Through the exercise, patients should have succeeded in experiencing the importance of attention in the perception of physical (mis)sensations. They should have become aware that what I pay attention to is perceived by me more strongly or more intensely. For example, if I focus my attention on my larynx, sensations in my feet will fade into the background.

7.1.3 Spotlight Metaphor

Attention works like a spotlight. The spotlight can be consciously directed to certain stimuli. Stimuli on which we concentrate and which are in the "light cone of attention" are perceived more strongly and more intensively than stimuli to which we pay no attention and which thus remain shadowy in the background. An example from everyday life (adapted from Pinel, 1997) can illustrate this connection: If you turn your attention to a possibly important announcement in a noisy airport, the probability that you will understand it increases. At the same time, however, you will probably not grasp the content of a remark made by your travel companion.

Now, when we have somatic symptoms and experience them as distressing, we often find it difficult to concentrate on anything other than the symptoms. The whole attention is directed to the symptoms, so that we no longer notice other things in our environment, not even the positive things or small joys of everyday life, because they are out of the spotlight. The aim should therefore be to make the "rusty spotlight of attention", whose light cone is always directed at the somatic symptoms, more flexible, so that pleasant things that give pleasure or enjoyment can also come into the spotlight. It is therefore a matter of finding things or activities that capture the attention in order to let physical complaints fade into the background.

7.1.4 Role of Attention in the Perception of Somatic Symptoms

In the following, the role of attention in the perception of somatic symptoms should be elaborated. The following information should be conveyed:

- Many processes take place in our body **unconsciously**. We are usually not aware of most of the body's processes. We only clearly perceive them when we consciously focus our attention to them, e.g., to our breathing.
- Attention **can be consciously focused**. Most of the time, however, the focus of our attention changes automatically, but not deliberately. This happens, for example, in moments of shock. If we hear a loud bang, we automatically turn our head towards the source of the noise. When we are afraid, our attention is automatically focused on the object we feel threatened by. We do not take our eyes off it. Or we hear our name. Then, too, our attention automatically turns in the direction of the one who has just called us.
- If more and more attention is paid to somatic symptoms, this can lead to them influencing our thoughts and feelings, to us no longer noticing positive things in our environment, to us limiting our leisure activities, to us neglecting social contacts and/or avoiding physical exercise.
- It is therefore important that patients learns to pay less attention to their somatic symptoms. Instead, they should pay more attention to what they enjoy, when they feel good, and what gives him pleasure and enjoyment. In this way they make their attention spotlight more flexible!

The patient is given Worksheet 7.1 (Characteristics of attention).

7.1.5 What Is Important to Us

If something seems important to us, then this is the focus of our attention and is therefore well "illuminated". We perceive what is important to us in a brighter light and thus more intensely than things that we find uninteresting or that "leave us cold". Again with the help of the method of "guided discovery", patients should find out what is important to them personally. The following questions and information can be helpful.

- What things are particularly important to you?
- Do you notice them more often or more intensely than other people around you?

7

Sometimes we overestimate the frequency with which things that seem important to us actually occur. Examples of this are:

- **Patients' car:** If patients own a car, ask them what model it is and what color it is; then ask them whether they can remember when they bought the car and also whether they encountered more or fewer cars of the same model on the roads after buying the car. Most likely, patients will answer that after buying the car they noticed more of the same models than before. How do patients explain this phenomenon? The car is important to them, so they more or less consciously focus their attention to it.
- **Strollers:** Women who want a child or already have children notice strollers more often than women who are not or do not want to become mothers.
- **Couples:** If you are single, feel lonely and would like to have a partner again, you often have the feeling that you are surrounded only by couples.

Perhaps patients have already had the following experience in their everyday life: They are reading an exciting book, are completely absorbed in their reading and are not aware of what is happening around them (e.g., ambient noise such as birdsong or street noise). Suddenly they hear a loud bang. They startle. At that moment, their attention automatically shifts. The book becomes uninteresting from 1 second to the next. They ask themselves, "What caused the bang? Did an accident happen, perhaps?" It is important for them to know what just happened.

We can block out things that are unimportant to us from our consciousness. For example, we hardly notice everyday noises such as the ticking of a clock or the hum of the refrigerator. We also do not usually pay much attention to body functions such as breathing or the heartbeat.

In order to increase the flexibility of the attention spotlight, thoughts are of great importance. With the help of **self-instructions** or "self-talk" patients can direct their attention and thus influence their well-being. Patients should be motivated to say something to themselves that will help them shift their attention away from their somatic symptoms. They should learn to consciously focus their spotlight to other areas of perception and sources of stimulation: "Determine the focus of the spotlight! Give the direction! By doing so, you will experience how you can influence and control your somatic symptoms to some extent."

7.1.6 Attention-Refocusing Strategies: The Fakir

The example of a fakir can be used once again to illustrate the importance of refocusing attention. The following information can be conveyed to the patient on this subject:

The patient may have read, heard or seen something about fakirs before. Fakirs deliberately expose themselves to a strong pain stimulus. They either make themselves "comfortable" on a board of nails, walk over broken glass or red-hot coals, or pierce their skin with nails, skewers, or hooks. In doing so, they apparently feel no pain. Fakirs are considered **masters of attention focusing**. They can control their sensation of pain by concentrating very hard on something other than the pain.

This ability to control and consciously direct one's attention is useful and meaningful in many situations. By directing our attention we manage to concentrate consciously on an activity without being flooded by the manifold sensory impressions that surround us. If physical discomfort can be intensified by concentrating on certain parts of the body, it should also be possible to reduce the previously perceived discomfort by refocusing attention to other things, i.e. to feel relief.

Sometimes the change to an unfamiliar environment leads to the discomfort no longer being perceived. For example, some people who are plagued by toothache report that the pain is suddenly blown away as soon as they are called into the treatment room. Perhaps a little fear in the treatment chair does the rest to "forget" the pain.

Finally, distraction strategies that the patient already uses (more or less consciously) should be collected with the patient. The following questions can be useful:

- Have you ever experienced that due to a change of environment or changes in your immediate surroundings you hardly or not at all noticed your somatic symptoms?
- What strategies do you already use to distract yourself from your physical discomfort? What have you tried so far? What other strategies do you think might be helpful?

The patient is given Worksheet 7.2 (Coping with physical discomfort through distraction).

7.1.7 Practice of the Week

Patients are given Worksheet 7.3 (My strategies for refocusing attention). The task is briefly discussed. Patients are asked to try different strategies in the sense of a behavioral experiment and observe their effects. Accordingly, they are to test and find out which strategies are helpful in coping with somatic symptoms.

7.2 Session 5

Contents and Materials of the 5th Session

- **Contents**
  - Discussion of the practice of the week
  - Behavioral experiment
  - Cold pressor task
  - Building motivation
  - Other strategies to refocus attention
  - Practice of the week: Worksheet 7.5 (Mindful walk)
- **Materials**
  - Worksheet 7.4: Attention spotlight
  - Worksheet 7.5: Mindful walk
  - Stopwatch (necessary for the behavioral experiment)

7.2.1 Discussion of the Practice of the Week

Patients should be encourage to report which strategies to refocus attention (Worksheet 7.3) they have tried in the meantime and what success they have had.

- Were there any difficulties in the implementation?
- What strategies did patients find helpful to shift their attention away from their physical discomfort?

7.2.2 Behavioral Experiment

The following instructional text is proposed for the behavioral experiment which is supposed to demonstrate the relationship between attention refocusing and the perception of bodily processes (adapted from Bleichhardt & Weck, 2011).

- **Instruction: Behavioral Experiment**

Today I would like to do another small practice with you. It is important that you extend your right arm horizontally in front of you as soon as I say NOW! Then please close your eyes. Keep your arm stretched out until I tell you that you can put it down again. As the exercise progresses, I will ask you to focus on specific things.—PAUSE (about 5 seconds)—NOW, please extend your right arm forward and close your eyes (the therapist will watch the stopwatch).—Continue to keep your arm extended.—Be aware of the physical tension required to keep your arm in this position.—Focus fully on the weight of your right arm.—Pay attention to how much strength and effort it may take to keep your arm extended.—Focus on how heavy your right arm feels.—You may also feel your arm being slowly pulled down due to gravity.

(As soon as 50 seconds have elapsed): Now rest your right arm back on the back of the chair or your thigh. Loosen it a little to release the tension. In a short while, we will repeat the exercise in a similar way with the other arm.—PAUSE (approx. 5 seconds)—NOW please stretch your left arm forward and close your eyes (the therapist again watches the stopwatch).—Now shift your attention to a nice memory, e.g., a holiday by the sea.—Try to imagine yourself lying in the soft and warm sand.—The sun is shining on your skin and warming you.—The fine sand shines brightly, and when you look out to sea, you can see glittering plays of light on the calm water.—A light, warm wind gently strokes your skin.—You smell the salty sea air and may even taste it on your tongue—You hear the sound of the waves and the chirping of birds that have made themselves at home in your neighbourhood.—(Once 50 seconds have passed): Now rest your left arm back on the back of your chair or your thigh. Loosen it a little bit to release the tension.—Now please open your eyes again!

The evaluation of the exercise can be done with the following questions:

- What differences did you notice between the two exercises?
- Which of the two exercises was more enjoyable?
- What do you think—how long did each of the two exercises take?

- Which exercise took longer?
- Which exercise *seemed* longer to *you*?

This exercise usually demonstrates that focusing on a sensation in a particular part of the body—in this case, the weight of the outstretched right arm—increases that sensation.

7.2.3 Cold Pressor Task

Following Basler and Kröner-Herwig (1998), the so-called cold pressor task can be discussed with the patient. The effectiveness of distraction techniques has also been studied and proven in scientific experiments. In the cold pressor task, volunteers are asked to immerse their hand in ice-cold water for maximum 3 minutes. It is observed that subjects endure the cold pain the longest when they are distracted. Subjects who are instructed to focus on the pain linger the shortest average time with their hand in the ice water. This experiment demonstrates the effectiveness of distraction. Refocusing attention or distraction increases pain tolerance.

What does this mean for patients practically? If they learn to pay attention not only to their somatic symptoms, but also to when they feel good or are happy about something, or if they learn to occupy themselves with something interesting despite their symptoms, then they can achieve to be less affected by the somatic symptoms. In order to learn this, they should get to know strategies that can help them to distract himself from their symptoms and to perceive and experience pleasant experiences more intensively.

7.2.4 Building Motivation

The aim should be to change the patients' attitude so that they focus their attention more on things other than the somatic symptoms. The "rusty" spotlight of attention should be made more flexible, so that other, pleasant things are also increasingly in the "light of attention". The somatic symptoms should increasingly fade into the background, quasi into the "shadow" of conscious perception. Everyone knows the phenomenon that an interesting conversation, an entertaining film or an exciting book captivates you to such an extent that you forget what is happening around you (including your perception of time).

The patient should be motivated to decide against a constant "control" of the somatic symptoms. With the following questions about the benefit of their previous behavior (focusing more attention on somatic symptoms), a change in the patients' thinking can be triggered.

? What do you gain from focusing attention to your body's discomfort (ask for benefits)?

The patient will probably answer: "I can detect changes early. I notice more quickly whether the complaints increase or decrease or whether they become more intense."

?
- What are the benefits of focusing more attention on your somatic symptoms?
- What are the disadvantages?

Possible answers: "The complaints are perceived more often and more intensely. I can no longer enjoy anything. I withdraw. I lie down in bed. I avoid physical activity. The discomfort dominates my life more and more."

The following instruction can be used to motivate the patient to redirect attention in everyday life:

Instruction: Guidance for Attention Refocusing in Everyday Life

Practice self-observation! If you notice that your attention is focused on your physical discomfort, say "Stop!" inwardly or out loud to yourself. Then say something to yourself that will help you shift your attention to something else. What phrase might be helpful? What could you say to yourself to consciously detach and shift your attention away from your body's discomfort?

At least one helpful sentence should be developed and written down!

7.2.5 Other Strategies to Refocus Attention

In the following, we will look at the strategies that the patient can use to consciously direct the spotlight of attention. One possibility, for example, is to strengthen our sensations (e.g., auditory or visual sense or our sense of touch). The patient is given Worksheet 7.4 (Attention spotlight). Suggestions for exercises can be found on the worksheet. In addition, the patient's own ideas should be asked for.

7.2.6 Practice of the Week

The therapist introduces the practice of the week with the following words:

Instruction: Mindful Walk

When we experience bodily discomfort, we tend to focus entirely on this discomfort. So we turn the spotlight of attention inwards, into our body. As a result, things that are happening around us or outside of us fade into the background. They literally fade away. However, if we learn to focus on our surroundings when physical discomfort is present, we have a strategy at our disposal to better cope with our discomfort. For this reason, your task now until the next session is to practice noticing your surroundings. For this purpose, take a so-called mindful walk!

The patient receives Worksheet 7.5 (Mindful walk). The task is briefly explained.

7.3 Session 6

Contents and Materials of the 6th Session

- **Contents**
  - Discussion of the practice of the week
  - Protective factors: What keeps us healthy?
  - Rules of pleasure and enjoyment
  - Exercise to strengthen our sensations
  - Stress management through more movement in everyday life
  - Practice of the week:
    - Keeping a journal: Worksheet 7.8 (Positive review of the day)
    - Worksheet 7.9 (List of pleasant experiences)
- **Materials**
  - Worksheet 7.6: Rules of pleasure and enjoyment
  - Worksheet 7.7: Bringing more movement into your everyday life
  - Worksheet 7.8: Positive review of the day
  - Worksheet 7.9: List of pleasant experiences
  - Chocolate

7.3.1 Discussion of the Practice of the Week

Session 6 begins with a discussion of Worksheet 7.5 (Mindful walk). The following questions are to be understood as suggestions:

?
- How well did the patient succeed in the "mindful walk"?
- What did the patient notice?
- Were there any difficulties in the implementation? If so, what were they?

7.3.2 Protective Factors: What Keeps Us Healthy?

The therapist explains to the patient that today's session will focus attention on the patient's resources. The therapist briefly explains the term. Resources are strengths, idiosyncrasies, habits, skills, attitudes, and goals brought by the patient that can be used specifically for the change process. Typical examples of resources are: Patient motivation, interpersonal relationships, hobbies, and interests. In the sense of resource activation, already existing abilities and skills that are beneficial to the quality of life and health should be explored and promoted.

Recreation is a balance to the daily stress experienced through work or other demands. Now, recovery means something different for each person (rest and relaxation, but also actively doing something or seeking new challenges). In addition, the patient should be made aware that we do not have to passively wait for recovery alone, but that we can actively shape the recovery process so that the desired recovery effect occurs. In addition, patients should be careful not to expose themselves to so-called leisure stress in his search for balance and recovery. Duties and pleasant leisure activities should be more or less in balance. Even during the week, on weekdays, patients should plan pleasant activities and not postpone everything to the weekend.

Patients should be motivated to discover individual resources. The therapist can support them with the following questions:

?
- What do you like to do in your spare time?
- What's good for you?
- In which activities do you experience fun or relaxation?
- What does recreation mean to you?

7.3.3 Rules of Pleasure and Enjoyment

The rules of pleasure and enjoyment were originally formulated by Lutz and Koppenhöfer (1983) in their publication *Kleine Schule des Genießens. The* basic idea is to promote positive experience and behaviodocr or well-being. The patient receives Worksheet 7.6 (Rules of pleasure and enjoyment). The individual rules are briefly explained. The therapist points out that attention should be directed more towards positive sensory stimuli. The therapist conveys to the patient that pleasurable experiences and actions are promoted by following these rules and ultimately serve to increase mental health.

7.3.4 Exercise to Strengthen Our Sensations

Now mindfulness exercise to strengthen your sensory channels is introduced. The therapist hands patients two pieces of chocolate. The following instruction is intended to guide patients to experience the chocolate with all their senses.

▪ **Instruction: Chocolate Exercise**

Put the first piece of chocolate in front of you and look at it. What's going on inside you? Do you want to put it in your mouth right away? Can you enjoy watching it? Try to silently describe the appearance of the chocolate.

Now place the chocolate on the palm of your hand. How does it feel? Now bring the piece to your nose—how does it smell? When was the last time you really noticed the smell of chocolate?

Now moisten your lips and gently rub the chocolate over them. How does the chocolate affect your lips? Now lick your lips to experience the flavor.

Although such a piece of chocolate is already very small, first only bite off a half of the piece. Do not start chewing, but leave this half in the front of your mouth until it starts to melt by itself. Now push the piece first into the right cheek ... then into the left cheek ... in front of the teeth ... under the tongue ... and find out where in the mouth the flavor or feeling is best. Do not swallow the remaining piece, but let it melt completely ... Now once again trace the path of the chocolate with your tongue back to all the places it came into contact with in your mouth.

Now take the second half of the chocolate piece in your hand and lick around all the corners first. Enjoy the texture of the chocolate. Then put the whole piece in your mouth and let it melt under your tongue. Explore it every now and then with the tip of your tongue. When it is soft enough, press it against your palate until it is all squishy. Spread the rest of the chocolate in the places you liked it best in the first part of the exercise.

The next piece of chocolate is not treated so gently. Pop it in your mouth and eat it as fast as you can while thinking about what else you have planned for tonight.

The following questions are for evaluating the exercise:

- What differences have you noticed between this exercise and your everyday experience with chocolate?
- Was there an experience that was new to you or stood out in particular?
- What did you particularly like about it?
- Do you have a sensory channel that you prefer?
- Which sense do you use the least/most in your daily life?

7

7.3.5 Stress Management Through More Exercise in Everyday Life

This intervention is based on a stress management program developed by Kaluza (2004). Physical activity can protect the organism from the damaging effects of chronic stress. Sports activities, but also more gentle movement in everyday life, improve fitness and are an effective method to counteract or prevent stress. Any regular physical activity that leads to an acceleration of breathing and is performed for at least 10 minutes has a health benefit. To promote compliance, it is very important here to motivate the patient to incorporate more exercise into his or her daily routine by asking specific questions.

- For example, what could you do in your everyday life to move more?
- Are there already activities in your everyday life that you could combine with physical activity in the future?
- What could you do to motivate yourself to exercise more in your daily life?
- Are there times when you could firmly schedule exercise into your daily routine?

The patient receives Worksheet 7.7 (Bringing more movement into your everyday life). The individual points are briefly discussed.

7.3.6 Practice of the Week

The patient receives Worksheet 7.8 (Positive review of the day) and Worksheet 7.9 (List of pleasant experiences). The tasks are briefly discussed.

7.4 Worksheets

These worksheets are also available for download online at Springer Extras (▶ extras.springer.com).

Worksheet 7.1	Characteristics of attention	◘ Figure 7.1
Worksheet 7.2	Coping with physical discomfort through distraction	◘ Figure 7.2

Worksheet 7.3	My strategies for refocusing attention	◘ Figure 7.3
Worksheet 7.4	Attention spotlight	◘ Figure 7.4
Worksheet 7.5	Mindful walk	◘ Figure 7.5
Worksheet 7.6	Rules of pleasure and enjoyment	◘ Figure 7.6
Worksheet 7.7	Bringing more movement into your everyday life	◘ Figure 7.7
Worksheet 7.8	Positive review of the day	◘ Figure 7.8
Worksheet 7.9	List of pleasant experi-ences	◘ Figure 7.9

◘ **Fig. 7.1** Worksheet 7.1: Characteristics of attention

Worksheet 7.1: Characteristics of attention

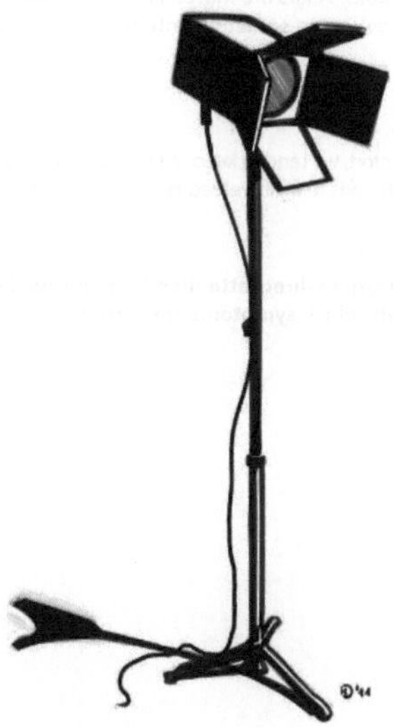

- Attention works like a spotlight. Things that are focused by the spotlight are perceived more intensively than the things that are outside the cone of light. If you focus your attention to your larynx, you will hardly perceive any sensations on your feet.
- In the focus of attention or spotlight, even the smallest changes in your body are perceived, which would otherwise may not stand out. If you pay attention to your feet then it will be much more likely that you will notice sensations in them than if you do not pay much attention to them.
- Many processes in our body happen without us being aware of them, i.e. we do not pay attention to them. However, we can focus our attention on certain areas of the body or on certain sensations. This has the consequence that we perceive them more intensely and clearly.
- Attention can be deliberately refocused. Often our attention shifts automatically (i.e., without us being aware of) to things that are important for us. Nevertheless, we can deliberately focus our attention on something.

7

Fig. 7.2 Worksheet 7.2: Coping with physical discomfort through distraction

Worksheet 7.2: Coping with physical discomfort through distraction

We experience our environment and our body with all our senses. However, it is impossible to experience our entire environment or our entire body at the same time, because our attention span is limited. We will hardly succeed in reading a book and driving a car or in looking after our feet and paying attention to our breathing at the same time. However, we can consciously shift our attention to things that are meaningful to us. What is in the focus of our attention will be perceived more intensely! What we do not pay attention to, becomes hardly perceived or not perceived at all. If we deliberately concentrate on our larynx, then this can lead to sensations in this part of the body. If we focus our attention on physical discomfort in our body, consequently this discomfort is perceived more intensely.

Conversely, by concentrating on other events or things, it is also possible to distract oneself from physical discomfort. By diverting attention to other things, relief from somatic symptoms can be experienced. Think of fakirs who seem to "get comfortable" on a bed of nails without feeling pain, walk over broken glass or burning coals or pierce their skin with nails, skewers or hooks. Fakirs are masters of controlling their attention. They can control their perception of pain by focusing their attention on something other than the pain.

When we have physical discomfort, we tend to keep our eyes on them. We direct the spotlight of attention to our body, which leads to an increased awareness of the discomfort.

Through practice, one can learn to direct attention from the inside to the outside or the environment. This can change the intensity with which symptoms are perceived.

■ **Fig. 7.3** Worksheet 7.3: My strategies for refocusing attention

Worksheet 7.3: My strategies for refocusing attention

For each day of the coming week, please make a resolution to use one or more strategies to direct your attention. Carry out activities that you think will distract you from your physical discomfort. Try to enjoy these activities deliberately with all your senses! Afterwards, make notes in your log about how successfully you have been able to distract yourself from your somatic symptoms.

Date	Which **strategy** do I try?	Which senses do I have focused on deliberately?	Evaluation 0 = no effect + = enjoyed strategy a little bit ++ = have enjoyed it very much and at the same time got distracted from my symptoms

Fig. 7.4 Worksheet 7.4: Attention spotlight

Worksheet 7.4: Attention spotlight

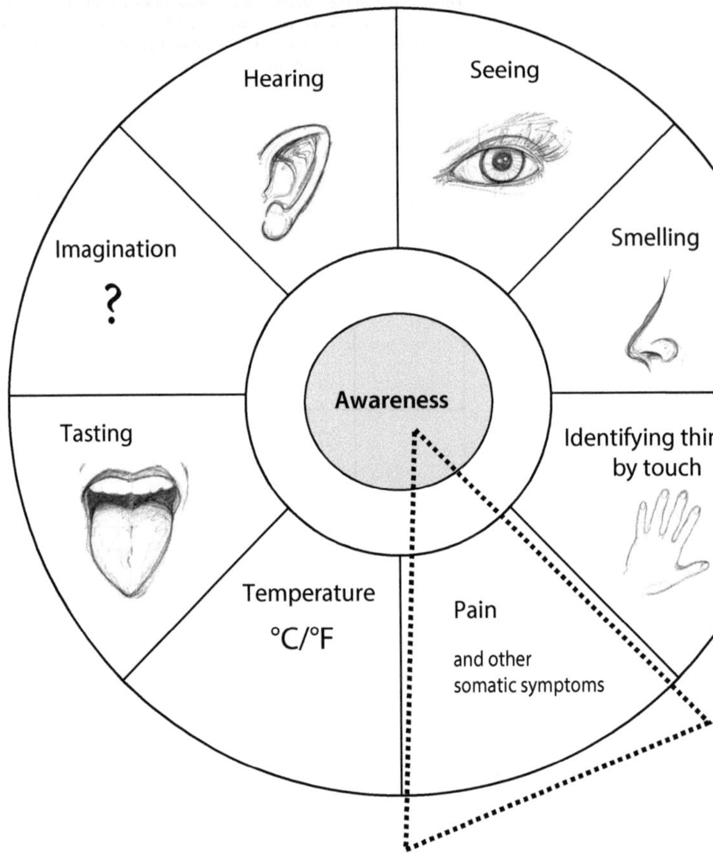

Try to exercise your senses, to make the spotlight of your attention more flexible!

- **Taste:** Try to deliberately enjoy your food and its flavor!
- **Smell:** Try to deliberately notice the smells in your environment!
- **Seeing:** Try to describe exactly what you see at the moment!
- **Touch, Feel:** Try to focus on the sensations of your skin while showering or bathing, or how it feels when you walk barefoot!
- **Listening:** Try to deliberately listen for common sounds, such as the noise of the refrigerator or birds chirping.

■ **Fig. 7.5** Worksheet 7.5: Mindful walk

Worksheet 7.5: Mindful walk

Take a walk in the upcoming days and write down your impressions and experiences!
Pay particular attention to the following points

- What do you see? What colors do you perceive? How do objects in the light differ from those in the shadows?

  ....

  ....

- What do you hear? Pay conscious attention for a while to all the sounds you encounter! What do you hear right around you? What sounds do you perceive in the distance?

  ....

  ....

- What do you feel on your skin? Focus on the wind, the air temperature and the temperature difference between areas in the sun and shady areas!

  ....

  ....

- What do you smell? What smells can you perceive?

  ....

  ....

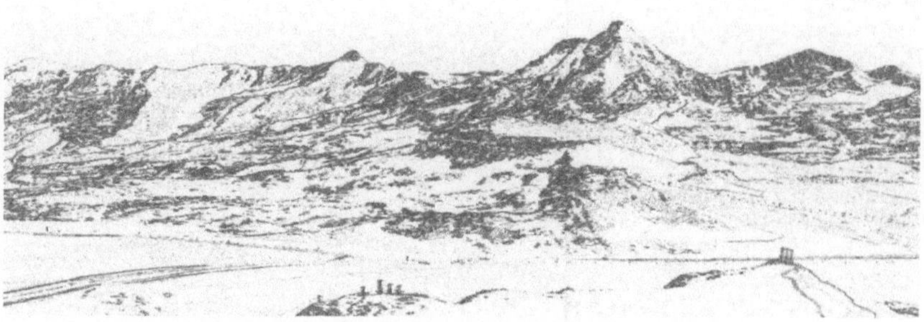

Fig. 7.6 Worksheet 7.6: Rules of pleasure and enjoyment

Worksheet 7.6: Rules of pleasure and enjoyment

1. **Enjoyment needs time!** Take time to enjoy. Enjoyment is not possible under time pressure.
2. **Enjoyment must be allowed!** Treat yourself with something. Do something good for yourself, without feeling shame or regret.
3. **Enjoyment is not something you can do on the side!** Enjoy deliberately. Be mindful. Focus your attention on enjoying. Try to avoid thinking about other activities, things of past or upcoming tasks, i.e., do nothing on the side.
4. **Be aware of what is good for you!** Find out what is good for you and what is not. Know your own preferences and interests and discover new ones.
5. **Less is more!** Enjoy rather little, but enjoy thoroughly. To experience pleasure it is not important to do much but to do things of high quality. Too much (of the good) has a saturating effect in the long run and causes boredom.
6. **Without experience there is no enjoyment!** Enjoyment needs a sensory perception. It comes down to the perception of nuances, i.e. small differences.
7. **Enjoyment can be part of your everyday life!** Learn to enjoy even the small things of your everyday life. Do not miss the small happiness while waiting for good fortune. It does not require extraordinary events or adventures to experience pleasure.
8. **Planning creates anticipation!** Don't leave pleasure to chance alone. Plan and prepare pleasant experiences into your everyday life.

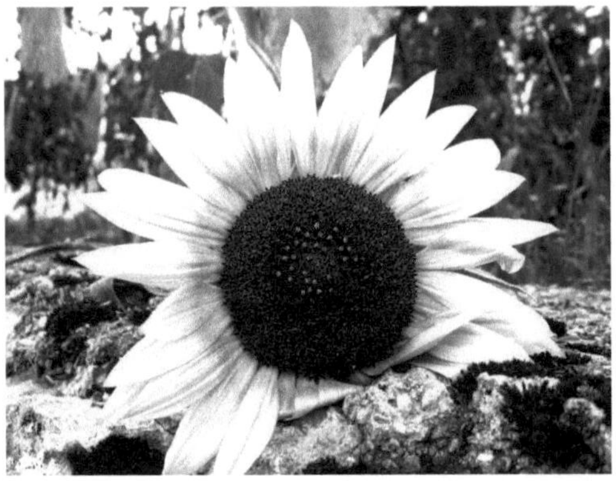

7

■ **Fig. 7.7** Worksheet 7.7: Bringing more movement into your everyday life

Worksheet 7.7: Bringing more movement into your everyday life

- **Combine necessary activities with movement!**
  - Do not take the bus or car to work, but walk or use the bicycle
  - Do not use the elevator, but climb stairs
  - Doing minor shopping or errands by bike or foot
  - When going on trips with the family, drive less and take shorter hikes instead, or go for a swim
  - Do not use machines (e.g., lawn mowers, leaf vacuums) when gardening and use your own muscle power more.

- **Increase the duration and intensity of physical activities!**
  - Walk more quickly, i.e. deliberately one step faster than usual.
  - Taking two steps at a time when climbing stairs
  - Take fewer breaks when gardening or doing housework
  - Walking the dog for longer
  - When using the bus or tram, get off one or two stops early and walk the rest of the way

- **Schedule regular exercise time (at least 10 min daily)!**
  - In the morning before breakfast 10 min of gymnastics
  - Take a little walk during lunch break
  - In the evening, before going to bed, take a walk to get some fresh air

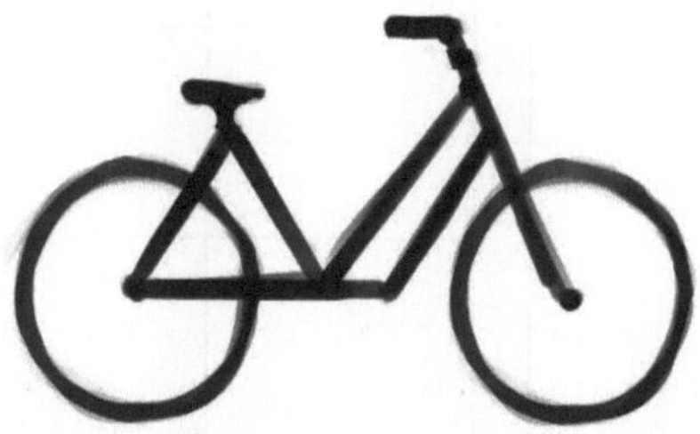

Fig. 7.8 Worksheet 7.8: Positive review of the day

Worksheet 7.8: Positive review of the day

Pleasure in your everyday life

In the coming days, please deliberately pay attention to beautiful things in your everyday life! What gives you joy? What do you find pleasant? What can you enjoy? These can be special events (e.g., celebration, winning the lottery, rare visit from a good friend), but also pleasant things and small pleasures in your everyday life (e.g., a relaxing Full bath, a beautiful sunset, the aromatic smell of freshly ground coffee). Pay attention to pleasant sensations coming from all your sensory channels (sense of vision, hearing, smell, touch and taste). Take a few minutes each day to reflect on your day and write down aspects of your day that you enjoyed most.

Date	Pleasant experiences or sensations of the day

Fig. 7.9 Worksheet 7.9: List of pleasant experiences

Worksheet 7.9: List of pleasant experiences

The following list includes a number of activities that many people find enjoyable and relaxing.
For each activity, please indicate how much you enjoy doing it and how often you do it! This is not a comprehensive list.
You also have the possibility to add your own ideas!

Activity	How much do you enjoy doing it?			How often?		
	not at all	somewhat	very much	never	rarely	often
SOCIAL ACTIVITIES						
Visiting friends, acquaintances, relatives	☹	😐	☺	☹	😐	☺
Inviteing friends, acquaintances, relatives	☹	😐	☺	☹	😐	☺
Playing with the children	☹	😐	☺	☹	😐	☺
Visiting a pub, restaurant	☹	😐	☺	☹	😐	☺
Going dancing	☹	😐	☺	☹	😐	☺
Activities, trips with the family	☹	😐	☺	☹	😐	☺
Parlor games	☹	😐	☺	☹	😐	☺
Charity work	☹	😐	☺	☹	😐	☺
What else?	☹	😐	☺	☹	😐	☺
What else?	☹	😐	☺	☹	😐	☺
HOBBYS						
Photography, filming	☹	😐	☺	☹	😐	☺
Collecting stamps or coins	☹	😐	☺	☹	😐	☺
Growing plants	☹	😐	☺	☹	😐	☺
Painting or drawing	☹	😐	☺	☹	😐	☺
Pottery	☹	😐	☺	☹	😐	☺
Handicrafts	☹	😐	☺	☹	😐	☺
Playing a musical instrument	☹	😐	☺	☹	😐	☺
Listening to music	☹	😐	☺	☹	😐	☺

From Kleinstäuber, M. et al: Cognitive behavior therapy for persistent somatic symptoms and somatic symptom disorders.

Fig. 7.9 (continued)

Activity	How much do you enjoy doing it?			How often?		
	not at all	somewhat	very much	never	rarely	often
Sing	☹	😐	☺	☹	😐	☺
Cooking something special	☹	😐	☺	☹	😐	☺
Puzzles, crosswords	☹	😐	☺	☹	😐	☺
Technical games (railway, computer)	☹	😐	☺	☹	😐	☺
Home improvement	☹	😐	☺	☹	😐	☺
What else?	☹	😐	☺	☹	😐	☺
What else?	☹	😐	☺	☹	😐	☺

Activity	How much do you enjoy doing it?			How often?		
	not at all	something	very much	never	rarely	often
CULTURE & EDUCATION						
Going to a concert	☹	😐	☺	☹	😐	☺
Visiting the theatre	☹	😐	☺	☹	😐	☺
Going to the movies	☹	😐	☺	☹	😐	☺
Listening to a lecture	☹	😐	☺	☹	😐	☺
Visiting a museum or exhibition	☹	😐	☺	☹	😐	☺
Reading a good book	☹	😐	☺	☹	😐	☺
Taking a continuing education class	☹	😐	☺	☹	😐	☺
Attending a reading	☹	😐	☺	☹	😐	☺
What else?	☹	😐	☺	☹	😐	☺
PHSYICAL ACTIVITY & MOVEMENT						
Walking, hiking	☹	😐	☺	☹	😐	☺
Trail running, jogging	☹	😐	☺	☹	😐	☺
Tennis, table tennis	☹	😐	☺	☹	😐	☺

Fig. 7.9 (continued)

Activity	How much do you enjoy doing it?			How often?		
	not at all	somewhat	very much	never	rarely	often
Swimming	☹	😐	☺	☹	😐	☺
Cycling	☹	😐	☺	☹	😐	☺
Skiing	☹	😐	☺	☹	😐	☺
Ball games	☹	😐	☺	☹	😐	☺
Gymnastics, aerobics	☹	😐	☺	☹	😐	☺
Attending games or tournaments	☹	😐	☺	☹	😐	☺
Gardening	☹	😐	☺	☹	😐	☺
What else?	☹	😐	☺	☹	😐	☺
NATURE EXPERIENCES						
Lying in the grass	☹	😐	☺	☹	😐	☺
Watching animals	☹	😐	☺	☹	😐	☺
Running barefoot	☹	😐	☺	☹	😐	☺
Gathering flowers	☹	😐	☺	☹	😐	☺
Sitting in the sun	☹	😐	☺	☹	😐	☺
Collecting mushrooms, herbs, berries	☹	😐	☺	☹	😐	☺
Enjoying a beautiful view	☹	😐	☺	☹	😐	☺
Sitting by the stove, looking into the fire	☹	😐	☺	☹	😐	☺
Sauna	☹	😐	☺	☹	😐	☺
Watching clouds, sunrise/sunset, stars	☹	😐	☺	☹	😐	☺
Fishing	☹	😐	☺	☹	😐	☺
Walking in water	☹	😐	☺	☹	😐	☺
Having a massage	☹	😐	☺	☹	😐	☺
What else?	☹	😐	☺	☹	😐	☺
What else?	☹	😐	☺	☹	😐	☺

Fig. 7.9 (continued)

Evaluation

Now please look at the completed list again! Are there any activities that you like to do, but that you only rarely or never do? Have you perhaps come across things you always wanted to do?
but have always put off until now? Are there any activities that you used to enjoy and that you would like to do again? Afterwards, please write down the pleasant things that you would like to do in the coming weeks as a balance to your everyday life duties and obligations!

- ....
- ....
- ....
- ....
- ....

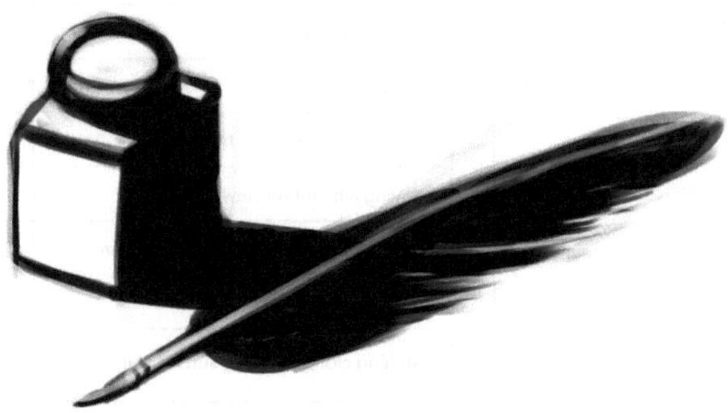

References

Basler, H.-D., & Kröner-Herwig, B. (1998). *Psychologische Therapie bei Kopf- und Rückenschmerzen* (2. Aufl.). Quintessenz.

Bleichhardt, G., & Weck, F. (2011). *Kognitive Verhaltenstherapie bei Hypochondrie und Krankheitsangst* (2. akt. Aufl.). Springer.

Kaluza, S. (2004). *Stressbewältigung: Trainingsmanual zur psychologischen Gesundheitsförderung*. Springer.

Lutz, R., & Koppenhöfer, E. (1983). Kleine Schule des Genießens. In R. Lutz (Ed.), *Genuss und Genießen. Zur Psychologie genußvollen Erlebens und Handelns* (pp. 112–125). Beltz.

Pinel, J. P. J. (1997). *Biopsychologie: Eine Einführung* (4. Aufl.). Springer.

Module 4: Cognitive Reappraisal

Contents

M. Kleinstäuber et al., *Cognitive Behavior Therapy for Persistent Somatic Symptoms and Somatic Symptom Disorder*, https://doi.org/10.1007/978-3-662-69726-9_8

8.1 Session 7

Contents and Materials of the 7th Session

- **Contents**
  - Discussion of the practice of the week
  - Lemon exercise
  - Teaching the "cognitive model": The ABC model of emotions
  - Illustration with an example: The spider in the bed
  - Practice of the week: My own ABC scheme (Worksheet 8.4)
- **Materials**
  - Worksheet 8.1: The four levels of behavior
  - Worksheet 8.2: ABC model of emotions
  - Worksheet 8.3: ABC example
  - Worksheet 8.4: My own ABC scheme

8.1.1 Discussion of the Practice of the Week

First, the "Positive review of the day" is evaluated (Worksheet 7.8), followed by the "List of pleasant experiences" (Worksheet 7.9).

- What did you experience positively?
- What little everyday things have you been able to enjoy?
- What activities do you enjoy and would like to do more often in the near future?

8.1.2 Lemon Exercise

The importance of evaluation processes is demonstrated with the help of a small guided imagery practice, the so-called lemon exercise.

Instruction: Lemon Exercise

In today's session and in the next sessions, we want to look at the influence of our thoughts on physical processes. To do this, I would like to start with a little guided imagery practice with you.

Now please sit down comfortably and relaxed.—If you wish, close your eyes, because most people find this exercise easier with their eyes closed.—Now imagine that there is an ordinary table in front of you.—On the table there is a lemon lying on a small board.—Next to the board is a knife.—Now take the lemon in your left hand.—Try to feel the surface of the lemon with both hands!—Do you feel any bumps?—Is the peel of your lemon rather soft or firm?—Now try to imagine the color of your lemon!—You perceive a bright and rich yellow of a ripe lemon.—Do you notice any spots or other blemishes on the peel of your lemon? Now imagine slowly bringing the lemon to your nose and smelling it.—You notice that it smells very lightly and discreetly of lemon.—Now imagine putting the lemon back on the board, taking the knife in your right hand and cutting the lemon in half.—As you cut it smoothly, some juice squirts out and runs over your fingers!—You will now clearly notice the sour smell of lemon.—Look at the juicy inside of your lemon halves, the chamber-like structure that is wet and shiny.—You notice that it now smells very strongly of lemon.—Now imagine cutting a slice from one lemon half.—You fold the slice and bring it to your mouth.—Meanwhile, lemon juice drips onto your clothes and runs down your hands.—Slowly bring the lemon slice to your mouth and bite into it without hesitation—after your teeth have penetrated the flesh, lemon juice spreads in your mouth.—You will now notice a very sour taste on your tongue and the roof of your mouth!—Imagine chewing the pulp slowly!—Even more lemon juice is released and slowly runs down your tongue, down your throat.

When you have tasted enough of your lemon, then finish our little guided imagery practice!—Put your lemon aside in your mind and open your eyes again!

To help patients reflect on their experience during the exercise, the following questions may be helpful:

- What changes did you notice in yourself during the exercise? ("Ideal" answer: increased salivation, contraction of facial features, lemon taste in the mouth—biting heartily into an imaginary lemon truly makes your mouth water).
- What do you learn from this?

This exercise shows that the imagination alone, i.e., a figurative thought, is sufficient to cause a physical reaction. We can influence physical processes with our thoughts alone!

8.1.3 Teaching the "Cognitive Model": The ABC Model of Emotions

There are situations in which most people react in the same way, such as braking at a red light in city traffic, rejoicing at winning the lottery, or grieving the loss of a loved one. However, there are also many events or situations in which people react very differently. A person can also behave differently in one and the same situation at different times.

With the help of the following questions, patients should be supported in explaining to themselves what can cause these different behavioral reactions in one and the same situation.

- How is that possible?
- Do you have an explanation for this?

If patients do not come up with the answer on their own, then the therapist's answer could be as follows: Depending on how one evaluates a certain situation or how one thinks about a certain event, this leads to different feelings and behaviors.

Before therapist and patient take a closer look at the connection between situation, thoughts and feelings, it should first be explained what exactly is meant by the term "behavior". The following instructional example can be used as an aid here.

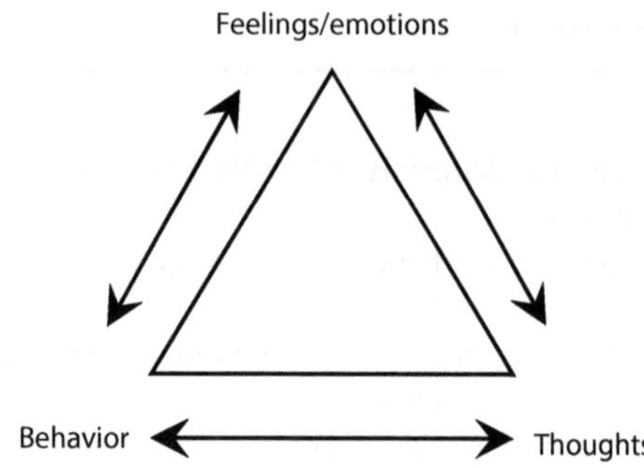

Fig. 8.1 Cognitive behavioral model of the relationships between feelings, behavior and thoughts

Instruction: Introduction to the Four Levels of Behavior

Behavior can be described on four levels.

1. *The cognitive level: This is where you find everything that goes on in your head—this includes thoughts or inner monologues or self-talk, perceptions, evaluations and interpretations, certain attitudes, convictions, norms and values that you hold; in addition, memories or pictorial ideas can also be found here.*
2. *The emotional level (based on Stavemann, 2001): By this we mean feelings and emotions: joy and affection (pleasant emtional states), indifference/calmness (neutral emotional states), fear, anger, shame, disgust and sadness (unpleasant emotional states). There are a variety of other terms used to describe emotional states, but ultimately they either represent hybrids of the emotional states mentioned or are used to describe the strength or intensity of the emotion. Emotions are accompanied by a greater or lesser degree of excitement, the so-called arousal level. The higher the accompanying excitement, the stronger the perceived intensity of the emotion.*
3. *The physiological level: Here you will find all physical reactions or accompanying symptoms, e.g., palpitations, sweating, change in respiratory rate, muscle tension, dry mouth, pain, dizziness, itching.*
4. *The behavioral and motor level: This includes everything that another person can observe about you in a certain situation. It is about overtly observable behaviors. For example, another person might notice that you cry, laugh, run away, avoid eye contact, shout, have a drink, ask questions or simply remain silent. It is true in this sense according to Watzlawick et al. (2000), "A person cannot not behave!" (respectively: "You cannot not communicate.")*

The distinction between these four levels should help you to observe and describe your own behavior in a differentiated way. In fact, the four levels are closely related to each other. They influence each other.

The patient is given Worksheet 8.1 (The four levels of behavior) as a summary.

In order to illustrate the connection between thoughts, feelings, physical reactions and observable behaviors in accordance with one of the basic models in cognitive behavior therapy (Fig. 8.1), the so-called ABC model has proven and established itself. It was developed in the 1950s by the American psychologist Albert Ellis. The following instruction can be used to explain the ABC model to the patient.

Instruction: ABC Model

I will first explain the individual components of the model. A means "activating event": This can be an event that is recognizable to everyone (e.g., the traffic light turns red or the phone rings) or can take place within the person (e.g., the heart beats faster or the thought that there is an exam tomorrow). You already know B. It stands for "belief": These are evaluations of situation A, i.e. thoughts in relation to A. They are the personal viewpoint of the person. It is the personal view of A. What conclusions do I draw? What consequences do I assume? What do I think? In principle, three assessments are possible here:

- *A is good for me (I see A as positive or challenging),*
- *A does not matter (I consider A to be neutral or harmless) or*
- *A is bad for me (I consider A to be harmful/dangerous/threatening).In order to arrive at an assessment, we more or less consciously draw on our prior knowledge and experience and evaluate our coping skills and options. Prejudices, values, and norms also influence our assessment of situation A. Important: thought processes can take place consciously and unconsciously! C should also sound familiar to you. C stands for "consequences." It is about the consequences that follow from our assessment of situation A. Our thoughts concerning A influence on the one hand our emotional life and on the other hand our physical processes as well as our behavior. The evaluation determines unambiguously and definitively with which*

feeling we react. One speaks of the so-called evaluation-feeling-logic. The behavioral consequences are different: You surely know from your own experience that you can "put a good face on it", that you can very well put on a smile and be friendly even though you don't feel like it. Even if we can hardly stand fear or are seething with anger inside, we can still behave in such a way that no one looks at our emotional turmoil. Feelings can be hidden. If the emotional pressure is too strong, it is better to change your B than to "let off steam" or behave according to your current feelings, because of the possible negative social consequences in your private and professional life!

The patienst receives Worksheet 8.2 (ABC model of emotions).

8.1.4 Illustration with an Example: The Spider in the Bed

After the theoretical explanation of the ABC model, the therapist should look with their patients for a specific everyday situations to which the model can be applied. We suggest the following example situation: Patients should imagine that when going to bed or throwing back the covers, they discover a palm-sized spider that has made itself comfortable on the bed sheet. Patients are given Worksheet 8.3 (ABC example). Using this example situation, patients should be familiarized with the various components of the ABC model by means of targeted questions.

❓
- What goes through your mind when you see the spider?
- What do you think of yourself?
- How do you feel?
- What are you going to do?

Patients enter their answers into the ABC model. The therapist helps by taking particular care not to confuse thoughts and feelings.

- **Possible Thoughts**

Ugh, spider! How disgusting! How interesting! But it has beautiful markings! What kind of spider is it? It must be dangerous! I can't let it out of my sight! It'll jump on me and bite me. It won't hurt me, it's probably more scared than I am! Oops, what an uninvited guest! She belongs back in nature! I can't sleep in a room with a spider like that. There are no poisonous spiders in our latitudes—this one is harmless! What am I supposed to do, I'm paralyzed!?

- **Possible Emotional Consequences**

Surprise, fear, disgust, curiosity, helplessness, etc.

- **Possible Physical Reactions**

Palpitations, sweating, restlessness, faster breathing, tremors, etc.

- **Possible Behaviors**

Scream for help, leave the room in a hurry, fix the spider with your eyes, get the vacuum cleaner, "rescue" the spider, step closer and take a closer look, turn into a pillar of salt, get an animal encyclopedia, beat it to death, etc.

❓
- What would another person think (spider lover, spider hater, arachnophobe)?
- How would this other person react in this situation?
- What would she feel and do?
- What would you have to think to face the spider calmly?

In conclusion: A certain event can lead to different feelings and behaviors depending on how the event is evaluated!

8.1.5 Practice of the Week

Until the next session, patients are given the task of creating their own ABC model. They should pick two situations which they have experienced themselves and in which they felt strong emotional reactions. It does not matter whether positive or negative feelings were experienced. Patients receive Worksheet 8.4 (My own ABC scheme).

8.2 Session 8

Contents and Materials of the 8th Session

- **Contents**
  - Discussion of the Practice of the Week
  - Illustration of the ABC model using the "story with the hammer".
  - ABC model applied to somatic symptoms: Back pain
  - Collecting thoughts about somatic symptoms
  - Reading out less helpful thoughts
  - Gathering helpful thoughts
  - Practice of the week: Find possible causes of headaches (Worksheet 8.7)
  - Relaxation practice according to Weitzmann

- **Materials**
  - Worksheet 8.5: The story of the hammer
  - Worksheet 8.6: ABC model: back pain
  - Worksheet 8.7: Causes of headaches

8.2.1 Discussion of the Practice of the Week

When discussing Worksheet 8.4 (My own ABC scheme), the therapist should pay particular attention to whether the patient has succeeded in keeping feelings and thoughts apart and not confusing them with each other. Once again, the basic assumption of the cognitive model is pointed out, namely that—depending on how a situation is evaluated—different feelings and behaviors occur!

8.2.2 Illustration of the ABC Model Using the "Story of the Hammer"

The therapist reads the following story (Watzlawick, 2007):

▪ **Instruction: "The Story with the Hammer"**

A man wants to hang a painting. He has the nail, but not the hammer. Therefore it occurs to him to go over to the neighbor and ask him to lend him his hammer. But at this point, doubt sets in. What if he doesn't want to lend me the hammer? Yesterday he barely spoke to me. Maybe he was in a hurry. Or, perhaps, he holds something against me. But why? I didn't do anything to him. If he would ask me to lend him something, I would, at once. How can he refuse to lend me his hammer? People like him make other people's life miserable. Worst, he thinks that I need him because he has a hammer. This has got to stop! And suddenly the guy runs to the neighbor's door, rings, and before letting him say anything, he screams: "you can keep your hammer, you bastard!"

This story illustrates how our thoughts and ideas influence our feelings. It also shows that sometimes we get in our own way by our thinking. That we talk ourselves into things, take our thoughts as facts and behave accordingly. It shows us that we sometimes use **less helpful thinking patterns**, for example by trying to look into other people's heads and read their thoughts, or by trying to predict the future, often in a negative way, so that we paint the devil on the wall or prophesy a catastrophe. In this sense, we often drive ourselves crazy by dabbling in superhuman abilities such as mind reading or clairvoyance.

Basically, one distinguishes appropriate from inappropriate thoughts or evaluations. With **cognitive reappraisal** my thinking is based on facts instead of opinions and speculations. It is focused on achieving my personal goals and causes only the emotional distress or upset necessary to do so. Appropriate thinking prevents unnecessary conflict with myself (e.g., in the form of intense emotional distress) or my environment. **Less helpful thinking** is based on speculation, misconceptions, prejudice, or unrealistic expectations or goals (e.g., "Everyone should like me! I can't make a mistake! I need 100% certainty!") and leads to severe emotional distress or other problems. Thinking patterns that are considered problematic include:

- Exaggerate or catastrophize,
- Generalizing or black and white thinking,
- Excessive demands or absolute demands on oneself, on others and on the world (some key words: should, must, absolutely, demand, must not),
- Low frustration tolerance (the belief that one cannot withstand pain, discomfort, disadvantage, deprivation, loss, inconvenience, or other adversity).

Our man from the "story with the hammer" believes he knows that his neighbour will refuse him the hammer (he therefore regards his thoughts as reality and says to himself: "That's the way it is and no other way!"), evaluates the neighbour's assumed refusal as impertinence, becomes correspondingly angry and snaps at his perplexed neighbour, who of course does not know what is happening to him. The patient receives Worksheet 8.5 (The story of the hammer).

8.2.3 ABC Model Applied to Somatic Symptoms: Back Pain

The ABC model is now explained to the patient with an example from the field of somatic symptoms, which can be done as follows:

? Now imagine the following situation, which may sound familiar to you. You wake up in the morning with back pain. What thoughts are going through your mind? What do you feel? What are you going to do?

The patient then receives Worksheet 8.6 (ABC model: back pain). Typical thoughts, feelings and behaviors are recorded on it.

8.2.4 Collecting Thoughts on Somatic Symptoms

Now typical thoughts of the patient are to be collected, which arise when somatic symptoms occur: "I would now like to collect together with you, which thoughts go through your mind when you have somatic symptoms (list symptoms of the patient!). Please try to remember exactly what typically goes through your mind when physical discomfort occurs!" The patient's answers are noted on the flipchart.

8.2.5 Reading Out Less Helpful Thoughts

Following the collection of thoughts on the flipchart, the therapist once again reads all the thoughts noted repeatedly and asks the patient to do the following: "I will now read these thoughts to you a few times. Please pay attention to how you feel as I repeatedly confront you with your thoughts!"

Patients are asked to report how they have been feeling. Usually, patients describe that thoughts (less helpful evaluations of physical discomfort) have a negative effect on their well-being. Here patients should again be pointed out to the connection between thoughts and feelings (following Basler & Kröner-Herwig, 1998): "As you may have just felt on your own body, such thoughts depress the mood, they lead to worry and fear, cause tension and even intensify the symptoms, e.g., pain. The aim of our work is not to prevent you from mentally dealing with your somatic symptoms. It is rather a matter of controlling broodings, which increase the feeling of helplessness, hopelessness and thus despair, better, i.e. of getting a grip on them better than before. It is therefore important for you to find realistic ways of replacing the less helpful thoughts that tend to intensify the symptoms with helpful thoughts that tend to alleviate the symptoms. An important prerequisite for this is that you are able to distinguish well between helpful and less helpful thoughts for coping with your somatic symptoms."

8.2.6 Collecting Helpful Thoughts

The next step is to collect helpful thoughts. For this it is necessary to question the less helpful thoughts. The following instruction can help here:

- **Instruction: Collecting Helpful Thoughts**

The thoughts we have just collected together can be true, but they do not have to be, because thoughts are not facts! Sometimes we have—without being aware of it—less helpful thought patterns. Then we assume, for example, that our thoughts reflect reality. Other less helpful thinking patterns that we often encounter will be discussed in more detail in a future session. If we regard our thoughts as facts, i.e. if we are very certain and strongly convinced that this must be the case, this has the disadvantage that we are more or less blind to other possibilities of evaluation and explanation and tend to neglect alternative ways of looking at things. Having just collected some of your thoughts, the next step is now for you to examine your thoughts for realism and practicality. Ask yourself if your way of thinking is appropriate, reasonable and realistic! Ask yourself if there is perhaps a less helpful thought pattern! Ask yourself if there are other ways of evaluating or explaining your symptoms! In order to practice this kind of examination or questioning of thoughts, your task now is to find alternative, helpful thoughts for your somatic symptoms!

In a next step, the patients should independently derive new helpful thoughts through "guided discovery" and targeted questions.

?
- What might you think of when somatic symptoms (name the patient's symptoms!) arise?
- What thoughts would be more appropriate or helpful to manage or alleviate your discomfort?
- What advice would you give to a good friend who suffers from similar ailments?

8.2.7 Practice of the Week

To practice collecting different possible explanations for a somatic symptom and disputing less helpful thoughts, the patient is given Worksheet 8.7 (Causes of headaches) as practice of the week.

8.2.8 Relaxation Practice According to Weitzman

Session 8 is rounded off with a relaxation practice according to Weitzmann (Goldfried & Davison, 1979).

- **Instruction: Weitzmann Relaxation Practice (Based on Goldfried & Davison, 1979)**

Note: The therapist should pause for about 5 seconds between each question!

Sit down comfortably and listen to me carefully. I would like to ask you a series of questions. Although each question could be answered either yes or no, it is not necessary for you to say "yes" or "no" or even to affirm or deny in your mind. Your own particular response to the question already constitutes the answer to the question. This will become quite clear in the course of our exercise. Just remember to listen to my questions. Don't be surprised if some of them seem a little unusual. Just allow the appropriate response to each question. It does not matter how you respond—it is always right. Because there is no wrong or right here.

- *Are you able to close your eyes?*
- *If they are not closed now, please close them now!*
- *Can you imagine the space between your eyes?*
- *Can you imagine the space between your ears?*
- *Can you imagine the space between your nostrils?*
- *Can you feel where your hair ends?*
- *Can you be aware of how close your breath comes to the back of your eyes when you take a breath?*
- *Can you imagine looking at something that is very far away?*
- *Can you consciously feel where your arms touch your body?*
- *Can you feel the ground under your feet?*
- *Can you picture in your mind's eye a beautiful flower floating in front of you?*
- *Can you be aware of the inside of your mouth?*
- *And is it possible for you to clearly visualize the position of your tongue in your mouth?*
- *Can you feel even the slightest breeze against your cheek?*
- *Are you able to perceive that one arm is more relaxed than the other?*
- *Can you detect any change in your body temperature?*
- *Can you feel like a rag doll?*
- *Can you imagine yourself floating on a cloud? Or do you feel much too heavy for that?*
- *Can you imagine where your tailbone ends?*
- *Can you visualize the texture of your larynx?*
- *Can you feel warm blood coursing through your veins?*
- *Can you imagine looking at something far away again?*
- *Can you feel your face getting all soft?*
- *Are you able to open your eyes now?*
- *And if you haven't opened it now, open it now.*

After the exercise there is a short discussion or evaluation:

❓
- Did the patient succeed in relaxing? (Assessment on the relaxation thermometer: 0–100)
- What changes has he noticed?
- Was there any trouble?

8.3 Session 9

Contents and Materials of the 9th Session

- **Contents**
  - Discussion of the practice of the week
  - Behavioral experiment: provocation of bodily sensations
  - See more ideas about behavioral experiments
  - Less helpful thoughts on somatic symptoms
  - Practice of the week: Helpful thoughts on somatic symptoms (Worksheet 8.9)
  - Relaxation practice: Guided imagery
- **Materials**
  - Worksheet 8.8: Less helpful thoughts on somatic symptoms
  - Worksheet 8.9: Helpful thoughts on somatic symptoms

8.3.1 Discussion of the Practice of the Week

The following examples can be used to evaluate Worksheet 8.7 (Causes of headaches): Weather change, flashes of light, glaring light, overloading of the muscles (back, neck) due to prolonged and one-sided physical strain (poor posture), certain foods and stimulants (red wine, chocolate, cheese, milk), a "hangover" after a night of drinking, certain medications, hormonal changes, everyday stress, etc. The therapist should emphasise (especially in patients with health anxiety) that a brain tumour or other serious illness is a very rare cause of headache. It is important to consider as many different causes as possible for each somatic symptom. It is very unlikely that there is a threatening disease behind the symptom.

8.3.2 Behavioral Experiment: Provocation of Somatic Symptoms

The patient should experience that somatic symptoms can be self-induced and do not necessarily have to be signs of a threatening disease or a less robust organism. Through this behavioral experiment, a correction of less helpful interpretations should be brought about or initiated.

Instruction: Provocation of Bodily Sensations

I would now like to do a little exercise with you. I would like to ask you to walk with me quickly up a few floors. We are on the third floor. We will walk to the ground floor and back up again as fast as you can! Be aware of any physical changes in your body. Let's go!

The following questions are intended to facilitate the evaluation of the exercise:

❓
- How have you been?
- Was it exhausting?
- What physical changes in your body have you noticed in yourself?

Ideally, the patient mentions symptoms such as rapid heartbeat and/or faster breathing, possibly sweating. The exercise is well suited for patients to be able to explain themselves and to feel on their own body how certain body symptoms arise or can be caused by themselves.

- How do you account for the occurrence of the symptoms you just told me about?
- Why did the symptoms appear?

The patient should answer that the symptoms were caused by physical stress or exertion and are therefore signs of physical activation and therefore harmless. A serious disease as the cause of the symptoms is very unlikely. Rather, the physical changes are reactions of a healthy body to physical exertion. A further explanation could be that there are many somatic symptoms that one can cause or provoke oneself.

Can you think of any other symptoms that you can bring on yourself?

For example, we can create **vertigo** when we spin around our own axis. Patients may know this game where you put your hand on a bottle that is on the floor and then you have to circle the bottle quite a few times without letting go of the bottle. When one tries to walk straight after this, dizziness usually occurs. However, patients may simply sit on a swivel office chair and spin around a few times. If they then stop abruptly, they will feel dizzy. **Sweating** can be deliberately induced by going to a sauna or putting on thick, overly warm clothing. This is also a normal reaction of the body. You can provoke **faster breathing** by sprinting a short distance. This would also lead to an **acceleration of the heartbeat**. Often, the heart also beats faster when one thinks of a loved one or is newly in love. In this case, a loss of appetite or a sinking feeling in the stomach area may also occur, which is often referred to as "butterflies in the stomach".

The following summary can be drawn: Body signals can be interpreted in different ways! A somatic symptom does not necessarily have to be a sign of a disease or a danger signal. Our organism is highly complex. It is quite normal that some body processes do not run perfectly from time to time.

It is important that patients check their evaluation of the symptom for appropriateness! The following imagination can clarify the context once again: "Imagine you live in a high-rise building with a siren on the roof. There is an alarm button on each floor that you are supposed to push when there is a fire. One night the siren wails. What does this mean? First of all, it means nothing more than that the alarm button has been pressed. Whether a fire has actually broken out or there is a danger must be checked, because after all it can also be a false alarm. In this case, fear and panic would be unfounded. In addition, the picture shows that before you press the inner alarm button yourself or scream ALARM! or DANGER! inwardly, you should check whether there is a real danger or not, in order not to stress yourself unnecessarily emotionally."

8.3.3 Further Ideas on Behavioral Experiments

Behavioral experiments with to induce bodily sensations can also be used to test other thoughts than just less helpful causal attributions of the patients. They can be applied to many different problematic cognitions (◘ Table 8.2) related to persistent somatic symptoms. An example would be fear-avoidance thoughts: in patients who report dizziness, the cognition that physical activation would increase their dizziness and make them feel progressively worse had become entrenched. In a behavioral experiment, this cognition could be challenged by having patients initially perform head movements that provoke dizziness. After initially sitting in a chair, they would be asked to stand up and then continue to move their head increasingly even though they felt dizzy. Patients would probably reflect on this exercise that they had initially felt bad due to increasing dizziness. However, this discomfort had been short-lived and with repeated performance of the exercise, the dizziness induced by the head movements and other body movements had diminished. Through this experience, the patient could learn to tolerate a slight dizziness with movement and to move more again.

Symptom-related socially anxious thoughts also lend themselves to being put to the test in the context of behavioral experiments. Patients with irritable bowel syndrome developed the thought that they could only travel to work on trains that had a toilet. As soon as they would feel perceptions in the intestinal region, they would develop a strong urge to go to a toilet immediately. Otherwise they would expect an "accident", which would be very embarrassing for them. First of all, they would practice at home to develop healthy habits regarding bowel movements (e.g., regular visits to the toilet always at the same time of day). When unpleasant body sensations occurred in the bowel area, they would suppress the urge to deviate from the schedule of they toilet visits and would experience that after about 20 minutes the perceptions receded by themselves. They successfully would extend their behavioral experiments to situations outside their household, e.g., on train journeys or visits to public places without a toilet.

These examples demonstrate that behavioral experiments with symptom provocation can be used in a very versatile way in cognitive work with patients with persistent somatic symptoms. It is crucial that the problematic cognition is explored in detail in its content and that the behavioral experiment or symptom provocation is tailored to the cognitive content or the content that is to be questioned. In the context of the latter two examples, it is important that the patient be adequately educated about the purpose of the exercise and that the patient and therapist jointly plan the symptom induction exercise to ensure that the patient is absolutely committed to do the behavioral experiment. It may also be necessary to discuss planned behavioral experiments with the patient's treating primary care physician to determine the extent to which contraindications exist. Further suggestions for behavioral experiments can be found in Bennett-Levy et al. (2004). Concrete ideas for inducing bodily sensation are compiled in ◘ Table 8.1.

◘ **Table 8.1** Ideas for provoking various bodily sensations in the context of behavioral experiments

Bodily sensation	Provocation exercise
Cardiovascular symptoms	Repeated brisk stair climbing/ergometer/squats/any other form of physical activity (increased heart rate, shortness of breath, increased respiratory rate, sweating) Breathing through a straw (shortness of breath, feeling of not being able to breathe) Consume a lot of caffeinated drinks Stress test (e.g., answer general knowledge questions as quickly and correctly as possible)
Drowsiness	Hyperventilation
Trembling	Physical exertion/repeated brisk stair climbing Holding something heavy for a long time with an outstretched arm After physical exertion, stretch out and tense the arm and hand and spread the fingers strongly under muscle tension Perform fine motor task with camera recording Therabands Sit on a stool with back against the wall, lift and hold legs
Lump feeling in the throat	Repeated swallowing and attention to larynx Eat something dry Wrap scarf around neck and concentrate on larynx when swallowing
Dizziness/balance problems	Sit on swivel chair and get spun Lie down and get up spontaneously, quickly Hyperventilation Hand on the floor and walk in a circle around the hand (without losing contact with the floor) Rapid circular head movements Hyperventilation Finding balance standing on one leg with eyes closed Walking on wobbly ground (e.g., wobbly slabs, suspension bridge) Head between the legs and then spontaneously move head up and stand up Rotate around your own axis while standing with your eyes closed
Tingling sensation in extremities	Place on hands or shins Extend hands vertically upwards in a sustained manner Lie on your back and stretch your legs upwards at a sustained 90° angle Hyperventilation Hands in cold water When the outside temperature is low, let your hands get cold and then let them warm up inside the warm room Touch nettles

◻ Table 8.1 (continued)

Bodily sensation	Provocation exercise
Gastrointestinal symptoms	Air swallowing (flatulence) Drinking carbonated drinks (belching) Eat foods that cause flatulence (e.g., cabbage, lentils, sauerkraut, grain bread) Eating spicy food Certain odors can cause nausea (e.g., ammonia, stale flower water) Eating an excessive amount of food once or eating a lot of sweet foods (feeling of fullness) Herbal laxative/flaxseed Prunes/salt sticks/dark chocolate/coke (constipation) Wearing a tightly buckled belt (abdominal pain) Passing up hunger and eating a large amount afterwards (flatulence, abdominal pain) Quickly eat different foods in a jumble (flatulence) Postponing a toilet Consume a lot of milk-containing (cold) drinks quickly (abdominal pain, diarrhoea, flatulence)
Chest tightness	Hyperventilation Wrap scarf tightly around the chest Lie on your back and put a book on your chest Push-ups Put Coolpack on chest Wear tight top made of strong textile

8.3.4 Less Helpful Thoughts on Somatic Symptoms

In the next step, typical, less helpful thoughts are again collected together with the patient when somatic symptoms occur. The following overview (◻ Table 8.2) shows that these are not necessarily just attributions of illness. On the contrary, the less helpful thoughts can encompass many other areas, such as body image, worries about the future, social anxiety. Some patients have difficulty accessing their thought world and putting their cognitions into words. In this case, you can also discuss such a list with your patients (Worksheet 8.8: Less helpful thoughts on somatic symptoms) and see to what extent patients can identify themselves with the listed thoughts. The list can be supplemented, for example, with the less helpful thoughts developed in the previous session.

8.3.5 Practice of the Week

Patients receive Worksheet 8.9 (Helpful thoughts on somatic symptoms [based on Basler & Kröner-Herwig, 1998]). Patients should mark those thoughts that they know about themselves. In addition, they should try to formulate other thoughts that are less stressful for them and that could possibly help them to cope better with their somatic symptoms. Here, too, we give the hint that the patient should refer to the last session, in which initial suggestions of helpful thoughts were already collected.

8.3.6 Relaxation Practice: Guided Imagery

At the end of session 9, a guided imagery for relaxation is performed with the patients. As part of the exercise, patients are asked to imagine themselves on the beach of a beautiful island.

■ **Instruction: Guided Imagery**

Now make yourself comfortable and close your eyes if you like! If not now, then perhaps at a later point in our little journey.—You are now slowly coming to rest.—Your hands and arms are getting heavy.—Your neck and shoulders are getting heavy.—Your feet and legs are getting heavy.—Your whole body is pleasantly warm.—Your breathing is calm and even.—Your face is completely relaxed, smooth and detached.—Your head is free and light.

Table 8.2 Collection of typical thought contents of patients with persistent somatic symptoms

Thought content	Sample thoughts
Health anxiety/beliefs	
Somatic symptoms as a sign of a serious/life-threatening illness	"My frequent *symptoms* are a sign of *illness X* or that something is wrong with me."
Somatic symptoms as a sign of approaching death	"I will die/be paralyzed/be disabled/ …" "I'm dying/dying/ …"
Somatic symptoms as a sign of an undetected or very rare disease	"There must be some explanation for my *discomfort*; I am probably suffering from some as yet undiscovered disease." "I suffer from a disease that no one or only an unknown specialist on the other side of the world knows about."
Somatic symptoms as a sign of an illness that has already occurred in the family/among acquaintances or that has been reported in the media	"My *symptoms* are very similar to *person X*'s. Everyone said it wouldn't be a bad *disease X*, but then he passed away from it. I may have the same disease." "My *symptoms* are quite similar to the *disease X* I heard about on the radio recently."
Other disease attributions	"My symptoms may be side effects of my medications. I should stop taking *drug X*."
Thoughts that support the patient's passive attitude	"The cause has to be found, then I can take a medication or get a treatment that will finally make me stop having *symptoms*."
Uncontrollability of the symptoms	"My *symptoms* come and go as they please. They do what they want to me." "I can't get my *discomfort under* control." "I feel at the mercy of my *symptoms*."
Lowered tolerance level with regard to symptom perception	"I can't take this anymore."
Symptom history	"My *symptoms* are getting worse. I'll never be *symptom-free* again." "I will be limited by the *discomfort for the rest* of my life." "I'll never be able to enjoy anything again." "I'm never all right. There's always something wrong with me." "The *symptoms* are always there."
Symptom-related prophecies/ clairvoyance	"By the time I get to place X at the latest, my symptoms will be more severe again." "If the symptoms start this morning, you're done for the day."
Expectations regarding symptom-related social assessments	"Other passersby think I'm drunk when I get dizzy." "The others find me repulsive because of my symptoms." "My symptoms make me embarrassing in public."
Forward-looking concerns	"I'm going to lose my job and I won't be able to support my family." "I won't be able to be a good father/mother." "I will be a burden to others. I will be dependent on others." "I'll be alone." "I'm going to let my family down." "My health insurance won't cover the cost." "Maybe my kids will have similar ailments. It's my fault they inherited this from me." "I won't be able to manage my daily life anymore." "I will never find a partner with these symptoms."
Assumptions of guilt	"There must be a reason why I, of all people, am suffering from these symptoms. I am being punished for something." (Thoughts can have religious background if necessary) "I did something wrong/misbehaved." "I haven't exhausted all treatment options."
Symptom as "scapegoat" for life problems	"The symptoms are destroying my life. Nothing is the same because of them." "If it weren't for the symptoms, my life would be everything I want it to be."
Thoughts on avoidance behavior, fear-avoidance thoughts	"If my symptoms get worse again, I should avoid certain foods." "Exercise will cause the symptoms to strengthen again." "If the symptoms come back, I could fall over and hurt myself badly." "If I ride my bike now, it could result in the discomfort getting worse again." "The discomfort is getting worse again, I need to rest for now." "I can't keep working like this. I need a pension." "I can't take the train because there are no train toilets there."

8

■ **Table 8.2** (continued)

Thought content	Sample thoughts
Thoughts on other safety and illness behaviors.	"The *discomfort* is so bad that I need to see a physician urgently." "I need a safe place." "I need someone with me." "I need to take blood pressure/check my skin for spots/ …" "I can't believe the physician, there must be a cause. I'm going to see another specialist."
Need for 100% security	"Even though my physician tells me there's nothing wrong with me, he can't give me a guarantee that it's not *disease X*." "Actually, I know there's nothing wrong with my body, but then when the *symptoms* get stronger, no one can rule out that it's something bad."
Thoughts on perseverance tendencies	"He who rests on his *symptoms* is lazy." "I need to function." "Get a grip." "Now more than ever! I'm not going to let my *symptoms* limit me and I'm going to fight them." "I can still function the same way I did before." "I don't want anyone on the outside to perceive that I'm impaired."
Body image/body function related thoughts	"My body is no longer functional. I can no longer trust it/rely on it." "I am very sensitive/weak/helpless." "I'm not resilient anymore." "My *symptoms* make me unattractive." "I'm not normal." "My clothes don't fit anymore." "I'm getting old."
Thoughts about reactions of the environment (including therapist or physiciant)	"No one takes me and my *symptoms* seriously." "I can't trust anyone." "The others have never experienced anything like this. "They can't relate to what I'm going through." "No one understands me." "No one can help me." "The others think I'm a malingerer."
Thoughts in relation to partnership	"I am so ashamed in front of my partner." "With my symptoms, I can't allow physical closeness." "I need a lot of attention and support."
Thoughts towards the therapist/ physician	"You are my last hope. If you don't help me, no one can help me." "I shouldn't tell my physician that new kinds of symptoms have come up, or he'll send me for more tests."
Concept of health	"Health to me means being completely symptom free."
Thoughts on the connection between somatic symptoms and quality of life	"Only when the symptoms are completely gone can I regain quality of life."
Loss of control thoughts	"I just pass out." "I'm going crazy."
Self-esteem related thoughts	"I can't function the way I used to. I'm a failure." "I'm a hypochondriac. I'm just imagining it."
Personalize the symptoms	"It always hits me. It's unfair."
Life weary thoughts	"If this keeps going on and the discomfort keeps getting worse, I don't want to keep living like this."
Paranoid thoughts	"Someone drugged me."

Now imagine that you are awakened one morning by the first rays of the sun on your closed eyelids.—You smell the cool air of the morning.—You hear seagulls above you.—When you open your eyes, you see that you are on a small island.—You're lying on warm, soft, pale sand.—You look out at the open, blue, calm sea.—The morning sun's rays are reflected on the water.—Small waves roll onto the beach, bringing a few shells with them.—You watch the waves come and go.—You watch the waves for a while—as they come and go again—You breathe in the clear morning air.—It's fresh and salty and tastes like a beautiful day.—You take a deep breath and straighten up.—You look around you at the island you have awakened to.—Near you, a few palm trees spread their leaves to give you shade.—You stroll over to the palm trees.—In one spot, the palm trees are particularly dense.—Other plants with large, fleshy leaves also grow there.—Between the plants you discover a small, bubbling spring, where you refresh yourself.—You will now walk a little over the island.—It is not very big.—You are alone.—No one disturbs your path.—You have the whole island to yourself.—All its beauty and loveliness is just for you.—You let your eyes wander, over the island, and the sea.—You enjoy the peace and quiet.—You feel comfortable and at ease and completely relaxed.—You now sit back down on the beach, dig your toes into the soft and warm sand, and look out over the calm sea for a while longer.—You now breathe deeply.—Now slowly open your eyes again.

Finally, an evaluation of the relaxation exercise should take place:

- How well did the patient manage to relax? (Assessment on the relaxation thermometer: 0–100)
- Was there any trouble?

8.4 Session 10

Contents and Materials of the 10th Session

- **Contents**
  - Discussion of the practice of the week
  - Typical less helpful thinking patterns and auxiliary questions
  - Example of cognitive reappraisal
  - Exercise on solidifying helpful thoughts
  - On the necessity of practice for behavior change
  - ABCZ model: Extension of the ABC model by helpful thoughts
  - Practice of the Week:
    - ABCZ model (Worksheet 8.11)
    - Characteristics of a healthy body (Worksheet 8.12)
- **Materials**
  - Worksheet 8.10: Questions to help checking less helpful thoughts
  - Worksheet 8.11: ABCZ model
  - Worksheet 8.12: Concept of health

8.4.1 Discussion of the Practice of the Week

Session 10 begins with a discussion of Worksheet 8.9 (Helpful Thoughts on Somatic Symptoms). The following questions may be useful:

- Which of the listed thoughts does the patient find helpful?
- Did he additionally formulate his own thoughts?

8.4.2 Typical Less Helpful Thinking Patterns and Auxiliary Questions

When reviewing less helpful thoughts, it is useful to ask yourself if you may have fallen into a "thinking trap". Less helpful thinking patterns that people often exhibit and that lead to emotional distress include the following:

- **Catastrophic thinking**: Here one imagines the worst or paints the devil on the wall in one's mind.
- **Low rating of one's frustration tolerance**: tendency to believe that pain, discomfort, inconvenience, or other adversity is unbearable.
- **Prophecy, clairvoyance**: Presuppositions are treated as facts, even though there is no clear evidence that they are true. Example: "I know exactly that I am good for nothing today!"

In order for patients to discover "thinking traps" in themselves as independently as possible, typical less helpful thinking patterns can first be described to them. The patients are then asked to give examples of their own. The following questions can now be helpful in questioning identified "thinking traps":

Instruction: Auxiliary Questions for Typical Less Helpful Thinking Patterns

Once you have identified your thinking traps or less helpful thinking patterns, you can directly create an ABC model. This way you can remind yourself of the connection between thinking and feeling. Collect and note down situations, thoughts and behaviors that typically occur in connection with somatic symptoms and lead to stressful feelings.

Afterwards, ask yourself if you are in a thinking trap: Am I exaggerating (excessively)? Is it really unbearable, horrible or catastrophic, or would life go on anyway? Am I practicing supernatural abilities by trying to predict the future or read other people's minds?

Ask yourself whether your evaluations or thoughts are logical and realistic: Is there objective evidence for my evaluation? How do I know that what I think I know is true? What is the probability that the consequence I fear will happen? How convinced am I (assessing the degree of conviction)? What is in favor (pro) of my assumption being true? What speaks against it (contra)? After considering all the pros and cons, how convinced am I now that my catastrophizing assumption is true? Is this assessment verifiable? What could I do to test my assessment?

Ask yourself about the utility of your evaluation: this is a strategy called "hedonic calculus", which is an essential part of "rational-emotive therapy" developed by Albert Ellis (Schelp et al., 1997). How will I feel and behave as long as I believe this? Will this thought help me in the long run? Does my thought help me to feel and behave the way I would like to? Does it help me to keep thinking about the possible consequences?

Role reversal, taking on a different perspective: How would someone evaluate these physical discomforts for whom such discomforts do not trigger fear or despair? What would this person have to say to him/herself? Imagine that a friend of yours had your discomfort. What advice would you give your friend? What words would you use to reassure him? Could this work for you too? If not, why not?

Auxiliary questions for exploring counterarguments in hypochondriacal beliefs (adapted from Rief & Hiller, 1998):

- *Could there be one person in this world where it is not as you fear?*
- *What causes other than a serious illness could be responsible for causing such discomfort?*
- *How often can such symptoms be attributed to these less threatening and catastrophic causes?*

The patient is given Worksheet 8.10 (Questions to help checking less helpful thoughts).

8.4.3 Example of Cognitive Reappraisal

In the following (◘ Table 8.3) we give you an example of the questions and cognitive interventions one might use to challenge a typical less helpful cognition of a patient with persistent somatic symptoms. In this example, it is a catastrophizing, body image-related thought.

◘ Table 8.3 Starting points for cognitive reappraisal of the body image-related thought: "I can no longer experience confidence in my body"

Category	Specific questions
Questions to concretize the patient's statement	What specifically does "no confidence in my body" mean? Is your entire body affected? Can you no longer experience confidence in certain body parts themselves or rather in the functioning of certain body parts? Are there parts of the body that still function well?
Questions about influencing factors	Is the functional capacity of these body parts always, i.e. consistently, impaired? Are there also phases in which you have experienced these body parts functioning again? If so, what is different in these phases? What do you do in the phases? How do you feel? Can you recall a specific situation? We can also take another look at your symptom diary and look for periods where there were fluctuations in your symptoms
Questions on the meaning of "trust" (elaboration of fears behind the loss of trust)	What does "trust" mean to you in concrete terms? What makes it so difficult for you to regain trust in your body? (Is it, for example, that patients experience a loss of control or feel at the mercy of their body)?
Questions about rebuilding trust in the body (especially if the loss of trust is based on loss of control)	What would have to happen for you to regain confidence in your body? What would be benchmarks for trusting your body again? I suggest that we gather again situations in which you find it easier to regain control over the function of certain parts of your body, compared to situations in which you find it harder to gain control What could you specifically do in the situations in which you have little control over the particular body part, so that you can nevertheless cope well with the situation and do not feel so strongly restricted or at the mercy of others? (Use external aids; use strategies that have already been worked out in therapy; identify less helpful strategies such as avoidance behavior as less helpful and more limiting, etc.) How can you manage the situation even though you may not have full control over your body? (Question the patient's standards for coping with the situation, such as allowing yourself more time for a task)

(continued)

Table 8.3 (continued)

Category	Specific questions
Validating to patients that it is difficult to accept that they can no longer function in some areas in the way that was originally possible	I imagine this frustrates/saddens/frightens you…when you can't function in certain areas the way you originally could How do thoughts about not being able to fully function in some areas, or not being able to fully trust your body, help you in the long run? With these thoughts, can you behave and feel the way you would like to?
Collect formulations for a helpful thought	Put yourself in the position, your best friend thinks in a similar way as you. What would you say to him? How would you try to calm him down?
Example of a helpful thought	"I have tried to function at a very high level for a long time. My body is now showing me that I can't sustain that in the long run. That's not easy for me to accept. But I want to take my body seriously. Plus, there are many areas where I function well and can have confidence in my body. For the areas where I have a hard time trusting my body or where my body is difficult to control, I approach it and try to use my learned strategies to manage the situation."

8.4.4 Exercise on Solidifying Helpful Thoughts

In the next step, a so-called devil's advocat (based on Basler & Kröner-Herwig, 1998) can be carried out. The exercise serves to anchor the positive, helpful thoughts already worked out in the patient's mind. The therapist assumes the role of the devil's advocat. The following instruction can be helpful in carrying out this exercise.

Instruction: Devil's Advocat

At the beginning of the exercise, patients are asked to briefly describe a real situation in which their somatic symptoms occur. The exercise can be based on the two lists (Worksheets 8.8 and 8.9).

Past sessions have focused on helping you understand the importance of helpful thoughts in coping with physical discomfort. Despite this realization, you may be asking yourself, "How can I manage to think in a more helpful way in a stressful situation?" Since this is really difficult, I would like to do an exercise with you. This is a little "conversational duel" between the two of us. I will confront or "attack" you with your typical less helpful thoughts. You should then try to counter this less helpful thought with a helpful one. Defend this thought! Be an advocate in your own cause! Subsequently, I will attack you again with an less helpful thought, which you are to defend again with the help of a suitable helpful thought!

The exercise should be briefly evaluated afterwards. The following questions can be useful:

- What impact did the thoughts you expressed have on how you felt?
- How well did you succeed in asserting or defending your helpful thought?

8.4.5 On the Necessity of Practice of Behavior Change

Especially in the methods for changing thinking habits, practice plays a special role. It is therefore advisable to introduce separate measures at this point in the therapy to make the patient aware of the need to practice. For this purpose, the aspects listed below should be addressed in the conversation.

Inappropriate assessments are often **patterns of thought** that are firmly rooted. In some cases, they have existed for years or even decades. They are usually formed through upbringing, socialization as well as through formative experiences that are gathered in the course of life. Through constant "use", patterns of thought are maintained or stabilized. For this reason, thinking patterns are usually difficult to change. Consequently, change cannot happen overnight. It requires a lot of effort and practice. You have to pay more attention to your evaluations than usual, question them again and again and correct them if necessary. If one neglects this kind of self-reflection, one quickly falls back into old thinking patterns, as is the case with other habits (e.g., certain drinking and eating habits, smoking). Especially in stressful situations, there is a great danger of automatically falling back into old patterns of behavior. If you want to learn a new sport or to play an instrument, this usually does not work from one moment to the next. Practice or training of new behaviors is an absolute prerequisite for establishing new behaviors!

Scientific studies show—the work of Craik and Lockhart (1972) is considered groundbreaking here—that **learning processes** are all the more effective the more channels of experience are involved (listening, reading, writing, execution), i.e. the deeper the processing or the broader the engagement with the material to be learned. For this reason, it is useful and helpful not to limit oneself to theoretical knowledge alone, but to try out one's newly gained insights and ways of thinking in reality ("learning by doing"). An old Chinese proverb supports the logic of this view: "I hear and forget. I see and retain. I do and comprehend." An example from everyday life: no one learns to swim without getting into the water 1 day. Having certain swimming techniques explained and shown to you, practicing the moves on dry land, reading about them, or watching swimming competitions on TV—all of these alone are not enough to learn how to swim. The proverbial courageous "jump into the deep end" is essential, but effective. Or, in the words of Erich Kästner (Kästner, 1950): "There is nothing good unless: you do it!"

Behavioral experiments are particularly suitable in order to gain experience with the new, helpful thoughts. Accordingly, the patient should repeatedly confront physical discomfort by consciously provoking it. Here are some suggested exercises for consciously provoking physical discomfort: Eating plenty of lentils, beans, cabbage or onions will cause flatulence. Spinning around your own axis several times provokes dizziness. Walking briskly up and down a few flights of stairs or doing 20 squats will help the heart beat faster and more forcefully, breathing will become faster and you may get "out of breath".

8.4.6 ABCZ Model: Extension of the ABC Model by Helpful Thoughts

The already known ABC model is now to be extended by a further component, namely Z, which in this context does not stand for targeted emotional and behavioral reactions as originally thought by Stavemann (2001), but for new target thoughts, i.e. **appropriate, constructive** and **helpful thoughts** as already elaborated in the previous sessions (What do I want to learn to think about my somatic symptoms in the future?).

Patients should further be encouraged to evaluate their somatic symptoms realistically and appropriately. To this end, they are to counter their less helpful thoughts and evaluations, which occur to them almost automatically or as the first thing that comes to mind, with thoughts that lead to less strong negative emotions and/or to a reduction in inappropriate behaviors such as brooding or passivity. Patients are given Worksheet 8.11 (ABCZ Model).

8.4.7 Practice of the Week

Patients are given two tasks: The first task is to fill in the Worksheet 8.11 (ABCZ model) just received with an example of their own until the next session. An important therapeutic goal in the treatment of persons with somatoform disorders is the development of a realistic concept of health (Rief & Hiller, 2011). Patients should thus develop a realistic concept of health. To this end, patients are given the task of noting in bullet points what they consider to be the characteristics of a healthy and functioning body. Patients receive Worksheet 8.12 (Concept of health).

8.5 Session 11

Contents and Materials of the 11th Session

- **Contents**
  - Discussion of the practice of the week
  - The concept of health
  - Behavioral experiments
  - Everyday phenomena of the body
  - Practice of the week: Provoke bodily sensations (Worksheet 8.14)
- **Materials**
  - Worksheet 8.13: Common phenomena of the body
  - Worksheet 8.14: Behavioral experiments

8.5.1 Discussion of the Practice of the Week

Session 11 begins with a discussion of Worksheet 8.11 (ABCZ model) and Worksheet 8.12 (concept of health). First, it is checked whether the patient has succeeded in formulating **helpful thoughts** with the help of the ABCZ model. In the second task, it is to be expected that **unrealistic attitudes** will emerge that require disputation, e.g., "A healthy body is free from discomfort/physical discomfort". Such less helpful assumptions should be challenged, e.g., as follows:

- Is that realistic?
- What speaks for it, what speaks against it?

Worksheet 8.10 (Questions to help checking less helpful thoughts) can be used to support this.

8.5.2 The Concept of Health

Health is often understood as the complete absence of disease and disease-related impairments. But defining health solely in terms of the absence of disease is not enough.

The World Health Organization (1946) defines health as a state of complete physical, mental and social well-being and not merely the absence of disease or infirmity. It would not be surprising if this definition irritates, since it corresponds to a utopia. For in reality, presumably no human being is ever perfectly healthy, at least in the sense of the strict-seeming WHO definition. This ideal (perfect) state formulated here is not attainable for most people, and if it is, then certainly only for a narrowly limited time. A person's state of health deviates from this ideal to a greater or lesser extent. From a general point of view, it seems sensible to take mental leave of the mutually exclusive categories "healthy" and "ill". More appropriate and realistic is the assumption of a dimension with the two poles of illness and health. Every person can now be classified on this dimension. Sometimes he is closer to one, sometimes he tends more to the other pole. In addition, it must be taken into account: Whether someone classifies himself as sick or healthy does not depend solely on a medical diagnosis, but also on the attitude of the person concerned. Thus, a person who has caught a simple cold may feel terminally ill, while another person with a broken leg or arm may feel completely healthy and lively (although obviously ill in the sense of injured).

8.5.3 Behavioral Experiments

In the following, the implementation of two small behavioral experiments (following Watzlawick, 2007) is recommended.

- **Instruction: Behavioral Experiments According to Watzlawick (Based on Watzlawick, 2007)**

Exercise 1

Now please sit comfortably—close your eyes and focus your attention on your feet and shoes.—It shouldn't take long and you may notice how uncomfortable it actually is to wear shoes. No matter how well they seemed to fit before.—You will now notice pressure points and suddenly become aware of other uncomfortable sensations in your feet, such as burning, a slight tingling, heat or perhaps cold.—Good, now please open your eyes again!

Exercise 2

Now sit down again comfortably.—Now please look through the window at the sky.—Soon you will notice numerous tiny, bubble-like circles in your field of vision, which slowly sink down when you keep your eyes still, but shoot up again when you blink.—Try to focus more on the circles.—Good, now please concentrate on me again!

After performing both exercises, the therapist should explore how the patient felt or what the experience was. For exercise 1, the following questions may be useful:

?
- What did you notice?
- Have you noticed any discomfort in your feet?
- Were you suddenly uncomfortable wearing shoes?
- What is your explanation?

The evaluation of the second exercise can be done with the help of the following questions:

? What did you notice when you focused on the circles?

Usually, this response from the patient is to be expected: the circles seem to become more numerous and larger the more you focus on them.

? How do you explain this phenomenon?

It is a harmless phenomenon called "mouches volantes" (French for "flying gnats"; English "floaters"; gnat-like appearing perceptions in the visual field).

8.5.4 Everyday Phenomena of the Body

This refers to everyday processes in our body that take place without us consciously controlling them. It is quite normal for our body to make certain sounds from time to time or to cause certain sensations without these being signs of a disease. Some such phenomena and their causes are listed below (partly based on Neudecker, 2006):

- **Stomach Growling**

Our body produces about 1.5 l of saliva and mucus per day. With every swallowing process, a little air also slips into the stomach. When food is not being processed there, the air is mixed with the mucus in the stomach and tumbled. These contractions of the empty stomach produce the typical growling sound. The emptier the stomach, the stronger the contractions. When we have eaten, on the other hand, the stomach works more slowly. It "calms down" again. The growling disappears.

- **Nausea**

This phenomenon originates in the vomiting center, which is located in the brain. It can be stimulated by numerous events and trigger the vomiting process: Poisoning, balance disorders, intestinal disorders or the sight of things that provoke disgust in us. Psychological stress (any kind of excitement) can also cause nausea.

■ **Sensation of "Pins and Needles" in Feet**

Postures that lead to this phenomenon are, for example, the so-called cross-legged seat or crossed legs. But also staying too long in a sitting position can lead to the characteristic tingling or the feeling of light pinpricks. The cause of this sensation is too much pressure exerted on nerves. If a muscle nerve is also affected, this causes slight signs of paralysis in the affected part of the body.

■ **"Hellish" Pain When Hitting the Funny Bone**

Contrary to the popular name, it is not a bone, but one of the three main nerves of the arm, the ulnar nerve, which causes the typical pain when you accidentally bump your elbow. The ulnar nerve is located so close to the skin at the elbow, and in a relatively narrow bony groove at that, that it can be easily bumped or irritated. When working at the computer for a long time, it is quite possible that the arm rests on this nerve for too long, which can lead to a slight feeling of numbness. You will know this from your own experience: When you bump it, the pain is sharp, almost hellish, and comparable to an electric shock. It shoots from the elbow to the tip of the little finger and can cause tingling and numbness for minutes.

■ **Uncontrolled Muscle Twitching When Falling Asleep**

Behind the phenomenon known as "hypnic jerks" are harmless muscle discharges that only occur during the sleep phase. The tension of the day subsides and the muscles relax. In this phase, activating muscle impulses can still assert themselves and lead to such a twitch. While the cerebrum already switches to rest when falling asleep, other areas of the nervous system still remain active. The interaction between the brain and the spinal cord briefly becomes unbalanced, and the nerve cells involuntarily fire signals to the muscles. These signals trigger reflexes, which the person falling asleep then perceives as muscle twitching.

The patient is given Worksheet 8.13 (Common phenomena of the body).

8.5.5 Practice of the Week

Patients are given Worksheet 8.14 (Behavioral experiments). They are asked to decide which unpleasant bodily sensations they would like to provoke in the coming days. Patient are to be motivated by this task to deal with bodily discomforts as often as possible. In this way, fear of the occurrence of physical discomfort should be gradually removed or reduced. A realistic evaluation of physical discomfort is encouraged.

8.6 Worksheets

These worksheets are also available for download online at Springer Extras (► extras.springer.com).

Worksheet 8.1	The four levels of behavior	◘ Figure 8.2
Worksheet 8.2	ABC model of emotions	◘ Figure 8.3
Worksheet 8.3	ABC example	◘ Figure 8.4
Worksheet 8.4	My own ABC scheme	◘ Figure 8.5
Worksheet 8.5	The story of the hammer	◘ Figure 8.6
Worksheet 8.6	ABC model: back pain	◘ Figure 8.7
Worksheet 8.7	Causes of headaches	◘ Figure 8.8
Worksheet 8.8	Less helpful thoughts on somatic symptoms	◘ Figure 8.9
Worksheet 8.9	Helpful thoughts on somatic symptoms	◘ Figure 8.10
Worksheet 8.10	Questions to help checking less helpful thoughts	◘ Figure 8.11
Worksheet 8.11	ABCZ model	◘ Figure 8.12
Worksheet 8.12	Concept of health	◘ Figure 8.13
Worksheet 8.13	Common phenomena of the body	◘ Figure 8.14
Worksheet 8.14	Behavioral experiments	◘ Figure 8.15

Fig. 8.2 Worksheet 8.1: The four levels of behavior

Worksheet 8.1: The four levels of behavior

1. **The cognitive or thought-related level – everything that happens in your head**
   Inner monologues or self-talk, perceptions, evaluations and interpretations, attitudes, beliefs, norms and values, memories or imagined images.

2. **The emotional level - feelings**
   Joy and affection (pleasant sensations), indifference/serenity (neutral sensation), fear, anger, shame, disgust and sadness (unpleasant sensations). Emotions can occur in numerous combinations and various levels of intensity.

3. **The physiological level – physiological reactions**
   Examples: Palpitations, sweating, acceleration of breathing, muscle tension, dry mouth, pain, Dizziness, itching, flushing.

4. **The motor level – everything you do and others can observe about you**
   Examples: crying, running away, avoiding eye contact, yelling, having a drink, asking questions, staying silent. Basically two behavioral tendencies are distinguished: Approach vs. Avoidance. The following applies: A person can do not not behave in a certain way!

8

Fig. 8.3 Worksheet 8.2: ABC model of emotions

Worksheet 8.2: ABC model of emotions

The ABC model was developed by Albert Ellis, an American psychologist.

A →	B →	C
What just happened?	What do I think about A? What does that mean to me? How do I find it?	How do I feel? Do I perceive physical sensations? What do I end up doing?

The components of the model at a glance

A = Triggering event or current situation
B = Belief or appraisal of A or thoughts in relation to A
C = Consequences to B: feelings, physiological reactions, and observable behaviors

Appraisal-emotion logic

Appraisal of A	Emotion/Feeling Consequence of B
Excellent! Great! Beautiful!	Joy
Of all the nerve!	Anger, rage
So what!	Indifference, serenity
Oh, dear! How embarrassing!	Shame
Too bad!	Disappointment
How awful! Danger!	Fear
It's hopeless!	Depression

Fig. 8.4 Worksheet 8.3: ABC example

Worksheet 8.3: ABC example

A Situation	B Belief	C Consequences: emotions/feelings, physiological reactions, behavior
You want to go to sleep and throw back the duvet. On your bed sheet you discover a palm-sized spider. 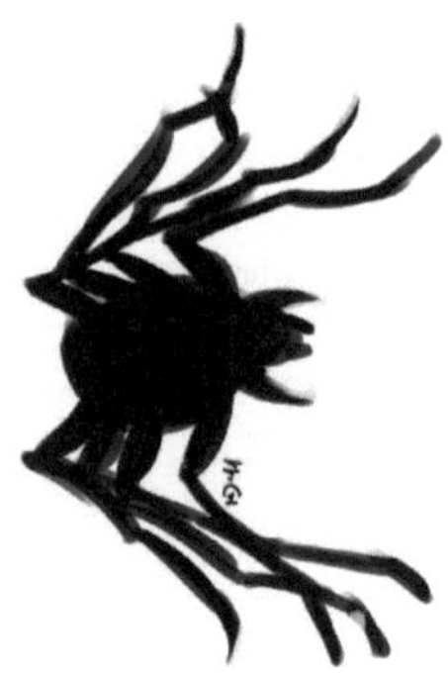		

Fig. 8.5 Worksheet 8.4: My own ABC scheme

Worksheet 8.4: My own ABC scheme

A Situation	B Belief	C Consequences
		1. Emotion/feeling: 2. Physiological reaction: 3. (Visible) Behavior:
		1. Emotion/feeling: 2. Physiological reaction: 3.(Visible) Behavior:

■ **Fig. 8.6** Worksheet 8.5: The story of the hammer

Worksheet 8.5: The story of the hammer

(Source: Paul Watzlawick 2007, "Guide to Unhappiness," pp. 37–38)

A man wants to hang a painting. He has the nail, but not the hammer. Therefore it occurs to him to go over to the neighbor and ask him to lend him his hammer. But at this point, doubt sets in. What if he doesn't want to lend me the hammer? Yesterday he barely spoke to me. Maybe he was in a hurry. Or, perhaps, he holds something against me. But why? I didn't do anything to him. If he would ask me to lend him something, I would, at once. How can he refuse to lend me his hammer? People like him make other people's life miserable. Worst, he thinks that I need him because he has a hammer. This has got to stop! And suddenly the guy runs to the neighbor's door, rings, and before letting him say anything, he screams: "You can keep your hammer, you bastard!"

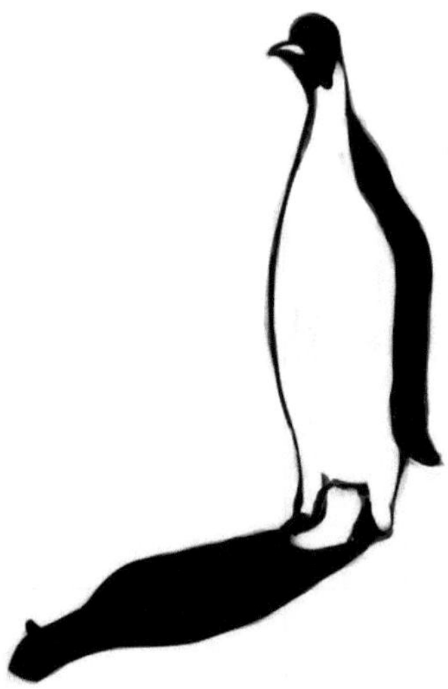

Fig. 8.7 Worksheet 8.6: ABC model: back pain

Worksheet 8.6: ABC model: back pain

A Situation	B Belief	C Consequences		
		Emotions/feelings	Physiological reactions	(Visible) behavior
I wake up in the morning with back pain. 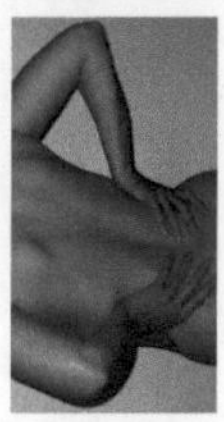	"When I wake up with backpain in the morning, then it's going to be like this all day." "I will maybe never have relief from my pain again." "I need to take it easy and have to avoid overexerting myself." "My body has not been resilient anymore."	Desperation, Sadness, Anxiety, Uncertainty, Loneliness	Persistent pain, Amplification of the pain	Staying in bed, Taking a lot of breaks, Taking relieving body posture, Cancelling meetings with friends, Withdrawal, Withdrawing from enjoyable activities

Fig. 8.8 Worksheet 8.7: Causes of headaches

Worksheet 8.7: Causes of headaches

It is important to have as many possible explanations for somatic symptoms as possible at hand or in the mind, in order to to be able to check for oneself whether the explanation first assumed is the only possible, realistic or most likely! Now try, to find as many possible explanations for headaches – a widespread somatic symptom – as possible and write down your answers! Also consider causes that seem less plausible to you! Try to find at least 10 possible explanations!

- ....
- ....
- ....
- ....
- ....
- ....
- ....
- ....
- ....
- ....
- ....
- ....

Fig. 8.9 Worksheet 8.8: Less helpful thoughts on somatic symptoms

Worksheet 8.8: Less helpful thoughts on somatic symptoms

Which of these thoughts (related to your symptoms) do you know yourself?

- "My frequent *symptoms* are a sign of *disease X*."
- "My frequent *symptoms* are a sign that something is wrong with me."
- "I will die/be paralyzed/be disabled/ ..."
- "I choke to death..."
- "There must be an explanation for my *symptoms*, I am probably suffering from an undiscovered disease."
- "I suffer from a disease that no one or only an unknown specialist on the other side of the world knows about."
- "My *symptoms* are quite similar to person *X*'s. Everyone has said that it is not a bad *disease*, but then they died of it. I may have the same disease."
- "My *symptoms* are quite similar to *condition X*, which I recently heard about on the radio."
- "My *symptoms* may be side effects of my medication. I should stop taking *drug X* take."
- "The cause has to be found, then I can take a medicine or get treatment, that's finally going to make me *symptom-free*."
- "My *symptoms* come and go when they want. They do what they want to me."
- "I can't get my *symptoms* under control."
- I feel at the mercy of my *symptoms*. I can't do anything about it anyway!"
- "My case is hopeless."
- "I am weak and suffer more than others."
- "I can't take it anymore."
- "My *symptoms* are getting worse and worse. I will never be *symptom-free* again."
- "I will be limited by the *discomfort* for the rest of my life."
- "I will never be able to enjoy anything again."
- "I'm never okay. There's always something wrong with me."
- "The *symptoms* are always there."
- "By the time I get to *place X* at the latest, my *symptoms* will be more severe again."
- "If the *symptoms* start this morning, the day is done."
- "I won't make it through the day."
- "Other people think I'm drunk when I get *dizzy*."
- "Others find me disgusting because of my *symptoms*."
- "I feel embarrassed because of my *symptoms* in public."
- "I will lose my job and won't be able to support my family."
- "I will not be able to be a good father/mother."
- "I will be a burden to others. I will be dependent on others."
- "I'll be alone."
- "I will abandon my family."
- "My health insurance won't cover the cost."
- "Maybe my children will have similar symptoms. It is my fault that they inherited this from me."
- "I won't be able to manage my daily life anymore."
- "I'll never find a partner with these *symptoms*."
- "There must be a reason why I, of all people, am suffering from these *symptoms*. I'm being punished for something."
- "I did something wrong/misbehaved."
- "Il wish I hadn't overexerted myself again."
- "I have not exhausted all treatment options."
- "The *symptoms* are destroying my life. Nothing is the same because of them."
- "If it weren't for the symptoms, my life would be the way I want it to be."
- "If my *symptoms* get worse again, I should avoid certain foods."
- "Exercise causes *symptoms to* strengthen again."

Fig. 8.9 (continued)

- "If the *symptoms* come back, I could fall over and hurt myself badly."
- "If I cycle now, it could result in the *discomfort* getting worse again."
- "The *discomfort* is getting worse again, I need to rest for now."
- "I can't keep working like this. I need a pension."
- "I can't take the train because there are no train toilets."
- "The *discomfort* is so bad that I need to see a doctor urgently."
- "I need a safe place."
- "I need someone with me."
- "I have to take blood pressure/check my skin for spots/ ..."
- "I can't believe what the doctor said. There must be a cause for my symptoms. I will see another specialist."
- "Although my doctor tells me that there is nothing wrong with me, they cannot give me a guarantee that is not *disease X* after all."
- "Actually, I know there is nothing wrong with my body, but then when the *symptoms* get stronger, no one can rule out that it's something bad."
- "People who lean back because of their *symptoms* are lazy."
- "I need to function."
- "Pull yourself together."
- "Now more than ever! I will not let my symptoms limit me and I will fight them."
- "I can still function the same way I did before."
- "I am no longer able to perform at all."
- "I am worthless, good for nothing."
- "No one should perceive to the outside world that I am limited."
- "My body is no longer functional. I can no longer trust it/rely on it."
- "I am very sensitive/weak/helpless."
- "I'm not resilient anymore."
- "My *symptoms* make me unattractive."
- "I'm not normal."
- "My clothes don't fit anymore."
- "I'm getting old."
- "No one takes me and my symptoms seriously."
- "I can't trust anyone."
- "The others have never experienced anything like this. They can't relate to what I'm going through."
- "No one understands me."
- "Nobody can help me anyway."
- "The others think I'm a malingerer."
- "I feel so ashamed in front of my partner."
- "With my *symptoms*, I can't allow any physical closeness."
- "I need a lot of attention and support."
- "You are my last hope. If you don't help me, no one can help me."
- "I should not tell my doctor that new kinds of symptoms have occured, or they will send me to further medical examinations and diagnostics."
- "To me, health means being completely symptom-free."
- "Only when the *symptoms* are completely gone can I regain quality of life."
- "I just pass out."
- "I'm going crazy. The symptoms are driving me to the edge of madness!"
- "I can't function the way I used to. I'm a failure."
- "I'm a hypochondriac. I'm just making things up."
- "It always hits me. It's unfair."
- "If this continues and the discomfort gets worse and worse, I don't want to live like this anymore."
- "I can't deal with that."
- "I give up."
- "Someone drugged me."

8

Fig. 8.10 Worksheet 8.9: Helpful thoughts on somatic symptoms

Worksheet 8.9: Helpful thoughts on somatic symptoms

Which of these thoughts (related to your symptoms) do you know yourself?

- I won't let it get me down!
- Don't panic – I'll get a handle on it!
- Others can do it too!
- Today I'm going to take it easy!
- I'm going to do something pleasant for now!
- This won't take all day!
- There are people worse off than me!
- Cheer up – I can do it!
- First of all, calm down!
- I'm distracting myself!
- Now I first think about what I can do step by step against my symptoms!
- I know it will get better too!
- I can take it – I am strong!
- I consider it a challenge!
- Il've handled situations like this before!
- I don't have to function 100% now!
- Things are looking up again!
- I take care of my body and respect my limits!
- Even if I have symptoms, I can do the following: ....!
- I do my job as best I can!
- I am aware of the healthy parts of my body!
- I actively search for solutions!
- I can have a positive effect on my symptoms!

Fig. 8.11 Worksheet 8.10: Questions to help checking less helpful thoughts

Worksheet 8.10: Questions to help checking lesshelpful thoughts

- Have I fallen into a thinking trap?
  - **Catastrophizing**
    Am I exaggerating? Am I assuming the worst possible outcome? Is it really unbearable, terrible or catastrophic, or would life still go on?
  - **Clairvoyance**
    Am I practicing supernatural abilities by trying to predict the future?
- Questions of **logic and reality**
  Is there any objective evidence for my appraisals? How do I know? Is it verifiable? How much am I convinced that my thoughts are true? What speaks for it (pro)? What speaks against it (contra)? What could I do to check my appraisals?
- Questions about the **benefits**
  How will I feel and behave as long as I believe these thoughts? Will this thought help me in the long run? Does my thought help me to feel and behave the way I want to? Does it help me to constantly think about the possible consequences?

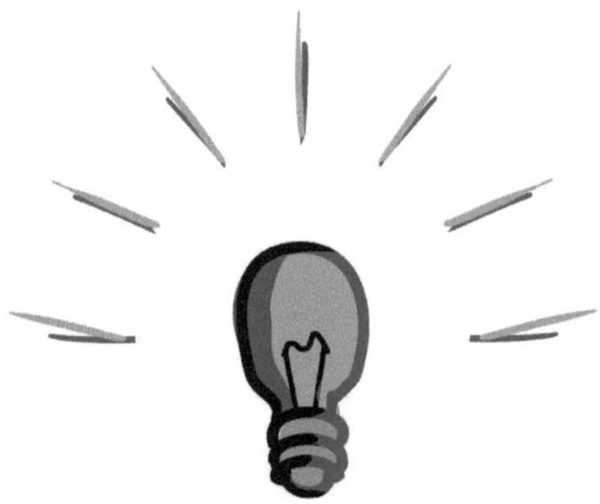

Fig. 8.12 Worksheet 8.11: ABCZ model

Worksheet 8.11: ABCZ model

A Situation What happened? Which was the symptom?	B Belief How do I feel about A? How do I evaluate what just has happened?	C Consequences How do I feel (having these thoughts listed under B)? Are there any somatic symptoms? What do I do in response? How do I behave?	Z Target thoughts Which constructive thoughts, i.e., helpful thoughts, come to my mind as an alternative to B - if negative?
		1. Emotions/feelings: 2. Physiological reactions: 3. (Visible) Behavior:	

Fig. 8.13 Worksheet 8.12: Concept of health

Worksheet 8.12: Concept of health

Make some notes.

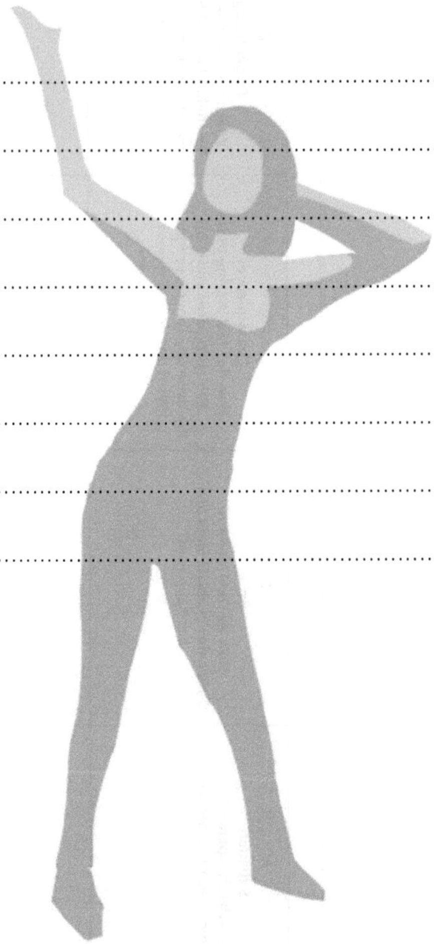

- ....

  ....
- ....

  ....
- ....

  ....
- ....

  ....

Fig. 8.14 Worksheet 8.13: Common phenomena of the body

Worksheet 8.13: Common phenomena of the body

- **Stomach growling:** Our body produces about 1.5 l of saliva and mucus a day. With each swallowing a little air also slips into the stomach. If there is not just food to be processed, the air together with the mucus is knead in the stomach. These contractions of the gastric cavity empty of food creates the growling. The emptier the stomach, the stronger the contractions. When we have eaten, on the contrary, the stomach works more slowly.

- **Funny Bone:** Contrary to popular myth, this is not a bone, but one of the three main nerves of the arm, the ulnar nerve. At the elbow this nerve lies so close under the skin and is located in a narrow bone groove that it can be easily bumped and irritated. When working at the computer for a long time it can happen that the arm rests too long on this nerve, which leads to a slight feeling of numbness.
You know it yourself, when bumped, the pain is sharp, almost hellish and comparable to an electric shock. It shoots from the elbow to the tip of the little finger and can cause tingling and numbness for minutes.

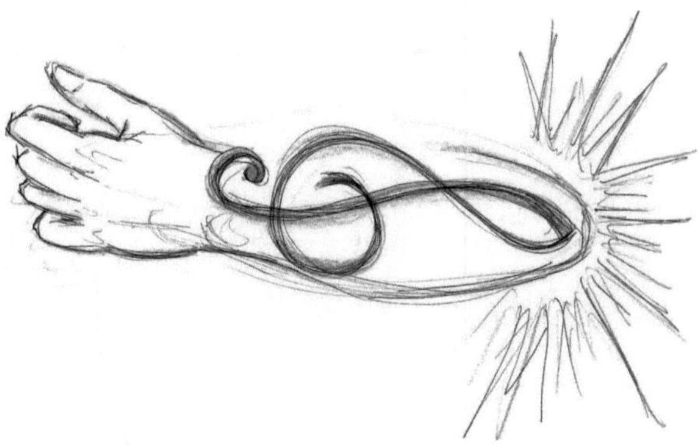

- **Nausea:** This phenomenon originates in the brain, in the so-called vomiting centre. It can be caused by numerous events and can trigger the vomiting process: Poisoning, balance disorders, intestinal diseases, seeing things that cause disgust in us, but also psychological stress.

- **Feet falling asleep:** Postures that lead to this phenomenon include cross-legged sitting. But also staying too long in one sitting position can lead to tingling and to the sensation of light pinpricks. The cause of this sensation is too long pressure exerted on nerves. If a muscular nerve is affected, this causes slight signs of paralysis in the part of the body concerned.

- **Uncontrolled muscle twitching when falling asleep:** Behind the phenomenon known as the sleep twitch are harmless muscle relaxations that only occur during the sleep phase: The tension of the day subsides the muscles relax. In this phase, however, activating muscle impulses can still prevail and lead to such a twitch. While the cerebrum already switches to rest when we fall asleep, other areas of the nervous system remain active.
The interaction between the brain and spinal cord is thrown out of balance. The nerve cells fire involuntary signals to the muscles. These signals trigger reflexes, which the person falling asleep then perceives as a muscle twitch.

Fig. 8.15 Worksheet 8.14: Behavioral experiments

Worksheet 8.14: Behavioral experiments

In the following days I will expose myself to the following somatic symptoms by deliberately inducing them:

- ....
- ....
- ....
- ....

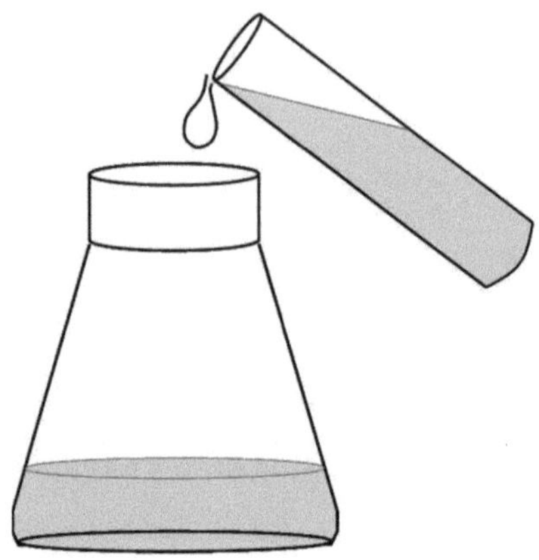

References

Basler, H.-D., & Kröner-Herwig, B. (1998). *Psychologische Therapie bei Kopf- und Rückenschmerzen* (2. Aufl.). Quintessenz.

Bennett-Levy, J., Butler, G., Fennell, M., Hackman, A., Müller, M., & Westbrook, D. (Eds.). (2004). *The Oxford guide to behavioural experiments in cognitive therapy*. Oxford University Press.

Craik, F. I. M., & Lockhart, R. S. (1972). Levels of processing: Framework for memory research. *Journal of Verbal Learning and Verbal Behavior, 11*(6), 671–684. https://doi.org/10.1016/S0022-5371(72)80001-X

Goldfried, N. R., & Davison, G. C. (1979). *Klinische Verhaltenstherapie*. Springer.

Kästner, E. (1950). *Kurz und bündig. Epigramme*. Atrium.

Neudecker, S. (2006, January 2). Körperphänomene: Hick und Hatschi. *ZEIT Wissen*, S. 1.

Rief, W., & Hiller, W. (1998). *Somatisierungsstörung und Hypochondrie* (Fortschritte der Psychotherapie Band 1). Hogrefe.

Rief, W., & Hiller, W. (2011). *Somatisierungsstörung* (Bd. 1, Fortschritte der Psychotherapie). Hogrefe.

Schelp, T., Gravemeier, R., & Maluck, D. (1997). *Rational-Emotive Therapie als Gruppentraining gegen Stress. Seminarkonzept und Materialien* (2. Aufl.). Huber.

Stavemann, H. H. (2001). *Im Gefühlsdschungel: Emotionale Krisen verstehen und bewältigen* (2. Aufl.). Beltz.

Watzlawick, P. (2007). *Anleitung zum Unglücklichsein. Vom Schlechten des Guten* (5. Aufl.). Piper.

Watzlawick, P., Beavin, J. H., & Jackson, D. D. (2000). *Menschliche Kommunikation – Formen, Störungen, Paradoxien* (10. Aufl.). Huber.

World Health Organization. (1946). *Constitution of the World Health Organization*. 29.05.2011. http://whqlibdoc.who.int/hist/official_records/constitution.pdf

Module 5: Illness Behavior

Contents

M. Kleinstäuber et al., *Cognitive Behavior Therapy for Persistent Somatic Symptoms and Somatic Symptom Disorder*, https://doi.org/10.1007/978-3-662-69726-9_9

9.1 Session 12

Contents and Materials of the 12th Session

- **Contents**
  - Discussion of the practice of the week
  - Patients' previous coping attempts
  - Avoidance or boom and bust behaviors and consequences
  - Avoidance or boom and bust behavior and a vicious circle model
  - Reduction of avoidance behavior/promotion of physical activity at a healthy level
  - Practice of the week
  - Avoidance /boom and bust behavior and consequences: Fourfold table (Worksheet 9.3a or 9.3b).
  - Avoidance/boom and bust behavior (Worksheet 9.4a or 9.4b)
- **Materials**
  - Worksheet 9.1a: What are the consequences of my avoidance behavior?
  - Worksheet 9.1b: What are the consequences of my attempts to "boom"?
  - Worksheet 9.2a: Avoidance behavior and somatic symptoms—a vicious circle
  - Worksheet 9.2b: Boom and bust behavior and somatic symptoms—a vicious circle
  - Worksheet 9.3a: Implementing more physical activity in the everyday life and consequences: Fourfold table
  - Worksheet 9.3b: Implementing healthy exercise in the everyday life and consequences: Fourfold table
  - Worksheet 9.4a: Practice of the week: avoidance behavior
  - Worksheet 9.4b: Practice of the week: boom and bust behavior

9.1.1 Discussion of the Practice of the Week

Session 12 opens with a discussion of Worksheet 8.14 (Behavioral experiments). The patient's experiences with various behavioral experiments are explored and evaluated:

- What physical discomfort has the patient faced?
- What was their experience?

9.1.2 Patients' Previous Coping Attempts

It can be assumed that in the course of the time patients have been dealing with their somatic symptoms, they have acquired strategies to deal with their symptoms in some way. By asking specific questions, the therapist should collect the previous coping strategies:

What have you done in the past when your symptoms occurred?

Possible answers include: taking it easy, avoiding physical exertion or stress, visits to the physician, examinations, taking medication, relaxation, avoiding certain foods, control behavior, observing oneself and one's own bodily functions more closely, increasing physical activities in order to prove to oneself that one is still functioning as before, etc.

From this collection of coping strategies, the next step is to identify typical avoidance behaviors or "boom and bust behaviors" (depending on where your patient's individual focus lies). In addition, the patient can be given further examples of corresponding behaviors.

Depending on which of the two behavioral categories—avoidance behavior or boom and bust behavior—is in the foreground with the patient, the content focus should be placed on the respective behavioral category at this point and in the further course of the session!

▶ Examples of Avoidance Behavior

- Avoid physical exertion
- Avoid certain postures or movements
- Overall less movement, stop training
- Sick leave
- Reduce or give up tasks at home or at work
- Hand over responsibility
- Cancel appointments (professional and private)
- Giving up social contacts, tasks and duties → social withdrawal
- Change breathing
- Avoid challenges
- Curtail leisure activities
- Avoid certain foods
- Avoid sexuality ◀

▶ Examples of "Boom and Bust"

- Continuation of physical exertion as in the period before the onset of somatic symptoms
- Intensification of physical activities

- Excessive workload
- Excessive activity in own household
- Excessive acceptance of responsibility
- Poor nutrition or fast food in between meals
- Efforts to get as much as possible under one roof
- Increase in sports activities
- „Getting through "sporting activities despite very pronounced somatic symptoms ◄

9.1.3 Avoidance Behavior or Boom and Bust Behaviors and Consequences

With the help of targeted questions, patients should now be supported in becoming aware of the short- and long-term consequences of their avoidance behavior. The focus should be on the short-term positive as well as the long-term negative consequences.

? What are the short-term consequences of these behaviors?

Short-term positive consequences include:
- Decrease in anxiety as symptoms do not worsen,
- Increased attention (family members, partners, friends, physicians),
- Avoidance of physical discomfort.

? What are the long-term consequences of these behaviors?

Long-term negative consequences include:
- Experience that the feared does not occur, is not made,
- Attention remains fixed on somatic symptoms and their negative evaluation,
- Quality of life decreases,
- Activities are restricted,
- Social withdrawal,
- Giving up independence leads to dependence,
- Deterioration of the general physical condition, which may cause further physical discomfort.

For patients who tend to overexert themselves and who show "boom and bust" tendencies, short- and long-term, positive and negative consequences can be derived in analogy to the examples for avoidance behavior. The consequences should be recorded on Worksheet 9.1a (What are the consequences of my avoidance behavior?) or Worksheet 9.1b (What are the consequences of my attempts to "boom"?).

9.1.4 Avoidance or Boom and Bust Behavior and a Vicious Circle Model

The patient is given Worksheet 9.2a/b (Avoidance/boom and bust behavior and somatic symptoms—a vicious circle). With regard to the avoidance behavior, the model illustrates the following: If we are acutely ill or injured, then we spare the affected body part so as not to jeopardise healing. For example, if an arm is broken, then it is immobilized by a cast so that the fracture can heal better. Taking it easy in the case of illness or injury has always been firmly anchored in us and therefore also has a biological meaning. Taking it easy is therefore a normal reaction to physical illness or injury.

In the case of long-term or chronic symptoms or illnesses, the question arises as to how long the affected parts of the body should be spared. We have already worked out that taking it easy has positive consequences in the short term (the symptoms are reduced), but in the long term it can lead to a worsening of the symptoms (frequency and intensity of the symptoms increase). New symptoms occur (e.g., as a result of a poorer general physical condition, the body becomes less resilient, in a state of poor physical condition even slight stress can lead to physical discomfort), activities are neglected or even abandoned and contact with other people is restricted. So this is where the vicious circle arises: Since I have somatic symptoms, I take it easy on myself, which reduces the performance or resilience of my body, which in turn leads to the fact that I will perceive physical discomfort more quickly or even at low levels of stress, which in turn leads to the fact that I judge my body to be sick and not very robust.

In terms of boom and bust behavior, instead of avoiding physical activity, there tends to be overexertion. Patients listen little to their own needs and want to prove to themselves that they still function the same way as they did when they did not experience any somatic symptoms. As a result, patients are constantly pushing their own limits and overtaxing their body. As a result, exhaustion may occur or patients may not feel as resilient as before. Somatic symptoms can be perpetuated by permanent overactivation.

9.1.5 Reduction of Avoidance Behavior/ Promotion of Physical Activity at a Healthy Level

A desired change in behavior—the refraining from the avoidance behavior—is often associated with a short-term worsening of the symptoms. In the same way, the attempt to bring one's own physical activation to a level appropriate to the circumstances can initially be experienced negatively in the short term, as one does not feel as resilient as before or has to make cutbacks and thus feels dissatisfied with oneself. In the long term, however, there is the chance of a better physical condition, which in turn leads to a reduction in somatic symptoms. In the following, patients have to find out in the sense of "guided discovery" how they themselves can break the vicious circle of avoidance behavior or holding out.

? How could you break out of the vicious circle?

The patient receives Worksheet 9.3a or 9.3b (Implementing more exercise in the everyday life and consequences: Fourfold table and Implementing healthy exercise in the everyday life and consequences: Fourfold table). Using the fourfold table shown on the worksheet, the patient and therapist jointly derive advantages and disadvantages that would result for the patient from more exercise and sport in everyday life or a healthy and tolerable level of exercise in everyday life. In collaboration with the therapist, the patient fills in the four boxes. Examples of both positive and negative long-term and short-term consequences are listed below.

▶ Examples of Short- and Long-Term Consequences of Exercise and Sport in Everyday Life

- Short-term positive:
  - Be satisfied with yourself
  - Feeling that you have done something for your fitness
  - Sense of control
  -
- Short-term negative:
  - Rapid exhaustion
  - Increased severity of somatic symptoms
  - More pain
  - Unusual pain
  - Worse mood
- Long-term positive:
  - Stamina gets better
  - Physical resilience becomes better
  - Pain threshold increases, i.e., one becomes more insensitive to pain.
  - Sleep quality improves
  - Better mood
- Long-term negative:
  - Long-term negative consequences should at best not arise at all ◀

Similarly, to reduce physical activity and sport to a reasonable level, short- and long-term, positive and negative consequences can be derived.

9.1.6 Practice of the Week

With the help of Worksheets 9.3a and 9.3b, patients should continue to consider the question of what they could gain if they had the confidence to reduce their avoidance behavior or to reduce their physical activity to an appropriate level. In addition, patients should think about the people who would notice if they would change their behavior and how they would react to it. The goal of the task is to build motivation for change by having patients focus on their thoughts on anticipated positive changes that would be associated with a reduction in their excessive behavior. Patients are given Worksheet 9.4a or 9.4b (Practice of the week: avoidance behavior or Practice of the week: boom and bust behavior).

9.2 Session 13

Contents and Materials of the 13th Session

- **Contents**
  - Discussion of the practice of the week
  - Brief review of the therapy rationale
  - Dealing with less helpful cognitions
  - Behavioral experiments
  - Implementing physical exercise and positive activities in patients' lives
  - Overcoming obstacles of the implementation
  - Practice of the week:
    - Conduct behavioral experiments
    - Record training
- **Materials**
  - Worksheet 9.5: Behavioral experiment: log
  - Worksheet 9.6: Instruction sheet for advanced physical exercise training
  - Worksheet 9.7: My plan of physical exercise and positive activities
  - Worksheet 9.8: My obstacles of implementing physical exercise and positive activities and what I can do about them ...

9.2.1 Discussion of the Practice of the Week

At the beginning of the 13th session, Worksheets 9.3a and 9.3b (Implementing more exercise in the everyday life and consequences: Fourfold table and Implementing healthy exercise in the everyday life and consequences: Fourfold table) and Worksheet 9.4a or 9.4b (Practice of the week on avoidance behavior or Practice of the week on boom and bust behavior) are discussed. In order to continue to promote motivation to change, the patient's focus should be directed in particular towards positive future changes that are associated with a reduction in avoidance or boom and bust behavior.

9.2.2 Brief Review of the Therapy Rationale

It is important to encourage the patient to reduce avoidance behavior or to build up physical fitness, as low fitness generally leads to a reduction in health. If fitness is low, there is a high risk of developing somatic symptoms even during low physical exertion, e.g., during everyday stress. Alternatively, depending on the focus of the content, it should be made clear to the patient again and again that too ambitious attempts to "boom" despite somatic symptoms is also not appropriate. Patients thereby repeatedly brings their own body to its own limits, which in the long term lowers stress tolerance and makes the body susceptible to illness.

9.2.3 Dealing with Less Helpful Cognitions

The fourfould table (Worksheet 9.3a or 9.3b) can be used to detect dysfunctional thoughts and assumptions that occur in the context of reducing avoidance behaviors or boom and bust behaviors. Attention should be drawn to the **perpetuating function of** these unhelpful thoughts. The following is a list of typical dysfunctional cognitions associated with avoidance behaviors or excessive attempts to "boom".

▶ Examples of Typical Dysfunctional Cognitions Associated with Avoidance Behavior

- Typical thoughts and assumptions concerning the **body** or **general bodily functions:**
  - If I move more, my somatic symptoms will get worse! → It should be noted here that this may well be the case in the short term if an untrained body is put under strain; in the long term, however, the body's state of fitness increases, which is accompanied by an improvement or reduction in symptoms.
  - If I don't take it easy, I won't make it through the day and I'll collapse!
  - My body won't stand for it!
  - If I have pain, it means that I have to limit my activities and take it easy, because „pain is a warning signal and therefore dangerous"!
- Typical thoughts and assumptions that affect **specific areas of the body** or **selected bodily functions:**
  - I can't move too much or exert myself too much or I will have a heart attack!
  - When I exercise, I tense my muscles; I'm sure I'll get an upset stomach and have to go to the bathroom right away! ◀

▶ Examples of Typical Dysfunctional Cognitions Related to "Holding Out" Behavior

- I have to hang in there and function as I always have!
- If my body can't take it, I can't take it!
- If I don't function the way I used to, everything falls apart!
- I have to prove it to myself that everything still works the way it did when I had no symptoms.
- I can't just "shut down" and do less now! ◀

The therapist should seek to change these usually stubborn beliefs through **disputation**, i.e. questioning and reviewing these evaluations. The helpful questions on thinking errors in session 10 (▶ Sect. 8.4) can be used for this purpose. Another method of restructuring unhelpful thoughts is behavioral experimentation, which will be discussed below.

9.2.4 Behavioral Experiments

Behavioral experiments have already been used in session 9 (▶ Sect. 8.3). It can be repeated here that they are another technique from the repertoire of behavioral therapy to change dysfunctional thoughts and assumptions of patients. With their help, patients should be given the opportunity to check whether their fears come true or whether their assumptions correspond to reality. However, the focus in this session should be primarily on the thoughts that specifically promote avoidance or boom and bust behaviors. In session 9, on the other hand, the focus was more on generally unhelpful thoughts related to patients' somatic symptoms.

The following example Illustrates"the behavioral experiment technique using the topic of vertigo (adapted from Bennett-Levy et al., 2004).

▶ Dizziness and the Avoidance of Head Movements

- Dysfunctional cognitions to review: "I can't stand vertigo. I am likely to fall over. When I get dizzy, I have to avoid moving my head or moving at all."

- Alternative, functional views: "I often feel dizzy, which shows that I can tolerate dizziness. If I avoid head movement, my vestibular organ will not be able to learn to adapt. By avoiding movement, I will not be able to learn to cope with the dizziness. My vertigo problem will get bigger and bigger as a result – it would be like a vicious cycle. If I dare to move more while having dizziness, my vestibular organ will get used to it and I will gradually get better."
- Patient's expectation regarding the behavioral experiment:" the more I move, the dizzier I'll get and the worse I'll feel."
- Behavioral experiment: Patients are asked to turn in a circle 10 times to induce dizziness. They should pay close attention to the dizziness. Patients should perform this exercise—if dizziness is a relevant symptom for them—daily for one week and record their experience. ◀

The patient receives Worksheet 9.5 (Behavioral Experiment: log).

In the sense of learning from the model, the therapist can participate in the behavioral experiment. Another suggested exercise to speed up heartbeat and breathing is to do 10 squats or "jumping jacks" 20 times. Following the exercise, the therapist should point out that faster breathing and a faster pulse are **normal responses to physical exertion** and should therefore be taken as signs of a healthy body.

In the event that patients do not show any avoidance behavior, but rather boom and bust behavior, a behavioral experiment can also be planned, which should then, however, be scheduled as practice of the week. For example, patients could be asked to consciously plan where they would like to reduce their activity level in the coming week; for example, they could decide to cut back on strenuous activities that are obligatory for them (e.g., cleaning the apartment) and instead plan a positive, relaxing activity that they enjoy. In the event that patients have problems with their time planning, the contents of session 17 (▶ Sect. 10.2) could be anticipated at this point.

9.2.5 Implementing Physical Exercise and Positive Activities in Patients' Lives

In this session, the focus is on building more movement into the patients' daily routine. For patients with pronounced avoidance behavior, the focus here is primarily on planning physical activities. However, if patients also have less "sporty" but positive activities in general (e.g., going to concerts, meeting friends), which they also avoid because of their symptoms, these should be taken into account later when drawing up the activity plan.

For patients with rather pronounced boom and bust tendencies, it is important to set up a program of physical activities that are restorative, healthy (but not too excessive) and good for them. Their previous excessive level of activity should be reduced to a healthy level. In doing so, not only sporting activities but also other positive activities that have been neglected recently should be consciously included. Indications of sporting or generally positive activities that patients enjoy or have enjoyed can be taken from the list in Worksheet 7.9.

To initiate the planning of sporting activities, the patient is given Worksheet 9.6 (Instruction sheet for advanced physical exercise training). The essential points are discussed. Physical activity improves **fitness**, increases **resistance** to stress and promotes mental **well-being** (feelings of invigoration, refreshment, balance or pleasant relaxation). Roughly summarized, physical performance can be increased in two ways (Kaluza, 2004): more movement in everyday life and regular exercise. For patients with "boom and bust tendencies", this leaflet is primarily intended to clarify what constitutes "healthy" sport.

In cooperation with the patient, an individual rehabilitation program is to be developed to improve the patient's physical fitness. The first step is to collect sports or physical activities that the patient currently performs. The second step is to collect athletic activities that the patient has enjoyed in the past and currently avoids. Below are some suggestions for incorporating more exercise into everyday life (Kaluza, 2004).

▶ Suggestions for Exercise in Everyday Life (Based on Kaluza, 2004)

- Gardening
- Brisk walking (deliberately walking one step faster than usual)
- Riding a bike instead of using a car or public transport
- Climbing stairs instead of using an elevator
- Shove snow, sweep leaves or street
- Walk the dog
- Gymnastic exercises
- Walks ◀

Any regular physical activity that at least leads to an acceleration of breathing and is performed for at least 10 min already promotes health. Patients should make sure to challenge themselves physically as much as possible every day, but at least 5 days a week. Patients should also make sure to consciously increase the intensity and duration of physical activities in their everyday life (e.g., take fewer breaks, take several steps at once when climbing stairs; Kaluza, 2004). The following is a summary of suggestions for regular exercise.

▶ Suggestions for Regular Sporting Activities (Based on Kaluza, 2004)

- Jogging
- (Nordic) Walking
- Swimming
- Cycling
- Cross-country skiing ◀

Patients should now be motivated by questions from the therapist to look for physical activities that would give them pleasure. They should be encouraged to think concretely about how they could implement these activities in their everyday life.

- What type of physical activity would you enjoy the most?
- In what environment would you most like to be physically active?
- Do you prefer to exercise indoors or outdoors?
- Would you prefer to do sports alone or together with others?

The patient's current physical capacity should of course be taken into account when planning and creating the build-up training. Lack of exercise leads to an underload of the body. Immediately overloading the body can lead to overstressing it. Both under- and over-exertion are harmful. As is so often the case, the dose of a behavior determines its effect.

As a rule of thumb to prevent overexertion, the following applies: You should still be able to talk during the sporting activity. To prevent overexertion, it is also important to take breaks. Other important tips: Only regular sporting activity brings long-lasting benefits. Regular means at least 3 times a week, for at least 20 min. In addition, warming up, loosening up and stretching, preparing muscles and joints for sporting activity should not be forgotten in order to prevent injuries. In addition, the patient should ensure sufficient fluid intake due to fluid loss through sweating (Kaluza, 2004).

In order to achieve a quick sense of achievement, you should start with simple or easily achievable exercises, e.g., short walks at the weekend. A gradual increase can be achieved on the one hand by increasing the intensity (faster performance of the activities) and on the other hand by increasing the duration (more activities or more frequent performance per week). Initially, it makes sense to increase the duration so that the activity can be carried out for at least 20 min with moderate intensity. Only then should the intensity be gradually increased, e.g., running or swimming faster (Kaluza, 2004).

The importance of **positive self-instruction,** or more generally the relevance of **reward** in establishing new behaviors, should be explained to the patient. It is considered scientifically proven that behavior that is positively reinforced or rewarded is exhibited more often and is more stable than behavior that is not reinforced at all. It is important to learn how to reinforce oneself. Accordingly, patients are instructed to "pat themselves on the back" each time they have performed a physical activity. In addition to positive words, other forms of self-reward are also possible. Patients can therefore be asked in what other form they could reward themselves when they have carried out agreed exercises.

After this important information has been collected and explained, a training plan is now drawn up together with the patient (Worksheet 9.7: My plan of physical exercise and positive activities). First of all, a sports workload for the coming week is to be compiled within the framework of the weekly plan. The aim is that the patient then maintains this plan for 2 weeks (until the end of therapy). The program can then be extended in the following weeks. For this purpose, two "incremental steps" should already be worked out on Worksheet 9.7. In addition to the sporting activities, other positive activities that the patient has neglected so far should also be entered in the plan.

9.2.6 Overcoming Obstacles of the Implementation

It should be made clear to the patient that the beginning of such a profound change in behavior is always difficult and that one will encounter resistance within oneself. This is quite normal. However, there are a few strategies that make it a little easier to overcome one's "own stubbornness", such as planning sporting activities together with another person, putting the sports bag in the car straight away or scheduling the activities at fixed times. Together with your patients, anticipate their possible obstacles, enter them on Worksheet 9.8 (My obstacles of implementing physical exercise and positive activities and what I can do about them ...) and think about solution strategies together.

9.2.7 Practice of the Week

Patients should carry out the agreed training program and behavioral experiments over the next week or more and record their experiences (including any difficulties encountered) on Worksheet 9.7 (My plan of physical exercise and positive activities).

9.3 Session 14

Contents and Materials of the 14th Session

- **Contents**
  - Discussion of the practice of the week
  - Experiences with somatic symptoms and illness behavior
  - Identify individual positive consequences associated with the sick role
  - Developing alternative behaviors that also lead to positive consequences
  - Practice of the week: How do I treat myself in a caring way? (Worksheet 9.10)
- **Materials**
  - Worksheet 9.9: Light and shadow of the sick role
  - Worksheet 9.10: How do I treat myself in a caring way?

9.3.1 Discussion of the Practice of the Week

At the beginning, Worksheet 9.7 (My plan of physical exercise and positive activities) is discussed: To what extent has the patient been successful in implementing the exercise program developed in the last session to increase fitness or physical resilience? Helpful questions for further evaluation can be:

- What difficulties were encountered?
- How did the physical stress affect the symptoms?

If necessary, revisions should be made to the training and activity plan (Worksheet 9.7). If unexpected obstacles have arisen, solutions should be sought together. In addition, the patient's experience with behavioral experiments should be explored:

- Have behavioral experiments been conducted?
- If so, with what success?

9.3.2 Experiences with Somatic Symptoms and Illness Behavior

As an introduction to the topic of gaining illness, the therapist should be aware of the following:

> Illness behaviors can also be thought of as behaviors learned through operant conditioning, especially in childhood. Reinforcers can be increased attention from other people, avoidance of unpleasant work or unpleasant social situations, and financial benefits. Furthermore, there is model learning, whereby children adopt the behavior of their parents. (Margraf et al., 1998)

The sick role is defined as a combination of obligations and privileges that come with being sick (Rief & Nanke, 2003). Today's session will focus on the benefits, privileges or positive consequences associated with the sick role. In this context, one also speaks of **"illness gain"**. This topic is a delicate one, as patients can quickly get the impression that they are perceived to be only faking their symptoms or presenting them in an exaggerated manner in order to intentionally benefit from them. The introduction to the topic should therefore be gentle. The following questions can be helpful, as they are based on the patient's experience and do not contain any insinuations.

- Has anyone in your family or close circle of friends or acquaintances been ill for a longer period (more than 3 months)?
- What did this person miss because of their symptoms or illness? Has he/she had to do without anything? (This is a question about disadvantages or limitations associated with an illness).
- How did other people react to the symptoms or illness? How did they behave towards the sick person?
- Did the sick person also have any benefits due to their symptoms?
- If so, which ones? (If the patient can't think of anything, give some examples).

In the next step, the focus is directed to your patients and their experiences with the sick role. A look is taken at childhood and adolescence.

- If you were ill as a child—how did your parents or other significant others react?
- Did you have to go to the doctor then and miss school as a result?
- Were you given more attention when you were sick?

9.3.3 Identify Individual Positive Consequences Associated with the Sick Role

It is often difficult to encourage patients to think about the personal positive consequences that may be associated with their role as a patient. The following instruction should be understood as an aid to get as therapist the "foot in the door" on this rather sensitive topic.

Instruction: Identification of Positive Consequences of the Sick Role

In the sessions so far, we have primarily dealt with the disadvantages or negative consequences associated with your somatic symptoms (list individual patient limitations at this point). Let us now try to look at the "other side of the coin". As we all know, there are always two. So if you look closely—are there perhaps also positive consequences that follow from your somatic symptoms? What could these be?

The patient receives Worksheet 9.9 (Light and shadow of the sick role). Positive consequences that can be associated with the sick role are, for example, the following:

- Increased attention, increased interest, more attention and care/comfort from other people,
- Avoidance or release from unpleasant tasks or usual obligations (work, school, household, annoying appointments),
- Avoidance of uncomfortable social situations,
- More consideration for the patient within the family (patient is spared, not unnecessarily burdened, conflicts are avoided),
- Financial allowance (sickness benefit, early retirement).

These positive consequences or objective advantages associated with the sick role are called "secondary gain". Assuming that the patient would be free of symptoms or healthy again, this would mean the loss of this "gain". Further questions on the subject of "gain from illness" are listed below.

?
- What benefits do you think you could lose if your symptoms improve?
- What would change in your environment?
- Can you imagine giving up the positive consequences associated with the disease?

9.3.4 Developing Alternative Behaviors that Also Lead to Positive Consequences

Now it is a question of considering together how identified positive sides could be achieved other than through the sick role. The sick role should therefore be made superfluous to a certain extent, but at the same time care should be taken to ensure that important needs of the patient can be met in other ways. The following question could help in this regard:

? How can you satisfy your needs (e.g., for more attention, more interest, fewer duties) without having to remain in the sick role?

9.3.5 Practice of the Week

Patients receive Worksheet 9.10 (How do I treat myself in a caring way?). Until the next session, they should consider what needs are being met by the current sick role (e.g., attention from others). In addition, they should consider how they can meet the identified needs in other ways. They should record the results of their reflections in writing. In addition, patients should continue to implement the training program (Worksheet 9.7).

9.4 Session 15

Contents and Materials of the 15th Session

- **Contents**
  - Discussion of the practice of the week
  - Previous experience with doctor visits and medical treatment
  - The ideal doctor
  - Practice of the week: Doctor visits (Worksheet 9.13)
- **Materials**
  - Worksheet 9.11: Seeking reassurance from doctors—a vicious circle
  - Worksheet 9.12: What you should know about visiting the doctor
  - Worksheet 9.13: Practice of the week on the topic "Doctor visits"

9.4.1 Discussion of the Practice of the Week

The aim is to check whether and how well the patient has succeeded in implementing the exercise program to increase fitness or physical resilience (Worksheet 9.7). Helpful questions for the evaluation of the practice of the week can be:

?
- What difficulties were encountered?
- How did the physical stress affect the symptoms?

If necessary, revisions should be made to the training and activity plan (Worksheet 9.7). If unexpected obstacles have arisen, solutions should be sought together. Patients should be advised at this point to hang up their training plan in a clearly visible place. From now on, they must motivate themselves to continue the physical and positive activities. Now that the first two weeks of training have passed, patients should be encouraged to move on to the next higher level of the training plan starting next week. Patients should again record their experience (Worksheet 9.7). In addition, Worksheet 9.10 (How do I treat myself in a caring way?) should be discussed.

9.4.2 Previous Experience of Visits to Doctors and Medical Treatment

First, for the therapist: A common feature of patients with somatoform disorders is **frequent use of medical services** (but this need not be the case; there are indeed patients who rarely or never consult physicians). Patients with somatoform disorders often have difficulty accepting that there is no sufficient organic medical cause for the somatic symptoms, which often leads to strains on the physician-patient relationship (on the patient side: frustration, disappointment, helplessness, breaking off the relationship; on the physician side: Frustration and disappointment at the lack of successful treatment, irritation, insinuation of simulation or aggravation of the symptoms, premature consideration of psychological conflicts and discouragement of diagnostic examinations) or to the patient demanding further organ-medical measures or frequently changing doctors ("doctor-shopping" or "doctor-hopping"). Important: Temporary organically unexplained somatic symptoms that do not become the cause of repeated visits to the doctor are part of normality and must not be confused with somatoform disorders that tend to become chronic.

In the sense of an introduction to the topic "Utilization of medical services", the patient's experiences to date with physicians and medical examinations and treatments can be explored.

9.4.3 The Ideal Doctor

In order to find out what the patients' idea of an "ideal doctor" is and what expectations they have of their "ideal doctor", the following questions can be helpful:

- What does an ideal doctor look like in your eyes?
- What do you hope for, what do you wish for, what do you expect from him?
- What qualities should an ideal type of doctor have?

The therapist and patient should then work out which needs are associated with each of the characteristics or expectations mentioned. Examples of these are given below.

▶ Examples of Needs that May Be Behind the "Characteristics of the Ideal Doctor" Are

- Need for security; to feel that they are in good hands; associated characteristics: The doctor should …
  - be competent
  - have a lot of expertise
  - inform myself thoroughly (test results etc.)
  - tell me everything is all right
  - can help me quickly and professionally
  - eliminate my pain
- Need to be taken seriously; feel involved in treatment; associated characteristics: The doctor should …
  - listen to me or listen to my problems
  - are interested in my explanatory approaches/hypotheses
  - want to cooperate with me
- Need to be cared for; to feel that the doctor cares for one; associated qualities: The doctor should …
  - have time for me
  - build me up, comfort me, give me courage
  - be warm, caring
  - to be empathetic, to be able to respond to me
  - be kind ◀

The need for **reassurance** about the harmlessness of the symptoms is usually particularly strong in patients with **illness anxiety.** If the patient also has illness anxieties, then the "vicious circle" of reassurance (short-term-consequence: fear reduction; principle of negative reinforcement) and maintenance of the illness anxiety (long-term-consequence) should be explained at this point.

Other **long-term consequences** of frequent visits to the doctor (based on Bleichhardt & Weck, 2011):
- Focus on disease,
- Increase in reassurance (due to experienced anxiety reduction),
- Dependence on feedback from the doctor,
- Ability to distinguish between harmless and serious symptoms decreases,
- Tolerance for fear decreases,
- Experience that one can help oneself or that the symptoms can disappear again without a visit to the doctor is missing,
- Different doctors have different opinions, so that uncertainty can arise in the patient,
- The doctor may examine less and less thoroughly the more often you come,
- It costs a lot of time and money,
- Examinations and medications also have unwanted side effects,

- You could catch it in the waiting room/hospital,
- Possibly a disease can be detected more quickly and thus treated more effectively (a positive long-term consequence).

Due to the numerous negative long-term consequences, a reduction in frequent visits to the doctor is the logical and desirable consequence.

The aim should be **time-contingent** (as opposed to **symptom-contingent**) doctor visits, i.e. the doctor consultation takes place at fixed intervals and not as quickly as possible, as soon as symptoms and illness anxiety increase. The time contingency is intended to take away the anxiety-reducing effect of doctor visits. Patients should be given the opportunity to cope with anxiety independently and to attribute the anxiety-reducing effect to themselves and no longer to the examination or the doctor's statement.

The patient receives Worksheet 9.11 (Seeking reassurance from doctors—a vicious circle). Subsequently, patients should be supported through guided discovery to find an appropriate level of doctor visits for them. The following questions can be useful:

?
- Which of the above is realistic?
- What can be fulfilled?
- What problems/symptoms can you handle yourself and with what strategies?
- When does it make sense for you to go to the doctor, when not?

With regard to the last question, the following should ideally be mentioned:

- In the case of already known somatic symptoms, own coping possibilities are selected and tried out.
- Visits to the doctor are particularly advisable in the case of new, massive and long-lasting somatic symptoms.
- It is better to go to the doctor at regular intervals (time-contingent, e.g., once a month) than every time when symptoms occur or when there is a general deterioration in well-being (this would be symptom-contingent behavior).

The patient is given Worksheet 9.12 (What you should know about visiting the doctor).

9.4.4 Practice of the Week

The patient receives Worksheet 9.13 Practice of the week on the topic "doctor visits"). The task is explained according to the information on the worksheet.

9.5 Worksheets

These worksheets are also available for download online at Springer Extras (► extras.springer.com).

Worksheet 9.1a	What are the consequences of my avoidance behavior?	◘ Figure 9.1
Worksheet 9.1b	What are the consequences of my attempts to "boom"?	◘ Figure 9.2
Worksheet 9.2a	Avoidance behavior and somatic symptoms—a vicious circle	◘ Figure 9.3
Worksheet 9.2b	Boom and bust behavior and somatic symptoms—a vicious circle	◘ Figure 9.4
Worksheet 9.3a	Implementing more physical activity in the everyday life and consequences: Fourfold table	◘ Figure 9.5
Worksheet 9.3b	Implementing healthy exercise in the everyday life and consequences: Fourfold table	◘ Figure 9.6
Worksheet 9.4a	Practice of the week: Avoidance behavior	◘ Figure 9.7
Worksheet 9.4b	Practice of the week: Boom and bust behavior	◘ Figure 9.8
Worksheet 9.5	Behavioral experiment: Log	◘ Figure 9.9
Worksheet 9.6	Instruction sheet for advanced physical exercise training	◘ Figure 9.10
Worksheet 9.7	My plan for physical exercise and positive activities	◘ Figure 9.11
Worksheet 9.8	My obstacles of implementing physical exercise and postive activities and what I can do about them …	◘ Figure 9.12
Worksheet 9.9	Light and shadow of the sick role	◘ Figure 9.13
Worksheet 9.10	How do I treat myself in a caring way?	◘ Figure 9.14
Worksheet 9.11	Seeking reassurance from doctors—a vicious circle	◘ Figure 9.15
Worksheet 9.12	What you should know about visiting the doctor	◘ Figure 9.16
Worksheet 9.13	Practice of the week on the topic of "doctor visits"	◘ Figure 9.17

Fig. 9.1 Worksheet 9.1a: What are the consequences of my avoidance behavior?

Worksheet 9.1a: What are the consequences of my avoidance behavior?

Please enter the consequences of your avoidance behavior in your everyday life!
Think about positive as well as negative consequences, in the short as well as in the long term!

	short-term consequences	long-term consequences
 positive	short-term/positive	long-term/positive
 negative	short-term/negative	long-term/negative

Fig. 9.2 Worksheet 9.1b: What are the consequences of my attempts to "boom"?

Worksheet 9.1b: What are the consequences of my attempts to "boom"?

Please enter the consequences of your attempts "boom" in your everyday life!
Think about positive as well as negative consequences, in the short as well as in the long term!

	short-term consequences	long-term consequences
☺ positive	short-term/positive	long-term/positive
☹ negative	short-term/negative	long-term/negative

Fig. 9.3 Worksheet 9.2a: Avoidance behavior and somatic symptoms—a vicious circle

Worksheet 9.2a: Avoidance behavior and somatic symptoms – a vicious circle

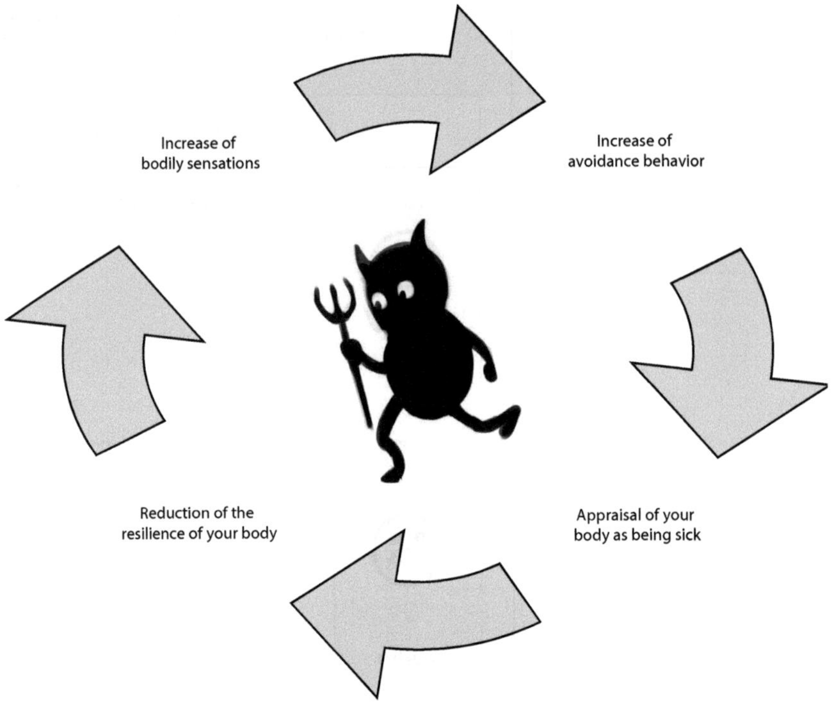

How can you break out of this vicious circle?

It is necessary to reduce the avoidance behavior, because this maintains the physical discomfort. You can reduce avoidance behavior by exposing yourself to more physical stress, despite existing somatic symptoms. It is important that physical performance is increased slowly and gradually. You can improve your physical shape, for example, by Nordic walking, cycling, or swimming. However, you should be prepared for the fact that the physical discomforts may worsen in the short term as a result of the increased physical movement and exercise. In the long term, however, you have with a reduction of the avoidance behavior the possibility to reduce your somatic permanently.

Fig. 9.4 Worksheet 9.2b: Boom and bust behavior and somatic symptoms—a vicious circle

Worksheet 9.2b: Boom and bust behavior and somatic symptoms – a vicious circle

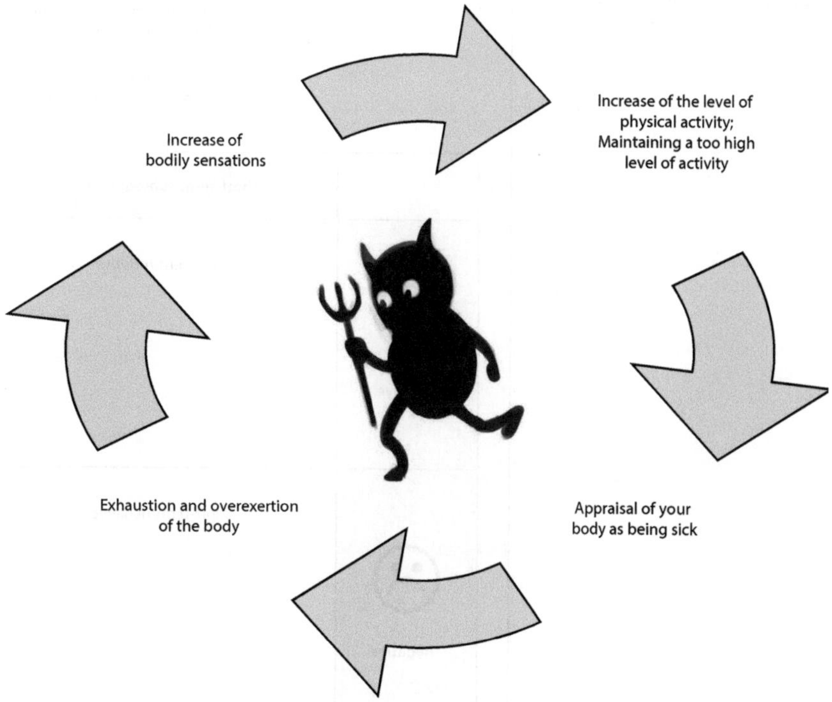

How can you break out of this vicious circle?

It is necessary to reduce your aspirations "to boom", because these maintain your somatic symptoms. You can reduce this rather obstructive behavior by trying to find an appropriate and reasonable level of physical activation. It is important that you increase your level of physical activity only slowly and gradually. While it is significant that you remain active despite your physical discomfort, you should do so only to the extent that it also does you good. It is important that you focus on activities that you have enjoyed so far. You should be prepared to feel dissatisfied with yourself in the short term, when you reduce your high levels of activity. In the long term, however, you have the opportunity to permanently reduce your somatic symptoms if you do not constantly push your body to its limits.

Fig. 9.5 Worksheet 9.3a: Implementing more physical activity in the everyday life and consequences: Fourfould table

Worksheet 9.3a: Implementing more physical activity in the everyday life and consequences: Fourfold table

What happens when I reduce my avoidance behavior and gain more and more confidence?

Enter the consequences of a change in behavior in the fourfold table below.

	short-term consequences	**long-term** consequences
☺ positive	short-term/positive	long-term/positive
☹ negative	short-term/negative	long-term/negative

Fig. 9.6 Worksheet 9.3b: Implementing healthy exercise in the everday life and consequences: Fourfold table

Worksheet 9.3b: Implementing healthy exercise in everyday life and consequences: Fourfold table

What happens when I reduce my attempts to "boom" and I get back to an appropriate level of physical activity?

Enter the consequences of a change in behaviour in the fourfold table below.

	Short-term consequences	**Long-term** consequences
☺ **positive**	short-term/positive	long-term/positive
☹ **negative**	short-term/negative	long-term/negative

Fig. 9.7 Worksheet 9.4a: Practice of the week: avoidance behavior

Worksheet 9.4a: Practice of the week: avoidance behavior

Who will notice that I have reduced my avoidance behavior, that I trust myself more and more and that I I've become more active? How will my environment react to this? How will people behave towards me?

....

....

....

....

....

....

....

....

....

....

....

....

....

....

....

....

....

....

....

....

Fig. 9.8 Worksheet 9.4b: Practice of the week: boom and bust behavior

Worksheet 9.4b: Practice of the week: boom and bust behavior

Who will notice that I have reduced my attempts to "boom", that I have become more attentive to my needs and that I get back to an appropriate level of physical activity? How will my environment react to this? How will people behave towards me?

....

....

....

....

....

....

....

....

....

....

....

....

....

....

....

....

....

....

....

....

Fig. 9.9 Worksheet 9.5: Behavioral experiment: log

Worksheet 9.5: Behavioral experiment: log

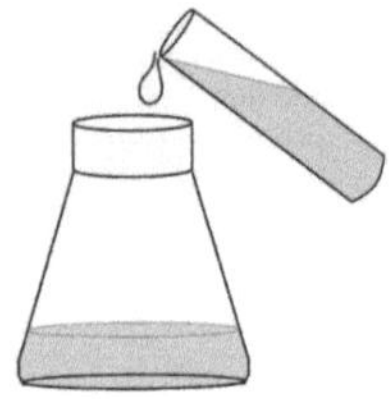

Day, time	
Somatic symptom that I want to expose myself to	
Expectation/prediction: What exactly do I expect will happen Probability that my expectation/prediction is correct? 0–100	
Experiment: What did I do to check my expectation/prediction against reality?	
Results: What actually happened? Was my expectation and prediction correct?	
What I'm learning from this: Has my expectation changed? Probability that the expectation is true (in the future)? 0–100	

Fig. 9.10 Worksheet 9.6: Instruction sheet for advanced physical exercise training

Worksheet 9.6: Instruction sheet for advanced physical exercise training

- If you are physically active on a regular basis, you will improve your fitness and increase your body's performance and resistance.
- In addition, regular physical activity promotes physical and mental well-being.
- To increase your fitness, you can move more in your daily life and/or exercise regularly.
- More exercise in your everyday life: You should be physically active as much as possible every day, but at least 5 days a week (acceleration of your breathing for at least 10 min).
- Exercise regularly: Consider your current physical fitness level! Both under- and overexertion is detrimental to your health. Keep in mind as a rule of thumb: You should be able to have a conversation while you exercise.
- Only regular physical activity provides long-lasting benefits; regular means at least 3 times a week for at least 20 minutes
- Take a break!
- Don't forget to warm up to prevent injuries!
- Make sure you drink enough fluids!
- Gradually increase the duration and only then the intensity of the physical activity!
- Reward yourself for your physical activity – either by praising yourself (e.g., for overcoming the obstacles that kept you from exercising more regularly in the past) or by giving yourself a treat!

Fig. 9.11 Worksheet 9.7: My plan for physical exercise and positive activities

Worksheet 9.7: My plan for physical exercise and positive activities

- for the next 2 weeks: ______________ [insert date] -

Increase your fitness and resilience by planning and implementing physical activities for the coming week! Also, think about other positive activities that you have neglected lately. Record your plans and experiences!

Weekday	What physical activity do I plan to do?	Did somatic symptoms occur? If yes, which symptoms and how severe? 0–10	Were there any difficulties in implementing the physical activity, e.g., less helpful and hindering thoughts? If so, which ones?	Did I reward myself afterwards? If so, how?	What other positive activities do I plan that I avoided in the past?
Monday					
Tuesday					
Wednesday					
Thursday					
Friday					
Saturday					
Sunday					

From Kleinstäuber, M. et al: Cognitive behavioral therapy for medically unexplained physical complaints and somatoform disorders.

■ **Fig. 9.11** (continued)

Worksheet 9.7 (continued): My plan for physical exercise and positive activities

- for another 2 weeks: ______________ [insert date] -

After the first 2 weeks of increasing your physical activity or positive activities, think about how you can further expand your program of physical exerice and positive activities.

Weekday	What physical activity do I plan to do?	Did somatic symptoms occur? If yes, which symptoms and how severe? 0–10	Were there any difficulties in implementing the physical activity, e.g., less helpful and hindering thoughts?	Did I reward myself afterwards? If so, how?	What other positive activities do I plan that I avoided in the past?
Monday					
Tuesday					
Wednesday					
Thursday					
Friday					
Saturday					
Sunday					

Fig. 9.11 (continued)

Worksheet 9.7 (continued): My plan for physical exercise and positive activities

- for a further 4 weeks: ____________________ [insert date] -

After the first 2 weeks of increasing your physical activity or positive activities, think about how you can further expand your program of physical exerice and positive activities.

Weekday	What physical activity do I plan to do?	Did somatic symptoms occur? If yes, which symptoms and how severe? 0–10	Were there any difficulties in implementing the physical activity, e.g., less helpful and hindering thoughts?	Did I reward myself afterwards? If so, how?	What other positive activities do I plan that I avoided in the past ?
Monday					
Tuesday					
Wednesday					
Thursday					
Friday					
Saturday					
Sunday					

Fig. 9.12 Worksheet 9.8: My obstacles of implementing physical exercise positive activities and what I can do about them …

Worksheet 9.8: My obstacles of implementing physical exercise and positive activities and what I can do about them...

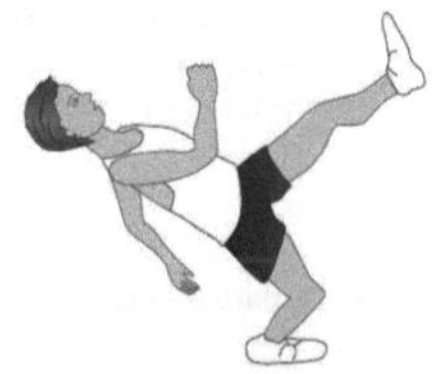

My obstacles of implementing physical exercise and positive activities	What can I do about my obstacles?

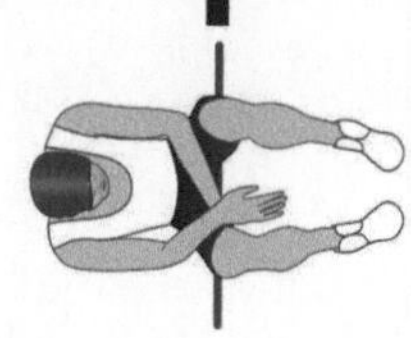

Fig. 9.13 Worksheet 9.9: Light and shadow of the sick role

Worksheet 9.9: Light and shadow of the sick role

On the one hand, being ill is associated with numerous disadvantages that you know all too well. On the other hand – and it sounds strange at times – there are, however, certain benefits associated with being sick. However they are not as obvious at first glance as the limitations. These advantages, which are associated with the sickness, are very important to consider, as they can play an important role in perpetuating somatic symptoms. Potential benefits of the sick role:

Potential benefits of the sick role:

- Increased attention, increased interest, care and comfort from other people
- Avoidance or release from unpleasant tasks or usual obligations (work, school, household, appointments)
- More consideration for a person (it is avoided to put unnecessarily burden on a person, conflicts are avoided), e.g., avoidance of conflicts in families
- Financial support (sickness benefit, early retirement)

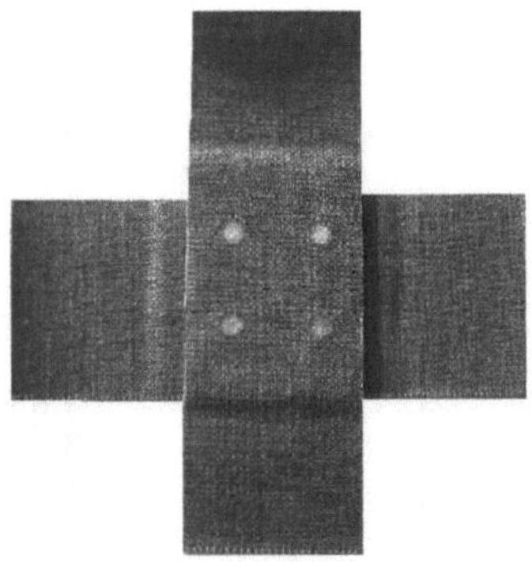

Fig. 9.14 Worksheet 9.10: How do I treat myself in a caring way?

Worksheet 9.10: How do I treat myself in a caring way?

My strategies of being more attentive to my needs

What is my need? What's important to me? What do I need?	How can I be more attentive to my needs?

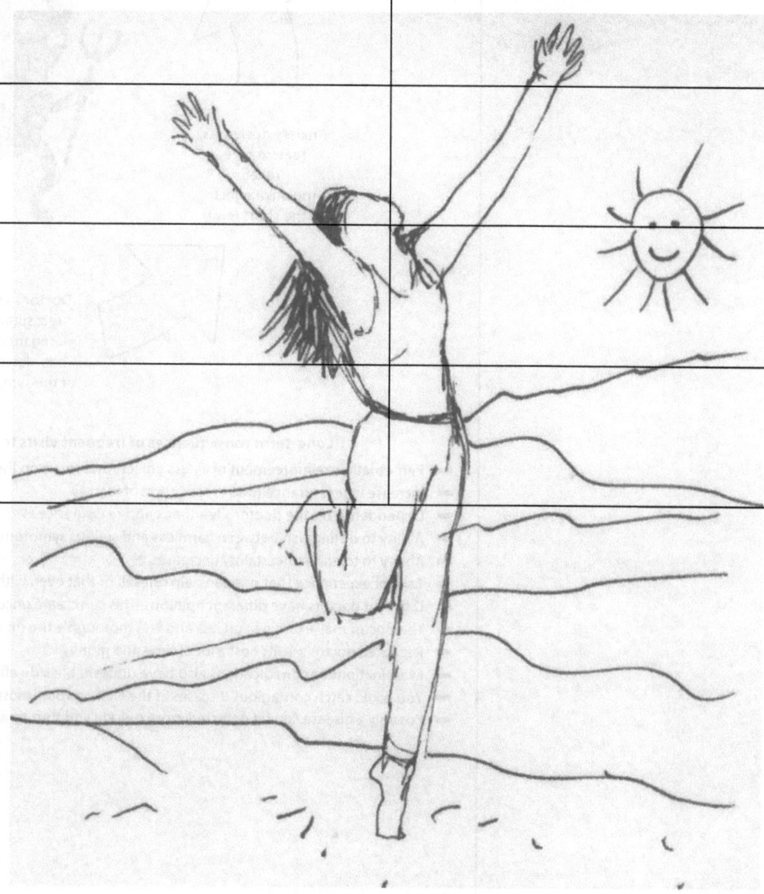

9

Fig. 9.15 Worksheet 9.11: Seeking reassurance from doctors—a vicious circle

Worksheet 9.11: Seeking reassurance from doctors – a vicious circle

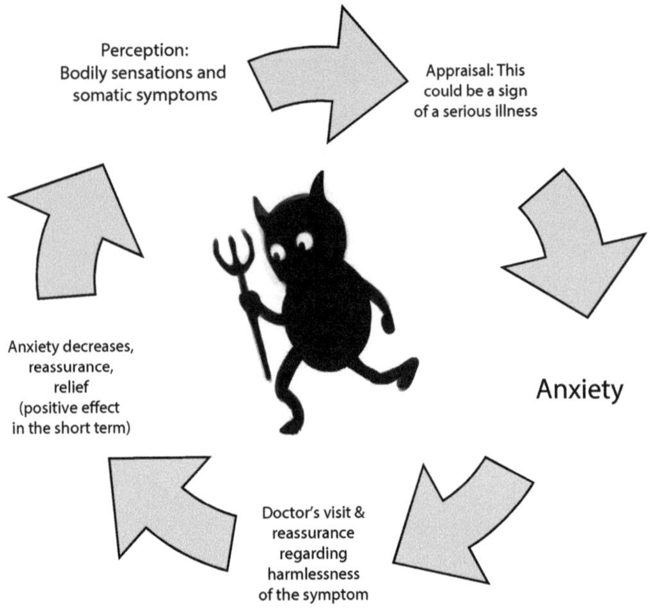

Long-term consequences of frequent visits to the doctor or seeking medical reassurance

- Perpetuation/reinforcement of illness anxiety and focus on the topic of illness ☹
- Increase in reassurance (due to reduction of fear) ☹
- Dependence on the doctor's feedback and reassurance ☹
- Ability to distinguish between harmless and serious symptoms decreases ☹
- Ability to tolerate uncertainty decreases ☹
- Lack of experience that one can help oneself or that even without a visit to the doctor the symptoms can remit ☹
- Different doctors have different opinions. This can create uncertainty for the patient. ☹
- The doctor may examine you less and less thoroughly the more often you have doctor's appointments. ☹
- Repeated doctor's visits cost a lot of time and money ☹
- Examinations and medications also have undesirable side effects ☹
- You could catch contagious diseases in the waiting room/hospital. ☹
- Possibly a disease can be detected more quickly and thus treated more effectively ☺

◻ **Fig. 9.16** Worksheet 9.12: What you should know about visiting the doctor

Worksheet 9.12: What you should know about visiting the doctor

Pain and other somatic symptoms often have a signalling function. They can alert us to injuries or diseases. Therefore, when new, unknown symptoms appear and do not go away on their own, it is important and reasonable to seek medical help. Careful medical examinations can help to discover possible medical conditions and the necessary treatments (e.g., pharmacological therapy) can be initiated.

However, somatic symptoms and bodily sensations do not always have to be an expression of an medical condition. They can be caused by various different things. Often they arise from the interaction of different factors (e.g., persistent daily hassles or stressful life events, an indiviudal's level of physical fitness, weather, age, vigilance towards body, illness). Repeated medical examinations usually do not help to completely explain the causes of the symptoms, as the focus remains solely on the body. Nevertheless many individuals who are affected by persistent somatic symptoms, repeatedly consult with doctors and hospital staff and go through extensive diagnostics, because they feel sick and helpless and hope to find ways of making their symptom completely diminish. Some patients embark on a veritable odyssey, wandering over years from doctor to doctor, from one expert to the next specialist. Others, however, rarely or never see a doctor. The individual reaction to less medically explained, persistent somatic symptoms can look very different – it ranges from the avoidance of medical services to an extensive utilization of medical services. Given that medicine is in a continuous process of development, research constantly reveals new findings, diagnostic methods and pharmacological agents, which constantly induces hope in patients to finally find explanations and treatments of their symptoms. Patients often take medications that promise short-term relief. Sometimes the prescription of a drug by a doctor can let patients feel confirmed that they suffer from a medical condition ("The doctor prescribes me with a medicine, so I have to be sick."). This can sometimes be fatal, if other possible explanations for the symptoms as well as active coping strategies are ignored. In addition, patients can develop less helpful expectations which induce passivity in patients (e.g., "Only a drug can help me!").

Frequent visits to the doctor should also be viewed critically, given that the actual developmental factors of the somatic symptoms remain undiscovered and the search for alternative possible explanations and alternative coping strategies can be hampered. As a patient with persistent somatic symptoms, one should therefore do not rely solely on medical action (medical examinations and diagnostics, prescription of medication), but patients should also become proactive and look for strategies of how they influence their symptoms by themselves. More or less medically explained, persistent somatic symptoms, do not have to be a significant problem. Many people have learned to cope with the discomfort. Although they also suffer from the symptoms, they learn to understand them and to take appropriate action to manage them.

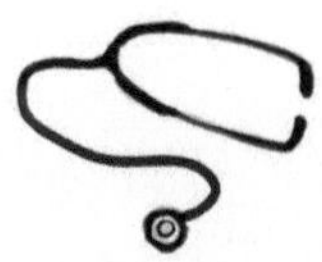

It is often helpful for patients with recurring somatic symptoms to set a fixed time schedule for doctor's visits, i.e.,to schedule regular doctor's visits (e.g., once a year or a month). If, in the meantime (between two scheduled doctor's appointments), your physical well-being changes or worsens, you should not automatically make an additional doctor's appointment, but first try to cope with the symptoms yourself. Also, on occasion, inform your doctor about your search for a better way of dealing with your symptoms, about your coping strategies, and about the progress you have made! Discuss with your doctor all the medications you are taking and talk about the benefits that you expect to have from taking them!

Fig. 9.17 Worksheet 9.13: Practice of the week on the topic "Doctor visits"

Worksheet 9.13: Practice of the week on the topic "Doctor visits"

1 When does it make sense to consult a doctor? What do I expect from a visit to the doctor? How realistic is it that the doctor will meet my expectations?

....

....

....

....

....

....

....

2 Which of my symptoms I can manage by myself? Which coping strategies do I have? Which coping strategies are available to me?

....

....

....

....

....

....

....

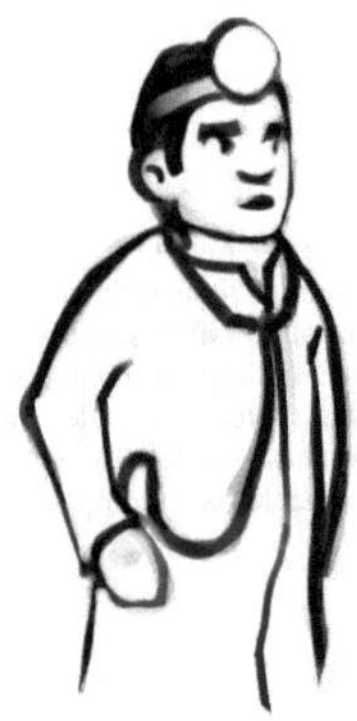

References

Bennett-Levy, J., Butler, G., Fennell, M., Hackman, A., Müller, M., & Westbrook, D. (Eds.). (2004). *The Oxford guide to behavioural experiments in cognitive therapy*. Oxford University Press.

Bleichhardt, G., & Weck, F. (2011). *Kognitive Verhaltenstherapie bei Hypochondrie und Krankheitsangst* (2. akt. Aufl.). Springer.

Kaluza, S. (2004). *Stressbewältigung: Trainingsmanual zur psychologischen Gesundheitsförderung*. Springer.

Margraf, J., Neumer, S., & Rief, W. (1998). *Somatoforme Störungen: Ätiologie, Diagnose und Therapie*. Springer.

Rief, W., & Nanke, A. (2003). Psychologische Grundkonzepte der Verhaltensmedizin. In U. Ehlert (Hrsg.), *Verhaltensmedizin* (S. 95–132). Springer.

Module 6: Stress and Stress Management (Part 2)

Contents

M. Kleinstäuber et al., *Cognitive Behavior Therapy for Persistent Somatic Symptoms and Somatic Symptom Disorder*, https://doi.org/10.1007/978-3-662-69726-9_10

10.1 Session 16

Contents and Materials of the 16th Session

- **Contents**
  - Discussion of the practice of the week
  - Outlook for the next four sessions and exercises
  - Daily hassles vs. critical life events
  - Transactional stress model by Lazarus and Launier (1978)
  - Types of stress management
  - Practice of the week: Individual stressors (Worksheet 10.4)
- **Materials**
  - Worksheet 10.1: Stressors: daily hassles and critical life events
  - Worksheet 10.2: When do I experience stress?
  - Worksheet 10.3: How can I cope with stress?
  - Worksheet 10.4: What do I personally experience as stressful?

10

10.1.1 Discussion of the Practice of the Week

Session 16 begins with a discussion of Worksheet 9.13 (Practice of the week on the topic "doctor visits").

10.1.2 Outlook for the Next Four Sessions and Exercises

In the next four sessions, we want to take a closer look at the topic of "stress" and ways of coping with it. Subjectively perceived stress can express itself in many different ways. It can, for example, weigh on the mind, cause headaches or hit the stomach. In any case, it is not uncommon for stress to manifest itself on a physical level and to cause or intensify physical discomfort. How close the connections are between sensitivities and bodily reactions becomes clear when we take a closer look at our speech habits. The following exercise serves this purpose (modified after Drexler, 2006).

Instruction: Exercise on Colloquial Phrases Related to the Body (Based on Drexler, 2006)

What colloquialisms can you think of that refer to an area of the body or specific organs (e.g., breathing, heart, head, stomach)?

- *Breathing: Something takes your breath away.*
- *Heart: It stops, flutters, races, breaks, skips a beat, the unhappy lover suffers from "heartbreak".*
- *Head: something is growing over one's head, something is giving one a headache, losing one's head.*
- *Stomach: A louse is running over your liver, you have a queasy, sinking feeling in the stomach area, you're scared.*
- *Other body sensations that occur during emotional turbulence: spine-chilling, your hair stands on end, you get goose bumps, cold sweat.*

10.1.3 Daily Hassles Versus Critical Life Events

Whether a person experiences stress depends on whether and how they perceive and evaluate the situation. What puts pressure and strain on one person can leave another more or less cold. Things that can trigger stress are called **stressors.** A distinction is made between internal and external stressors, whereby the former take place inside a person, while external stressors are outside the individual or can be observed and measured by others:

- Examples of external stresses: Injury, intense heat or cold, noise, extreme physical stress, spatial confinement, sensory deprivation.
- Examples of internal, emotional stresses: Deadline pressure, conflicts with other people, excessive or insufficient demands.

In addition to the differentiation between internal and external stressors, another distinction is common and helpful. This is the concept of **"daily hassles"**. This refers to recurring or persistent burdens and annoyances of everyday life (microstressors or also called "minor life events"). Some of them may be small things in themselves, but in total—depending on the day's mood—they can sometimes "get on your nerves" and drive you to despair (e.g., being stuck in a traffic jam, missing the bus, standing in the "wrong" queue at the supermarket, bill in the letterbox, trouble with the neighbour). These everyday adversities are contrasted by so-called **critical** or **drastic life events,** which tend to happen rarely, i.e., not on a daily basis (e.g., death of a close person, loss of job, serious accident, divorce or separation from partner, own serious illness or that of a relative, birth of a child, marriage, retirement, experience of violence). Scientific studies suggest that everyday worries are probably more relevant to health than critical life events. In addition to the "size" or "weight" of the stressor (i.e. everyday worry vs. deeply impacting event), there are other criteria of a stressor that influence the course of a stress reaction or the organism. These are temporal proximity, duration, controllability, predictability, and personal relevance.

The patient is given Worksheet 10.1 (Stressors: daily hassles and critical life events) to work on.

10.1.4 The Transactional Stress Model by Lazarus and Launier (1978)

According to the transactional stress model of Richard Lazarus (important American psychologist, 1922–2002), stress is generated less by the situational demands themselves than by their subjective interpretation and the type of coping strategies employed. The stress model according to Lazarus explains the occurrence or the experience of stress as follows:

- The affected person perceives a situation or an event and the so-called **primary appraisal** as follows. The person asks themselves what the event means for their well-being: Does the event affect me? Does it have any meaning for me? The following answers are possible: the event is either irrelevant/significant, relevant/favorable/positive, relevant/stressful/negative (if an actual or anticipated damage or a significant loss is perceived, a feeling of threat or challenge follows; in addition, expectation of positive consequences when coping).
- This is followed by the so-called **secondary appraisal**. The person asks themselves whether they are able to cope with the situation: Do I have the skills? Do I have the possibilities? Do I feel that I can cope with the situation? Do I experience it more as a challenge? If I feel that I am helpless in the face of the situation, then I am more likely to see it as a threat. Logically, primary and secondary evaluation processes influence each other.
- Finally, a **reappraisal** is carried out on the basis of the experience made or coping with the situation, which influences future evaluation processes when similar situations occur.

Simplified according to Rettenbach (2007), **coping** can be defined as the effort to cope with difficulties and stressful events. In the first analysis step of the primary appraisal, the situation is evaluated, for example, as a threat or challenge. In the secondary appraisal, one's own possibilities are assessed. Coping mechanisms are then chosen as a result of accounting for these two components. According to Lazarus and Launier (1978), coping includes: information seeking, direct action (e.g., escape or removal of the threat), action inhibition (e.g., silence), and intrapsychic changes (e.g., not seeing the threat, self-deception, denial, repression). Coping changes the appraisal of the stressful situation. Ehlert (2003) defines coping as a coping response that requires effort and effort is distinguished from automated behaviors for adaptation. Coping includes both behavioral (overtly observable) and intrapsychic responses. Included are all responses aimed at active mastery of the situation (consequently, including such responses as endurance, tolerance, avoidance, and denial). Coping serves the goal of coping with the demands placed on us. It is not defined by its success.

The decisive factor is cognitive processing, not the nature of the situation or stimulus. Basically, two types of coping can be distinguished according to the transaction model:

- **problem-focused coping:** Attempts to change the situation itself or own characteristics, e.g., goals, values, attitudes;
- **emotion-focused coping:** Attempts to influence negative emotions such as fear, anger or guilt without changing the situation, e.g., acting out or controlling emotions.

Further differentiation possibilities are: overtly observable vs. intrapsychic coping, attention (changing or eliminating the stressor) vs. avoidance, avoidance (turning away from the problem, denial, withdrawal). When these strategies are combined with those mentioned in the previous paragraph, the following coping strategies can be identified:

- **cognitive attention:** making sense of, reassessing or positively reinterpreting the situation;
- **open attention:** take direct action, seek support, solve the problem;
- **cognitive avoidance:** denial;
- **open avoidance:** flight, evasion, resigned acceptance of the situation.

It is important to convey to the patient in this psychoeducational therapy session that there is no generally effective standard strategy for coping with stress. The patient is given Worksheet 10.2 (When do I experience stress?).

10.1.5 Types of Stress Management

There are countless possibilities and strategies for dealing with stress, i.e. with the demands that are placed on us. We use many of them without being aware of them. There is no perfect stress management strategy that is effective in all situations. As is often the case, the effectiveness of a strategy depends on many factors.

At this point, patients can be prepared to be introduced to various stress management options or coping strategies in the coming sessions. Patient and therapist can then look together at which strategies the patient have already been used, which ones they have become familiar with in the course of therapy, and which strategies they could best benefit from in their current life situation. First, however, patients should be given an overview of three main ways of coping with stress. For this purpose, patients are given Worksheet 10.3 (How can I cope with stress?).

10.1.6 Practice of the Week

As practice of the week, patients are asked to write down events and situations that they experience as stressful. Patients are given Worksheet 10.4 (What do I personally experience as stressful?).

10.2 Session 17

Contents and Materials of the 17th Session

- Contents
  - Discussion of the practice of the week
  - Problem-solving stress management strategies
  - Time management
  - Social support
  - Practice of the week: Social support (Worksheet 10.6)
  - Guided imagery "Tree"
- Materials
  - Worksheet 10.5: Thoughts on the use of time
  - Worksheet 10.6: Social support

10.2.1 Discussion of the Practice of the Week

At the beginning of the session, Worksheet 10.4 (What I personally experience as stressful) is discussed. The patient should have succeeded in identifying individual stressors.

10.2.2 Problem-Solving Stress Management Strategies

The development of problem-focused stress management strategies should be done with targeted questions. The patient should be encouraged to become aware of different ways of coping with stress.

- Do you have any influence over some of the things that you feel are a burden?
- Can you change it?
- Do you want to change it?
- Would it be worth the effort and expense involved to you?
- If so, how might the requirement be addressed?

A large group of coping strategies is based on the stress-triggering situation or the associated evaluation processes. Attention is focused on the problem, the requirement or on relevant thoughts. If the situation is controllable and can be influenced, the problem can be tackled directly, e.g., by making an effort to eliminate the stressor, handing over the task, managing time better or seeking help to solve the problem. However, if the situation is beyond one's control, i.e., cannot be changed by one's own efforts, one way to cope with it is to reappraise the situation (for example, by positively reinterpreting it, attempting to make sense of the event, reevaluating the meaning of the event, or appraising one's own abilities). According to the theory of radical constructivism (von Glaserfeld, 1997), there is no reality independent of the observer. Each person invents or constructs his or her own reality. Even though this statement may seem shocking at first, at the same time it contains a helpful, if not comforting thought, because if realities are always constructions, it opens up the possibility for the individual to decide for himself, i.e. on his own responsibility, for a reality (Watzlawick, 2005). Consequently, an event can be viewed in different ways. The personal view is only one of many possible ones and has no claim to truth or correctness.

Instruction: Change of Perspective

One possibility, then, is to change perspective in order to arrive at new possible solutions. The French writer Antoine de Saint-Exupéry expressed this in his book "The Wisdom of the Sands" (1948, respectively "Die Stadt in der Wüste", 2009) as follows: "For to see clearly, changing one's perspective is often enough.". You will also know from previous sessions that certain thoughts, attitudes and evaluation processes can also cause or intensify the experience of stress. These can be changed to enable better coping with the situation. In general, it is better to face a problem than to repress it (deny it, don't want to see it), because—and you will know this all too well from your own experience—you don't forget what you repress, and what you put off (usually) doesn't take care of itself.

10.2.3 Time Management

Many people complain about having too little time, being constantly under time pressure, feeling rushed and often falling into a hectic state. Often they say "I don't have time, I have to go". In both professional and private life, there is a tendency for many to get as much done as possible in a short time and to rush from one appointment to the next. Those who take a break are considered lazy. On the other hand, those who accomplish a lot and are constantly busy are considered important, powerful, successful and often enjoy a high reputation. Rest usually occurs as a compulsion, for example, when one falls ill or becomes unemployed.

At this point, patients can be asked whether they are possibly familiar with the fairy tale novel "Momo" ("Momo or The Curious Story about the Time Thieves and the Child Who Returned the People's Stolen Time") by Michael Ende (1973). It is a story about time that is not only suitable for children and that makes them think about their own handling of this precious commodity. The "Grey Gentlemen" try by all means to get people to save time and persuade them to open accounts at the Time Savings Bank. They talk people into wasting their time on useless things (like meeting up with friends or caring for a sick person). Instead, they should focus on the most important thing in life, which is making money and becoming famous. The "Gray Lords" are very persuasive. Soon people are falling into hectic schedules, "forgetting" their friends and trying to save time wherever they can. At the beginning of the story, the orphan girl Momo also feels this when more and more friends have no time for her. In truth, however, people are being cheated out of their time. Because while they try to save time for later, they forget to live in the present. Because time cannot be saved, like money, for example.

In the following, patients' handling of the time available to them can be explored first:

- How do you deal with time?
- What comes to mind when you hear the term boredom?

French philosopher Blaise Pascal on boredom (1979):

> Nothing is so unbearable to man as to be in a complete silence, without passions, without business, without distraction, without devotion. He then perceives his nothingness, his abandonment, his inadequacy, his dependence, his impotence, his emptiness. Immediately, from the bottom of his soul, boredom will rise, gloom, sadness, sorrow, vexation, despair.

What comes to mind when you hear the term leisure?

By leisure is meant the time which a person has at his disposal for his own use, in which he "refreshes and edifies himself".

What comes to mind when you hear the term waste of time?

Time wasting is a popular expression for the use of time for activities that (apparently) do not serve a clearly defined goal and are therefore considered pointless. In this sense, an activity can also be recognised as a waste of time in retrospect if it has not led to the desired success. Often activities are wrongly called a waste of time when a benefit exists but is not recognised by the person making the judgement. Patients receive Worksheet 10.5 (Thoughts on the use of time).

10.2.4 Social Support

Another form of stress management is to talk to other people and ask others for help. Many people experience the attention of others alone as a relief. Social contacts are considered by many people to be important for mental well-being and mental health. The importance of social contacts for patients or their satisfaction with their current social relationships should be explored with the help of the following questions.

- Are you satisfied with the number of social contacts you have?
- Do you have someone you can turn to in confidence when something is bothering you?
- How important are social contacts to you?
- What do you experience as positive about social relationships?
- To what extent can social relationships help you cope better with stress/problems?

Social support has numerous forms of expression. For example, Diewald (1991) distinguishes the following forms of social support: work assistance (renovating, repairing, caring, e.g., babysitting), material support (lending money or goods), settling a dispute, providing information (e.g., about job vacancies or eligibility for social benefits), counselling (e.g., about job vacancies or eligibility for benefits) or personal advice, social activities, recognition (acceptance and appreciation), orientation (models of behavior and social norms), sense of belonging (being needed, taking responsibility for others), expectation of help (one hand washes the other), place to acquire social skills, security (feeling safe, stability), love, affection, motivational support (encouragement, protection). Sources of social support can be the following: partners, relatives, friends and acquaintances, neighbours, others (priest, teacher, salesman, innkeeper, etc.).

10.2.5 Practice of the Week

As practice of the week, patients are asked to think about which people in their life they experience as a reliable source of social support. They will receive Worksheet 10.6 (Social support) to work on.

10.2.6 Guided Imagery "Tree"

At the end of the session, the patient is invited to attend a guided imagery practice. The following instruction can be used. This is a slightly modified version of the authors Scharfenstein and Basler (2004).

Instruction: Guided Imagery "Tree" (Modified after Scharfenstein & Basler, 2004)

Sit comfortably and close your eyes if you like! Now observe your breathing without changing it … Just watch how you inhale and exhale … This happens all by itself, this inhaling and exhaling … Just watch your breath … Now emphasize the exhaling … with each exhale release some of your tension so that with each exhale you go deeper into relaxation … with each exhale you go deeper into relaxation … further and further … deeper and deeper … as far as you like … as it is comfortable for you …

Now imagine a tree … any deciduous tree that just appears in your imagination … Look closely at this tree … What kind of tree do you see? … How tall is it? … In what surroundings is it standing? … Now take a closer look at the surroundings of your tree … What do you see there? … Now look at your tree again … Look at its branches … its leaves … its bark … Take a closer look at the trunk … the bark … Is it rather smooth or rough … or even torn by deep furrows? …

Now imagine the roots of your tree … how they reach deep into the earth … and branch out more and more … Feel the support they give the tree … How it is firmly rooted with them in the earth … Now imagine how the tree absorbs water from the soil with its roots and transforms it into a nutrient fluid … Feel the power that slowly rises through the nutrient fluid in the tree … how it flows through the roots … through the trunk … through the branches … into the leaves …

Now imagine that it is spring … Watch the last of the snow melt … the first buds sprout … the sun becomes a little warmer … and life awakens around your tree … Notice the chirping of the birds … the fresh spring landscape … Imagine your tree in spring … its trunk … its branches … the fresh, bright green leaves … the bursting buds … and the fresh, delicately scented blossoms … Now say goodbye to spring …

The season is changing and it is summer … Now imagine your tree in summer … It is getting warmer … The sun is high on the horizon … It is a hot and sunny day … Look around you … What does the landscape around your tree look like? … What does the sky look like? … What does your tree look like? … its trunk … its branches … its leaves … Is there any fruit hanging from your tree? … Now slowly say goodbye to summer …

It's getting autumn … It's getting colder … The days are getting shorter … Stormy winds are blowing across the country and blowing through the leaves of your tree … But its firm roots give it a secure hold … The leaves are beginning to wilt … They are slowly changing colour … First they turn yellow … then brown … The wind blows off a few leaves and whirls them around … Look how the leaves fall from the tree … and how they remain lying all around the tree … What does your tree look like now? … its trunk … its branches … its leaves … What is the weather like? … Look at the landscape around your tree … Now slowly say goodbye to autumn …

Now imagine it is winter … There is snow … It is freezing cold … There is an icy wind … Imagine your tree in winter … Its trunk … Its bark … Its branches … Are there perhaps icicles hanging from the branches of your tree? … Is it covered with snow? … Look at the sky … What does it look like? … What does the landscape around your tree look like? … Now say goodbye to winter …

Now slowly come to the end … Feel your breath … Breathe deeply in and out a few times … Perceive the space you are in in your imagination … Keep your eyes closed for a little while longer and move a little … First stretch your legs … then your arms … Now slowly come back into this space and open your eyes.

The relaxation exercise should be followed by a short evaluation, which can be done with the following questions:

- How well did you manage to relax (on a scale of 0–100; the higher the score, the more relaxed)?
- What tree did you have in mind?
- Were there any difficulties? If so, what kind?
- Can you imagine calling the tree you have just imagined back into your consciousness during relaxation phases?
- Could you imagine this tree becoming a kind of resting image for you?

10.3 Session 18

Contents and Materials of the 18th Session

- **Contents**
  - Discussion of the practice of the week
  - Less helpful thoughts
  - Acknowledging your own strengths
  - Practice of the week: Your strengths (Worksheet 10.9)
- **Materials**
  - Worksheet 10.7: Attitudes and expectations that increase stress
  - Worksheet 10.8: My strengths
  - Worksheet 10.9: Practice of the week: my strengths

10.3.1 Discussion of the Practice of the Week

Session 18 begins with a discussion of Worksheet 10.6 (Social support). Which people in the patient's environment are reliable sources of social support?

10.3.2 Less Helpful Thoughts

There is a whole range of attitudes and expectations that are typically human, but can lead to putting oneself under unnecessary pressure. Often these are unreasonable demands and expectations of oneself or others, or inadequate ideas about how the world should be. Usually these expectations are too high, i.e. "the bar is raised to unattainable heights". If one recognizes these unfavorable expectations and beliefs and questions them self-critically, there is a chance to reduce stress by correcting these beliefs.

One way of reducing stress is therefore to lower one's own expectations or to lower the bar or to bring one's own ideals down from the "high horse" (Potreck-Rose, 2007). The patient receives Worksheet 10.7 (Attitudes and expectations that increase stress). The individual points of the worksheet should be discussed thoroughly with the patient. The following explanations may be helpful.

Inner Drivers and Critics

- **Be perfect!** Behind this is an excessive desire for success, self-affirmation and recognition by others through performance, as well as a pronounced fear of failure and one's own mistakes. The claim is: "I must not make a mistake and must always find the right, perfect solution." However, we are neither God nor a computer, but distractible and sometimes unfocused. To err is part of human nature and mistakes are therefore unavoidable.
- **Be popular!** Behind this is a very strong desire for belonging, acceptance and love, as well as a pronounced fear of rejection, criticism and rejection by others. The aspiration is: "I want to please everyone, and I want everyone to like me." This is also an unrealistic goal, since tastes, opinions, preferences, and goals are different. Consequently, there is no chance of pleasing everyone.
- **Be strong!** Behind this is an excessive desire for personal independence and self-determination as well as a pronounced fear of dependence on others, one's own need for help and weakness. This demand sometimes becomes visible in a lone wolf mentality.
- **Be on your guard!** Behind this is an excessive desire for security and control as well as a pronounced fear of loss of control, wrong decisions and aversion to risk. There is the conviction that whoever does not look forward cannot be disappointed, or whoever assumes the worst can at best be positively surprised. The goal of this attitude of entitlement is to protect oneself from unpleasant surprises. Negative consequences can be: Displeasure, dissatisfaction, fear of the future, self-esteem problems, passivity, withdrawal up to social isolation.
- **I can't!** Behind this is an excessive desire for one's own well-being and a comfortable life, as well as a pronounced fear of unpleasant feelings and of effort, and attitudes of one's own helplessness and low frustration tolerance. Typically, this belief manifests itself in a victim attitude.

Catastrophizing

Situations, persons or things are judged as terrible, unbearable, horrible, unbearable or catastrophic. Usually there is an unrealistic exaggeration behind it. Possible consequences of this kind of thinking are: resignation, giving up, letting things hang, lamenting, struggling with fate, lamenting, adopting a victim attitude. Since catastrophes cannot be influenced, the feeling of absolute helplessness can be awakened. Consequently, one practices alarmism and freezes in passivity. If, on the other hand, one assesses the same situation as "only" unpleasant or very bad, there is at least the possibility of checking whether one can do something about it, i.e. bring about a decision.

Must-Thinking

These are entrenched, fixed, rigid ideas. Examples: "It is a disaster if things are not or the world is not as it should or ought to be." Words like "absolutely, demand, must, must not, oblige, insist upon, claim, should, or require" are expressions of this way of thinking. From a desire comes an absolute demand, an unrelenting desire. If we then do not get what we think we absolutely have to have, if others do not do or do not do what they should do or do not do, then this results in anger, hatred, rage, frustration and aggression. Behind this is usually an unrealistic, unfounded demand on the environment, on others or on fate: something should be, must be or must not be. Generally valid norms and laws are set up, behind which the following justification is found: "Because I want it that way or because one does it that way." The assertion of having to do something suggests having no choice or influence over the situation (which is rarely the case). The goal is to learn to accept unpleasant realities.

10

- **Generalizing**

Inferring from one part to the whole, from one to all, from today's experience to future events. Examples: something fails → "I NEVER succeed at anything!"; a person is considered good or bad as a whole; metaphor with the fruit basket: "In front of you is a basket filled with numerous fruits. All the fruits are crisp, fresh and clean. Then you discover a rotten cherry. You say, 'It's all crap!' and immediately throw the entire basket and its contents into the trash."

- **Self-Praise Stinks! Does It Really?!**

Who says so? On what grounds? One should not expect others to praise one for progress. Instead, one should learn to inwardly "blow one's own trumpet" when one has done or achieved something purposeful. Self-praise is a necessary condition to be satisfied with oneself, to become independent of the opinion of others and to become more self-confident.

- **Self-Fulfilling Prophecies (Pygmalion Effect)**

All too often we perceive what we want to perceive. We often interpret our experiences in such a way that they confirm our preconceptions about ourselves and the world over and over again. Is it really possible, then, that expectations placed on a person influence his or her behavior in such a way that that person ultimately behaves unconsciously according to those expectations? First studied by Rosenthal and Jacobson (1986), the Pygmalion effect—as a phenomenon in school teaching—describes the effects of teachers' expectations on the behavior of their taught students. If a teacher already has an (anticipated) view of the students (such as student A is stupid, student B is highly gifted, student C is a troublemaker, etc.), this view will be confirmed later on. This is made possible by the teacher's ability to communicate his or her expectations to students in subtle ways, such as by waiting for a student response, by frequency and strength of praise or reprimand, by paying more or less attention to students, and by varying levels of performance demands. Another example: When news of an impending gasoline shortage circulates in the media and, as a result, everyone who calls a motorized vehicle their own rushes headlong to the gas station to grab some more of the soon-to-be precious and rare commodity, a shortage of gasoline does indeed quickly occur. An expectation is regarded as an imminent fact (in order to be able to say later that one knew it). For example, it is enough to assume—whether it is factually justified or groundless is irrelevant—that the others are whispering about you and secretly making fun of you. In view of this "fact", common sense suggests that one should not trust one's fellow men and, since the whole thing naturally takes place under a holey veil of concealment, pay close attention and consider even the slightest circumstantial evidence. It is then only a matter of time before one can catch the others whispering and laughing secretly, winking conspiratorially and nodding at each other. The prophecy has come true (Watzlawick, 2007).

The phenomenon of "panic buying", already explained above on the basis of prophesied gasoline shortages, can be explained in this way. "The prophecy of the event leads to the event of the prophecy" (Watzlawick, 2007).

- **Mind Reading**

Make assumptions about what other people think. No scientific evidence exists that this is possible.

- **Externalizing the Positive, Internalizing the Negative**

Here, one blames oneself for the bad events in the world. The following situation can be given as an example: A rainstorm dampens the mood at a garden party. However, the host does not attribute the dampened mood to the weather, but blames himself and looks for reasons that lie in his person. A different pattern can be seen when explaining a positive event, such as passing an exam. The person in question attributes the success to external factors, e.g., the supposed ease of the task, or says to himself "I was just lucky.". Failure is typically explained in terms of one's own inability in the thinking style described here. The cause of failure is therefore attributed to the individual. External explanations are ignored or not taken into account.

As the patient should already know from previous sessions, stress largely originates in our own mind. How we assess situations and evaluate our competencies has a great influence on whether we experience stress or not. Consequently, an important way of coping with stress is to discover and change stress aggravating thoughts. This is often easier said than done. Questions to ask yourself to check whether you have fallen into a thinking trap can be reviewed with the patient at this point. As a refresher, a few auxiliary questions can be mentioned again, which serve to discover stress-promoting thoughts and attitudes:

❓
- Am I only looking at the negative sides of the situation?
- Are there also positive sides?
- Am I overgeneralizing?
- Do I have too high or wrong expectations?
- What does someone who is less burdened by the situation than I am think?
- How will I feel about it later, in a month or a year?
- What would happen at worst?
- What would be so bad about that?

- How likely is that?
- What would be worse than this situation?
- Have I ever mastered a similarly difficult situation? If so, how?
- What would I say to a friend for support if they were in a similar situation as me?
- What would a good friend tell me or advise me to do in this situation?
- How important is this thing really to me?

10.3.3 Acknowledging Your Own Strengths

Now the focus should be on the patients' own strengths. What do the patients find good about themselves? These can be qualities, attitudes, skills, talents, knowledge and certain experiences. Experience has shown that many people find this task difficult. They have inhibitions to praise themselves and often hide their light under a bushel due to pronounced modesty. Patients should be taught that it is important to be aware of one's own qualities in order to increase self-confidence. Patients are given Worksheet 10.8 (My strengths) and are asked to work on it, i.e. to tick off those qualities which they think are strong in them. In the following, some hints and information for the discussion of the worksheet are given.

Peterson and Seligman as founders of "Positive Psychology" (Peterson & Seligman, 2004) describe a catalogue of 24 character strengths and 6 virtues. The authors have based their classification on various philosophical, religious and psychological sources from different cultures. As universal virtues the authors name:
- Wisdom and knowledge (associated strengths include creativity, originality and resourcefulness, curiosity, eagerness to learn, judgement, social intelligence, vision),
- Courage (e.g., bravery, perseverance and persistence, persistence, integrity),
- Love/humanity (e.g., capacity to love, bonding ability, philanthropy, generosity),
- Justice (e.g., belonging, teamwork and loyalty, fairness, leadership),
- Moderation (e.g., willingness to forgive, forgiveness and grace, self-control, humility), and
- Spirituality and transcendence (e.g., sense of beauty, reverence and gratitude, optimism, humour, enthusiasm).

10.3.4 Practice of the Week

As part of the practice of the week, patients are encouraged to take a closer look at their strengths and write them down. They are given Worksheet 10.9 (Practice of the week: my strengths).

10.4 Session 19

Contents and Materials of the 19th Session
- **Contents**
  - Discussion of the practice of the week
  - Palliative and regenerative stress management
  - Our general inner level of stress and tension
  - Mindfulness
  - Practice of the week: Journal of well-being (Worksheet 10.12)
- **Materials**
  - Worksheet 10.10: Our general inner levels of stress and tension
  - Worksheet 10.11: A story about mindfulness
  - Worksheet 10.12: Journal of well-being: How have I been today?

10.4.1 Discussion of the Practice of the Week

At the beginning of the 19th session, Worksheet 10.9 (Practice of the week: my Strengths) is discussed.

10.4.2 Palliative and Regenerative Stress Management

Another type of stress management is the **regulation** and **control of** the physical stress response. A distinction is made between two types:
- **Palliation:** coping attempts that serve short-term relief and relaxation, attenuation of an acute stress response;
- **Regeneration:** Coping attempts that serve long-term and regular recovery and relaxation.

It cannot be prevented that stress reactions occur again and again. Therefore, the following section will focus on how mental and physical agitation can be dampened or reduced. The following strategies are conceivable:
- regular use of a relaxation techniques,
- regular exercise,
- healthy, varied diet,
- maintaining extra-occupational social contacts,
- regular compensation through leisure activities and hobbies,
- learn to enjoy the little things in daily life,
- sufficient sleep,
- structured daily routine with integrated breaks.

10.4.3 Our General Inner Level of Stress and Tention

The patient is given Worksheet 10.10 (Our general inner level of stress and tension). The graph is explained. In order for a physical stress reaction to be initiated, the triggering stimuli must exceed a certain threshold. For example, if a dangerous animal runs towards us, the physical stress reaction is only activated when the animal falls below a certain distance and/or behaves in a certain way (e.g., growling, snarling, jumping) in order to avoid wasting energy. The threshold to activate a physical stress reaction varies from individual to individual. It is partly genetic, partly determined by experience. External circumstances also influence the height of the threshold. For example, it is lower at night than during the day (imagine walking in dark alleys at night and hearing footsteps behind you; now imagine the same situation during the day when the alleys are busier).

Depending on the general inner level of stress and tension, stress or stressful events can exceed the threshold, which leads to the triggering of a physical stress reaction. Certain influences can lower the threshold. The higher the general inner stress and tension level and the lower the threshold, the less additional stress is needed to activate a physical stress reaction.

Through "guided discovery" patients should now find out what they can do themselves to lower their general level of tension.

? What can you do to lower your overall tension level to become more calm and balanced overall?

10.4.4 Mindfulness

Mindfulness means to be attentive in a special way and to concentrate completely on the present moment, i.e. on the present, the so-called here and now. This should happen without evaluation and without active action. It is about pausing and perceiving what is right now. The pressure to act and change should be taken away.

The concept of (inner) mindfulness is often associated with Buddhism or Dialectical Behavioral Therapy for Borderline Personality Disorder, in which it is a central element.

Saving oneself from certain stress by focusing one's attention more often and consciously on the present moment is a popular idea that can also be found in the writings of some philosophers. For example, Blaise Pascal (1979) expresses himself as follows:

> Let each one examine his thoughts; he will find them all occupied with the past and with the future. We think almost nothing of the present... Thus we never live, but hope to live; and while we always prepare ourselves to be happy, it is inevitable that we never are.

Arthur Schopenhauer (1976) recommends:

> Instead, then, of being exclusively and perpetually occupied with plans and cares for the future, or of indulging in longing for the past, let us never forget that the present alone is real and alone certain; while the future is almost always different from what we think it will be; indeed, the past, too, was different; and in such a way that both, on the whole, have less to do with them than they seem to us.

The patient is given Worksheet 10.11 (A story about mindfulness). The patient can be asked to read out the story on the worksheet (Far Eastern wisdom, based on Grün, 2001). The meaning of the story for the patient can be made clear by asking questions:

?
- Do you recognize yourself in the story?
- Do you find it difficult to be mindful?
- Can you imagine practicing this, for example, while brushing your teeth every day?

10.4.5 Practice of the Week

The last practice of the week is to keep the journal of well-being again (as already at the beginning of the therapy) for one week. The patient receives (assuming that the next session will take place in one week) 7 copies of Worksheet 10.12 (Journal of well-being: How have I been today?).

10.5 Worksheets

These worksheets are also available for download online at Springer Extras (► extras.springer.com).

Worksheet 10.1	Stressors: Daily hassles and critical life events	◘ Figure 10.1
Worksheet 10.2	When do I experience stress?	◘ Figure 10.2
Worksheet 10.3	How can I cope with stress?	◘ Figure 10.3

Worksheet 10.4	What do I personally experience as stressful?	◘ Figure 10.4
Worksheet 10.5	Thoughts on the use of time	◘ Figure 10.5
Worksheet 10.6	Social support	◘ Figure 10.6
Worksheet 10.7	Attitudes and expectations that increase stress	◘ Figure 10.7
Worksheet 10.8	My strengths	◘ Figure 10.8

Worksheet 10.9	Practice of the week: My strengths	◘ Figure 10.9
Worksheet 10.10	Our general inner level of stress and tension	◘ Figure 10.10
Worksheet 10.11	A story about mindfulness	◘ Figure 10.11
Worksheet 10.12	Journal of well-being: How have I been today?	◘ Figure 10.12

◘ Fig. 10.1 Worksheet 10.1: Stressors: Daily hassles and critical life events

Worksheet 10.1:: Stressors: Daily hassles and critical life events

Scientific research has shown that recurring or persistent stressful events in our everyday life, so-called **"daily hassles"** (hassle = anger, difficulties, arguments), have a greater impact on health than single **critical life events** (e.g., death of a close person, loss of job, serious accident, divorce or separation from your partner, your own serious illness or that of a relative, birth of a child, marriage, retirement, experience of violence, etc.).

Which daily hassles do you face? The following is a list of typical "daily hassles" which you can add onto. Check stressors that you experience yourself in your everyday life!

- Time and deadline pressure
- Family responsibilities: Doing household chores, caring for relatives, dissatisfaction with the distribution of the housework
- Social commitments: Activities in the community or organizations
- Health problems with myself or others
- Boredom
- Commuting and long journeys to work or long business trips
- Marital or partnership conflicts
- Problems with the children: Education, school
- Financial worries
- Fear of job loss
- High responsibility at the workplace
- Dissatisfaction with working hours or working conditions
- A poor social climate or atmosphere at the workplace
- Disturbances and constant interuptions in the daily work
- Various requirements at work that cannot be met at the same time
- Too much or too little work
- Excessive demands or too difficult work tasks
- Unclear targets
- Too little say
- Introduction of new technologies or working methods
- Personal tensions at work with colleagues, superiors or customers
- Lack of recognition or feedback of work performance
- Disagreements among relatives
- Frequent recurring disputes with other people: Tenants, landlords, neighbors
- Dissatisfaction with the living situation: too narrow space, too noisy
- Fear of an imminent deterioration of the existing living situation
- ....
- ....
- ....
- ....
- ....
- ....

Fig. 10.2 Worksheet 10.2: When do I experience stress?

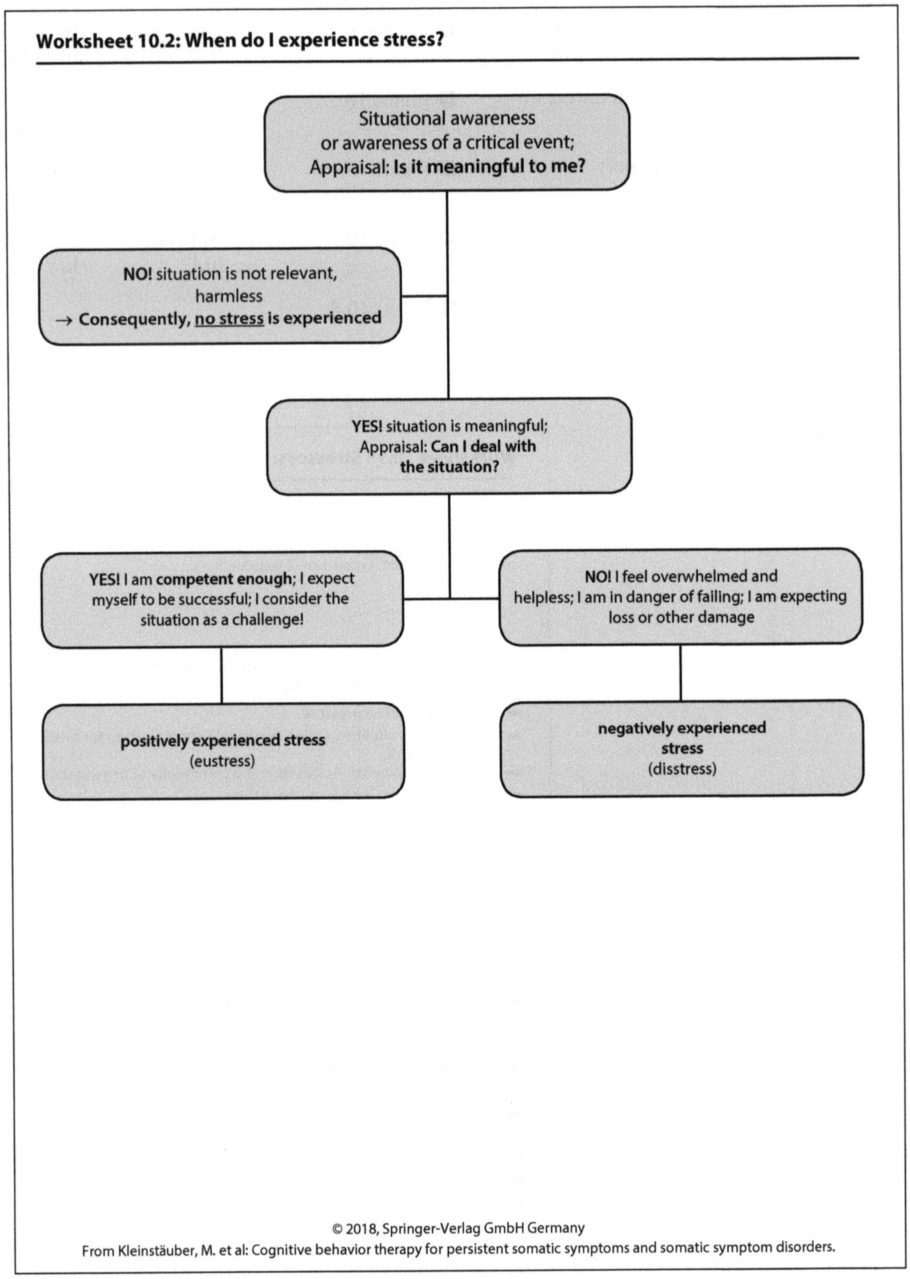

Fig. 10.3 Worksheet 10.3: How can I cope with stress?

Worksheet 10.3: How can I cope with stress?

1. **Problem-focused coping**

   (a) Attempts to change the situation, to eliminate the problem (the focus is *outside* the person)
   (b) Attempts to change own appraisals, attitudes, or expectations (the focus is *within* the person)

2. **Emotion-focused coping**
   Attempts to improve one's own emotional state and reduce unpleasant emotions

People deal with stress in very different ways. The goal is always to cope with the challenges of the situation, i.e., managing stress.

It is helpful to recognize whether or not the situation that is bothering you can be changed by you.
The following sentence by the theologian Friedrich Christoph Oetinger may clarify this:

"Give me the **serenity** to accept things that I *cannot change*. Give me **the courage** to *change the things that I can change*. Give me the **wisdom** to *know the difference*."

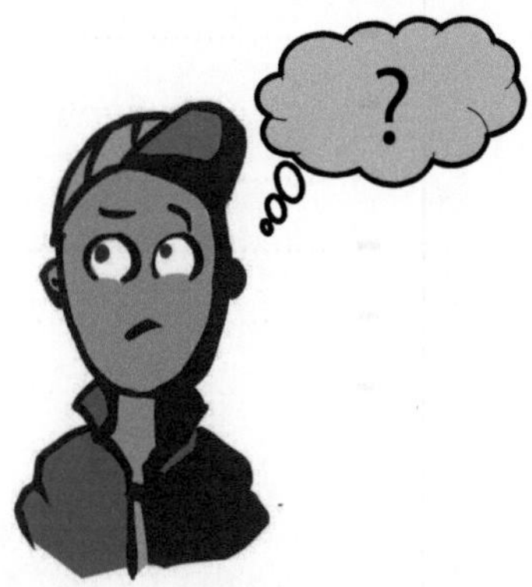

Fig. 10.4 Worksheet 10.4: What do I personally experience as stressful?

Worksheet 10.4: What do I personally experience as stressful?

Make notes of events, circumstances or situations that cause you stress in your daily life!

- ....
- ....
- ....
- ....
- ....
- ....
- ....
- ....
- ....
- ....
- ....
- ....
- ....

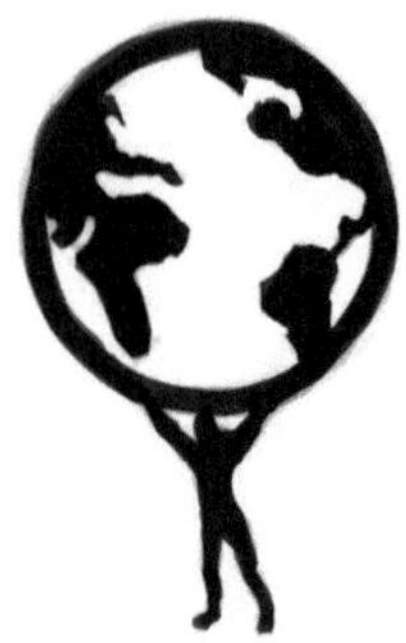

Fig. 10.5 Worksheet 10.5: Thoughts on the use of time

Worksheet 10.5: Thoughts on the use of time

Really, he was indispensable! *by Wilhelm Busch (1832–1908), from: "Criticism of the Heart"*

Everywhere, where something happened
For the good of the community,
He was active, he was there.

Shooting match, casino balls,
Horse racing, juries,
Singing societies, fairs,
Without him, there was no way.

Nothing could be done without him,
Not an hour did he have free.
Yesterday, when they buried him,
Was he right about that, too.

Wilhelm Busch (1874)
Critique of the Heart.
Friedrich Bassermann, Heidelberg.

Memento mori *by Eugen Roth (1895–1976)*

A man overwhelmed by work,
while time is running out,
has a lot to do, and comes,
they say, into the throng.

In the midst of all the fidgeting
he gets thunderstruck, and he's dead.
What just appeared so important yet,
falls down: What remains of the appointments?

Just this one last:
He'll be buried on Wednesday -
and look, he keeps it on time,
because he has time to be now.

Eugen Roth (2000)
The Miracle Doctor (3rd ed.).
Carl Hanser, Munich;
courtesy of
by Dr. Thomas Roth

Fig. 10.6 Worksheet 10.6: Social support

Worksheet 10.6: Social support

For many people, social contacts and relationships are a source of support and important to maintain their mental well-being.

The forms of social support are manifold and range from help with repairs to material support, giving information, giving advice, settling a dispute, providing a sense of security, or confidence through encouragement.

Which people in your life represent a reliable source of support?

- ....
- ....
- ....
- ....
- ....

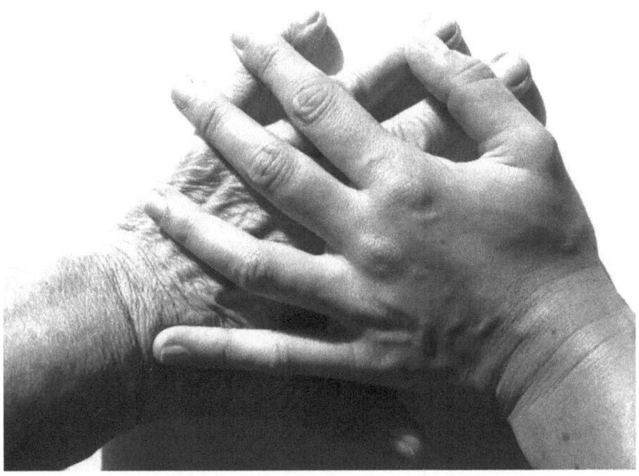

■ **Fig. 10.7** Worksheet 10.7: Attitudes and expectations that increase stress

Worksheet 10.7: Attitudes and expectations that increase stress

- **Inner drivers and inner critical voices**
  - **Be perfect!**
    Desire for success, self-affirmation and recognition by others over achievement, and fear of failure, Failure and own mistakes
  - **Be popular!**
    Desire for belonging, acceptance and love as well as fear of rejection, criticism and rejection by others
  - **Be strong!**
    Desire for personal independence and self-determination and fear of dependence on others, own neediness and weakness
  - **Keep your powder dry!**
    Desire for security and control as well as fear of losing control, making wrong decisions and shying away from risks
  - **I can't!**
    Desire for own well-being and comfortable life, as well as fear of unpleasant feelings and effort

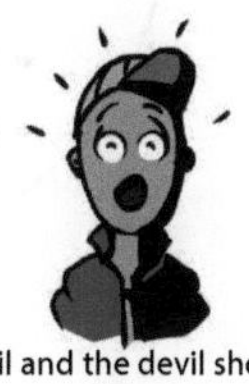

- **Catastrophizing thoughts**
  Exaggerate excessively, "speaking of the the devil and the devil shows up"
- **Must-thinking**
  Wishes turn into demands which, if not fulfilled, lead to anger and frustration
- **Generalizing way of thinking**
  To infer from a part of something to the whole, from one to all, from present experience to future events.
- **Self-praise stinks!**
  Does it really?! Self-praise is a necessary condition to be satisfied with yourself, to be independent from the opinion of others and become more self-confident
- **Self-fulfilling prophecies**
  Often we perceive what we want to perceive, and we interpret our experiences in such a way that they confirm our prejudices about ourselves and the world over and over again; moreover, our expectations influence not only our perception, but also our behavior
- **Mind reading**
  Making assumptions about what other people are thinking
- **Externalize the positive, internalize the negative**
  In case of success: that was luck, the task was easy; in case of failure: own inability, blame oneself

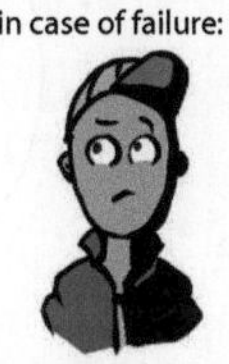

Fig. 10.8 Worksheet 10.8: My strengths

Worksheet 10.8: My strengths

Look at the following character strengths and virtues! Check traits that you think are your strengths! Which aastrengths characterize your person?

Wisdom, knowledge

- Creativity
- Curiosity
- Eagerness to learn
- Social intelligence

Spirituality and Transcendence

- Sense of beauty
- Gratitude
- Optimism
- Enthusiasm
- Humor

Courage

- Bravery
- Endurance

Love, Humanity

- Capacity for love
- Capacity for bonding
- Kindness
- Generosity

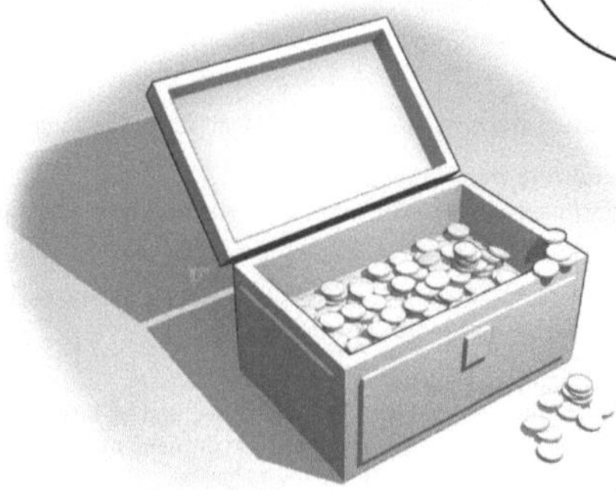

Moderation

- Self-control
- Modesty
- Forgiveness

Justice

- Affiliation
- Teamwork
- Fairness and sense of justice

Fig. 10.9 Worksheet 10.9: Practice of the week: My strengths

Worksheet 10.9: Practice of the week: My strengths

Top up your "treasure chest"! What do you find good about yourself? Name at least seven (more are welcome) traits, attitudes, skills, talents, knowledge, or specific experiences that you have gained over the course of your life. Many people find this task difficult. But overcome your inner inhibitions to praise yourself!

- ______________________________
- ______________________________
- ______________________________
- ______________________________
- ______________________________
- ______________________________
- ______________________________
- ______________________________
- ______________________________
- ______________________________

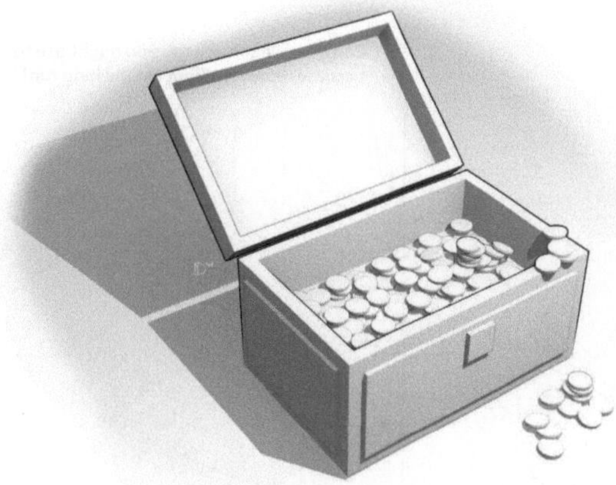

◘ Fig. 10.10 Worksheet 10.10: Our general inner level of stress and tension

Worksheet 10.10: Our general inner level of stress and tension

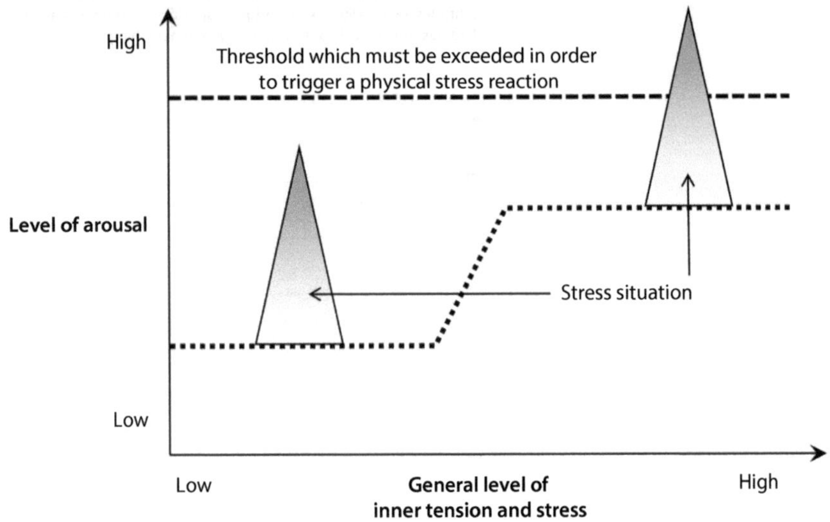

In order to trigger a physical stress response, the triggering stimuli must exceed a certain threshold.
The level of the threshold varies interindividually. Partly it is genetic, partly it is determined by experience.
Stress or stressful events and situations can, depending on how high your general level of tension is pronounced, lead to the threshold being exceeded, which in turn triggers a physical stress reaction. On the other hand, there are influences that can *lower* the threshold. The higher your general level of inner tension and stress and the lower the threshold, the less additional stress is needed to trigger a physical stress reaction.

Consider what methods you might use to reduce your general level of inner tension and stress, in order to become more "resilient" in the long run!

Fig. 10.11 Worksheet 10.11: A story about mindfulness

Worksheet 10.11: A story about mindfulness

Be happy

A man was once asked why he could always be so happy in spite of his many occupations.
He said:

"When I stand, I stand,

if I go, I go,

When I sit, I sit,

When I eat, I eat,

when I love, I love…"

Then the person who asked the question jumped in and said, "So do we, but what do you do beyond that?"
He said again:

"When I stand, I stand,

if I go, I go,

if I …

Again, the person who asked the question said, "But we do that too!"

But he said to them:
"No –
if you are sitting, then you are already standing,
If you're standing, you're already walking,
if you run, you're already there."

Far Eastern wisdom, based on Grün (2001)

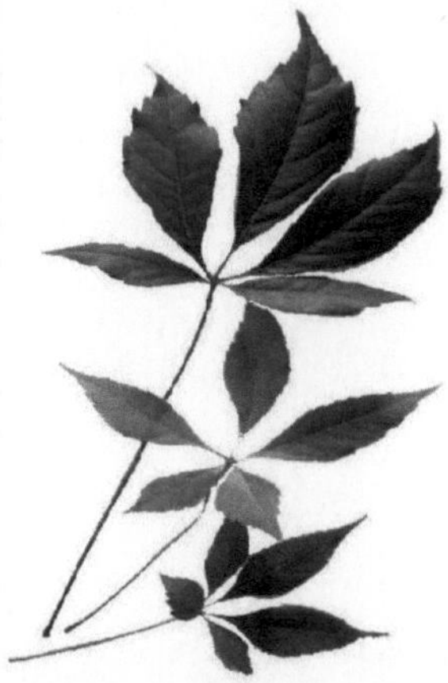

◘ **Fig. 10.12** Worksheet 10.12: Journal of well-being: How have I been today?

Worksheet 10.12: Journal of well-being: How have I been today?

Name/patient code:______________________ Date/Time:______________

1. **Tension/stress:**: How tense or under pressure or stress did you feel today?

   Please mark the amount of tension or inner pressure you felt today:

   I felt very calm. 0 1 2 3 4 5 6 7 8 9 10 I felt very tense and under pressure.

2. **General mood**: How was your mood in general today?

   On the following scale, please mark how you felt in general today:

   My mood was very bad. 0 1 2 3 4 5 6 7 8 9 10 My mood was very good.

3. **Efficiency**: How efficient did you feel today?

   Please mark on the following scale how fit and efficient you felt today:

   I've felt weak and not efficient. 0 1 2 3 4 5 6 7 8 9 10 I've felt in good shape and efficient.

4. **Physical condition:**

   (a) Have I experienced any physical discomfort or symptoms today?

   Please mark the extent of your physical discomfort that you have experienced today, on the following scale:

   I had no symptoms at all. 0 1 2 3 4 5 6 7 8 9 10 I had very severe somatic symptoms

   (b) Which somatic symptoms have I experienced today?

   Please name below the symptoms you experienced today:

   1.______________ 6.______________

   2.______________ 7.______________

   3.______________ 8.______________

   4.______________ 9.______________

   5.______________ 10.______________

5. **Fear of physical discomfort**: Have you experienced fear today that your somatic symptoms could be a sign of a serious illness?

   On the following scale, mark the extent to which you fear that your somatic symptoms could be a sign of a serious illness:

   I have no fear of being critically ill. 0 1 2 3 4 5 6 7 8 9 10 I have very intense fear of being critically ill.

From Kleinstäuber, M. et al: Cognitive behavior therapy for persistent somatic symptoms and somatic symptom disorders.

Fig. 10.12 (continued)

6. **Coping:**

(a) Did you have the impression that you were able to cope with or manage your somatic symptoms today?

Please indicate on the following scale how well you are coping with or managing your somatic symptoms today:

I was not able to cope with my somatic symptoms at all.	0	1	2	3	4	5	6	7	8	9	10	I was able to cope with my somatic symptoms very well.

(b) What have you done to manage your symptoms?

Please list below all the things that you have done today to cope with your symptoms:

1.________________ 4.________________

2.________________ 5.________________

3.________________ 6.________________

7. **Daily activities:** What did I do today?

Please list below all the activities that you did today, regardless of your somatic symptoms. These include professional, social, private, physical, and any other other activities. Also, using the time scale, mark the times at which you want to carry out the activities by blackening cells in the following graph. In the last line you can record the course of your somatic symptoms. Blacken the cells according to the periods of time when your symptoms worsened, and enter a circle when your symptoms improved.

Time / Activities	1	2	3	4	5	6	7	8	9	10	11	12	13	14	15	16	17	18	19	20	21	22	23
1.																							
2.																							
3.																							
4.																							
5.																							
6.																							
7.																							
8.																							
9.																							
10.																							
Somatic symptoms:																							

References

de Saint-Exupéry, A. (2009). *Die Stadt in der Wüste* (1. Aufl.). Karl Rauch.

Diewald, M. (1991). *Soziale Beziehungen: Verlust oder Liberalisierung? Soziale Unterstützung in informellen Netzwerken*. Edition Sigma.

Drexler, D. (2006). *Das integrierte Stress-Bewältigungs-Programm ISP*. Klett-Cotta.

Ehlert, U. (2003). *Verhaltensmedizin*. Springer.

Ende, M. (1973). *Momo* (20. Aufl.). Thienemann.

Grün, A. (2001). *Das kleine Buch vom Glück*. Herder.

Lazarus, R. S., & Launier, R. (1978). Stress-related transactions between person and environment. In L. A. Pervin & M. Lewis (Eds.), *Perspectives in international psychology* (pp. 287–327). Plenum Press.

Pascal, B. (1979). *Größe und Elend des Menschen*. Insel.

Peterson, C., & Seligman, M. E. P. (2004). *Character strengths and virtues: A classification and handbook*. Oxford University Press.

Potreck-Rose, F. (2007). *Von der Freude, den Selbstwert zu stärken* (5. Aufl.). Klett-Cotta.

Rettenbach, R. (2007). *Die Psychotherapie-Prüfung*. Schattauer.

Rosenthal, R., & Jacobson, L. (1986). *Pygmalion in the classroom*. Holt, Rinehart & Winston.

Scharfenstein, A., & Basler, H.-D. (2004). *Schlafstörungen: Auf dem Weg zu einem besseren Schlaf. Trainerhandbuch*. Vandenhoeck & Ruprecht.

Schopenhauer, A. (1976). *Aphorismen zur Lebensweisheit*. Insel.

von Glaserfeld, E. (1997). *Radikaler Konstruktivismus: Ideen, Ergebnisse, Probleme* (7. Aufl.). Suhrkamp.

Watzlawick, P. (2005). *Vom Unsinn des Sinns oder vom Sinn des Unsinns*. Piper.

Watzlawick, P. (2007). *Anleitung zum Unglücklichsein. Vom Schlechten des Guten* (5. Aufl.). Piper.

Module 7: The Explanatory Symptom and Treatment Model

Contents

M. Kleinstäuber et al., *Cognitive Behavior Therapy for Persistent Somatic Symptoms and Somatic Symptom Disorder*, https://doi.org/10.1007/978-3-662-69726-9_11

11.1 Session 20

Contents and Materials of the 20th Session

- **Contents**
  - Discussion of the practice of the week
  - Making up a balance of the therapy
  - Summary: explanatory symptom and treatment model
  - Helpful strategies for the future
  - Obtain feedback
- **Materials**
  - Worksheet 11.1: My therapy successes
  - Worksheet 11.2: Explanatory symptom and treatment model
  - Worksheet 11.3: Future coping strategies

11.1.1 Discussion of the Practice of the Week

The final session begins with the evaluation of the journal of well-being (Worksheet 10.12). The following questions can be helpful here:

11

- Were there any difficulties in processing?
- How frequent, how intense were the symptoms, or what was the extent of the distress?
- Has anything changed in the diary entries compared to the beginning of therapy? If so, what do these changes mean for the patient?

11.1.2 Making Up the Balance of the Therapy

The journal can be used as a transition to the balancing of the therapy. Patient and therapist together reflect on the course of therapy. The following questions are to be understood as a suggestion in this regard:

- What has changed for you?
- What have you learned and achieved with the help of therapy?
- Have your somatic symptoms changed?
- What do you think helped you the most?
- How will you be able to maintain or even build on progress?

Patients receive Worksheet 11.1 (My therapy successes). They should enter the original therapy goals and evaluate the extent to which these have been achieved.

11.1.3 Summary: Explanatory Symptom and Treatment Model

The therapy is now to be rounded off with a summary of the explanatory and treatment model. Patients are given the opportunity to integrate all the experiences they have gathered during the therapy into an overall model. The following instruction can be helpful here.

Instruction: A Summary of the Explanatory Symptom and Treatment Model

In the course of therapy, you have become acquainted with essential mechanisms or factors that play a role in the development and maintenance of your symptoms. Today, let us repeat, summarize and present in a diagram what you have learned in the course of treatment. At the same time, you should receive a plausible explanatory model for your symptoms.

It is very obvious and normal that when somatic symptoms occur you first think of a (physical) illness as the cause and act accordingly, i.e. take it easy and see the doctor. However, a somatic cause is only one of many possible factors that can play a role in the development of a disorder.

Cognitive behavior therapy assumes that numerous influences play a role in the development of mental disorders (and also somatoform symptoms). Research findings support this assumption. Factors that contribute to the development of a disorder are usually divided into three groups. A distinction is made between predisposing, triggering, and maintaining conditions.

***Predisposing factors** are understood to be genetic influences, biological processes, and formative experiences that one has gathered in the course of one's life, especially in childhood and adolescence. This is therefore the individual learning history (e.g., traumatic or stressful experiences, atmosphere in the parental home, upbringing). The personality of an individual is also a predisposing factor (peculiarities in information processing, early acquired thinking styles). Of particular relevance here is the "interoceptive perceptual style" or the concept of "somatosensory amplification"* (▶ Sect. 2.1). *This perceptual style, which also plays a significant role in the maintenance of the disorder, describes the tendency to experience bodily changes as intense, harmful and impairing, to pay particular attention to unpleasant sensations and to regard them as pathological signs rather than normal physiological reactions. Studies have shown that patients with persistent somatic symptoms observe their bodily functions more intensely and anxiously and are more prone to misinterpret them as signs of illness. Generally speaking, predisposing factors influence a per-*

son's risk of developing a mental disorder. They form the breeding ground, so to speak, and determine the susceptibility to developing a disorder.

Triggering or preceding conditions can be*: stress, problems or "the straw that breaks the camel's back", prolonged everyday stresses (e.g., double burden, constant pressure of deadlines and time, chronic physical illnesses and somatic symptoms), changes in lifestyle habits and adaptation situations to new stages of life and problems, such as professional reorientation, family changes (e.g., children leaving home), processes of physical changes in the body (e.g., menopause), stressful individual events (e.g., illness, accident, bereavement, divorce, relocation, change of job), also primarily positive events, such as marriage, pregnancy or birth, fall under this category, as they are also associated with stress and require adaptation to a changed situation.*

Maintaining conditions *lead to the fact that the disorder does not cease, but becomes more intense and frequent.*

Two "vicious circles" in particular are essential for the perpetuation of the problem:

1. *an internal **vicious circle** (not recognizable from the outside, takes place inside the affected person): increased attention to physical processes and changes or sensations, false evaluation of the symptoms;*
2. *an external **vicious circle** (observable from the outside, for others): Illness behavior (usually prolonged, often chronicized).*

For most mental disorders, such vicious cycles can be identified that perpetuate the problem. Often, the person's appraisals of the symptoms or the behaviors they take to control the symptoms contribute to their perpetuation. Treatment is then about breaking these vicious cycles.

After this initial theoretical explanation, the patient receives Worksheet 11.2 (Explanatory symptom and treatment model). The individual components are discussed together and validated using individual examples from the patient. The individual model components are explained below.

▪ Trigger

Physiological arousal, information (e.g., from the media, heard from acquaintances), minor illnesses or ailments, physical changes in the body.

▪ Perception and Attention

Physical reactions are perceived (they move into the spotlight) due to conscious or also spontaneous attention control. This can already lead to a more intense perception of the symptom—for example, one can think of the shoes that start to press as soon as one consciously focuses on one's feet.

▪ Misinterpretation of Body Signals as Threatening Signs of Illness

In most cases, the perceived symptoms are misinterpreted as dangerous and catastrophic, which leads to a build-up of symptoms. When one evaluates something as threatening, one naturally focuses one's attention more on it and is alarmed. For this reason, one's attention is increasingly focused on internal bodily processes, which is accompanied by increased physiological or physical arousal. Thus the vicious circle closes. As an illustrative example, the following situation can be addressed: "You wake up in the morning and feel listless. You might think to yourself: I feel weak because I pulled an all-nighter. Perhaps a cold is coming on. Here, the symptom of weakness is judged to be relatively harmless. You will remain calm. However, if you say to yourself, oh dear, I must be seriously ill, have multiple sclerosis, or something else bad!, this triggers great discomfort, if not anxiety, which in turn can cause a physical stress response or lead to an increase in physiological arousal." Misperceptions can also stem from unrealistic attitudes about health and how the body functions (e.g., "A healthy body is always symptom-free," "Pain in the arm signals an impending heart attack," "A doctor must always be able to find the right diagnosis and treatment").

▪ Illness Behavior

With so-called illness behaviors, affected persons try to control their symptoms or to alleviate or cure them with the help of medical services. In other words, the aim is to reduce the symptoms. In the long term, however, this leads to exactly the opposite, namely to a stabilization of the symptoms. For example, one visits the phsyician and demands medical examinations. If the findings are inconspicuous, doubts are raised and further physicians and specialists are sought out. This behavior, the excessive use of medical services, is also called "doctor shopping". Also among the illness behaviors are self-examinations and functional checks, so-called checking behaviors. For example, redness of the skin may be exacerbated by constant palpation of the affected area, or a lumpy feeling in the throat may be triggered by constant swallowing movements. In addition, many sufferers develop excessive avoidance behavior. Physical exertion or sporting activities are avoided for fear of worsening symptoms. In the long term, however, physical rest weakens physical resilience, condition and muscle strength, so that observable physical changes or sensations occur even at low levels of exertion. Attention is often drawn to the discomfort or to related information. Some sufferers buy medical reference books, watch health programs in the media or find no other topic than the somatic symptoms in conversations with family and friends, which in turn can put a strain on interpersonal relationships in the long term. Another illness behavior is taking unnecessary or medically unindicated medication. Here there is the danger that new symptoms are triggered (side effects). In addition, an organ-medical understanding of illness is supported ("Whoever is prescribed medication must also be ill"). Long-term negative consequences: Development of dependence, physical consequential damage.

- **Sick Roll**

Often the sick role is associated with certain "advantages". In this case, one speaks of „(secondary) gain from illness" or operant reinforcement. Possible advantages for the patient: increased attention from family, partner or physician, omission/avoidance of unpleasant private or professional duties, financial advantages (pension payment).

11.1.4 Helpful Strategies for the Future

Now that all the important factors that can contribute to the development and maintenance of somatic symptoms have been discussed, all the strategies for dealing with symptoms that the patient would like to use more in the future should be summarized with the patient. The patient is given Worksheet 11.3 (Future coping strategies).

11.1.5 Obtain Feedback

Finally, patients should be asked to report what they liked and disliked about the treatment. It is also helpful to ask patients which units they felt benefited them the most, or what they found most helpful about the therapy.

11.2 Worksheets

These worksheets are also available for download online at Springer Extras (► extras.springer.com).

Worksheet 11.1	My therapy successes	◘ Figure 11.1
Worksheet 11.2	Explanatory symptom and treatment model	◘ Figure 11.2
Worksheet 11.3	Future coping strategies	◘ Figure 11.3

11

Fig. 11.1 Worksheet 11.1: My therapy successes

Worksheet 11.1: My therapy successes

Therapy goal	Did I reach my goal?			
	not at all	a little	almost	very much

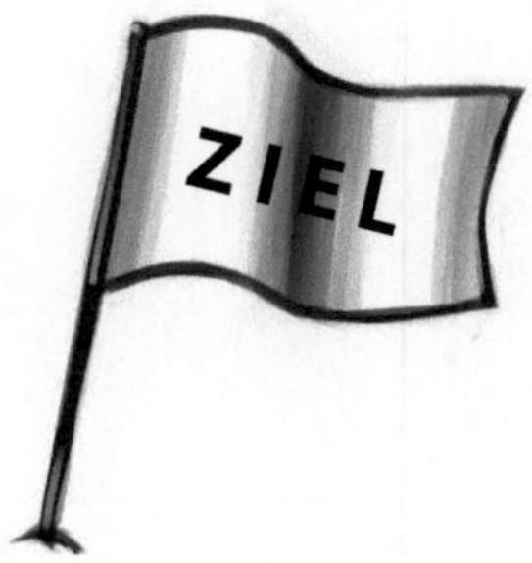

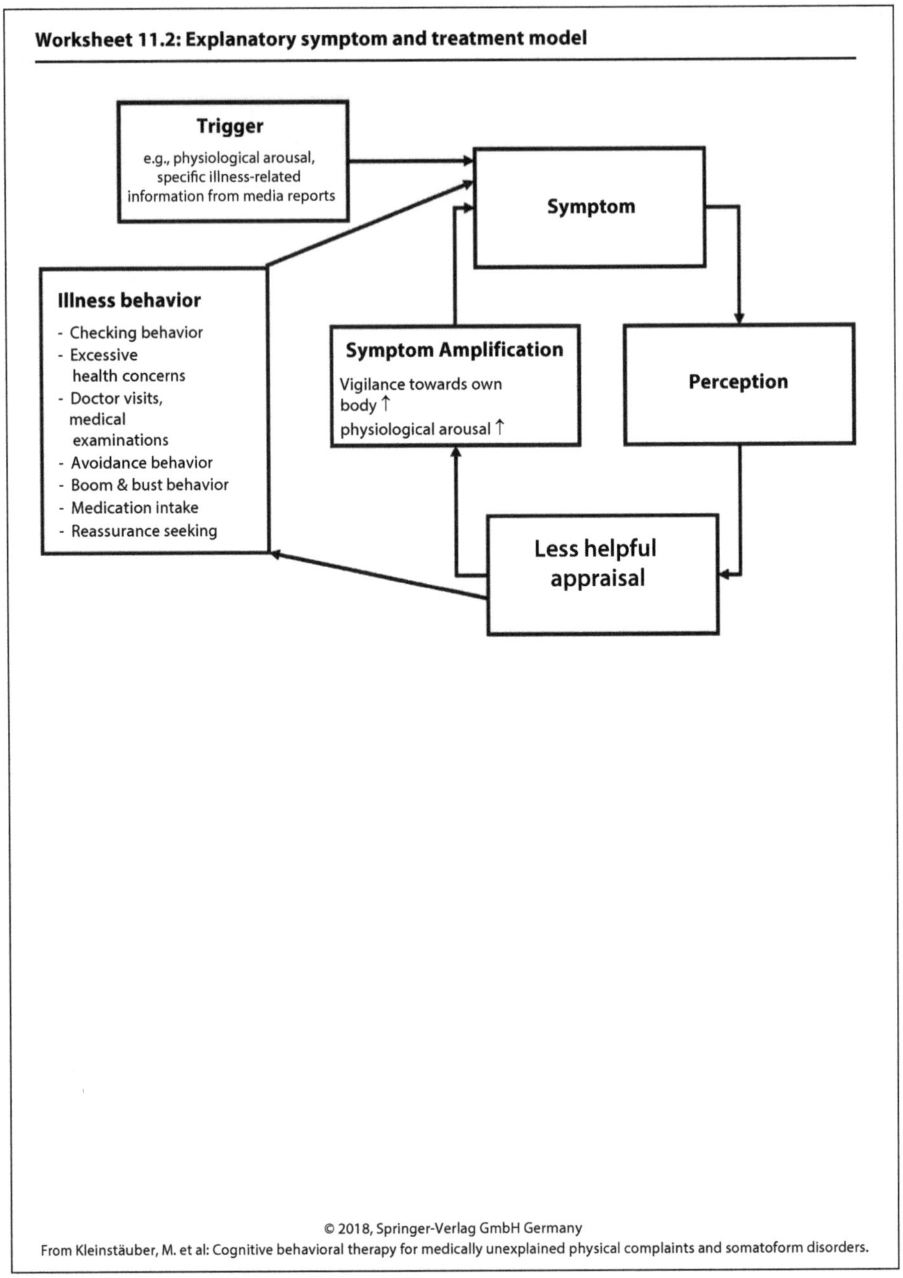

■ **Fig. 11.2** Worksheet 11.2: Explanatory symptom and treatment model

Fig. 11.3 Worksheet 11.3: Future coping strategies

Worksheet 11.3: Future coping strategies

What coping strategies do I want to use in the future when my somatic symptoms will be present?

1. ....
2. ....
3. ....
4. ....
5. ....
6. ....
7. ....
8. ....

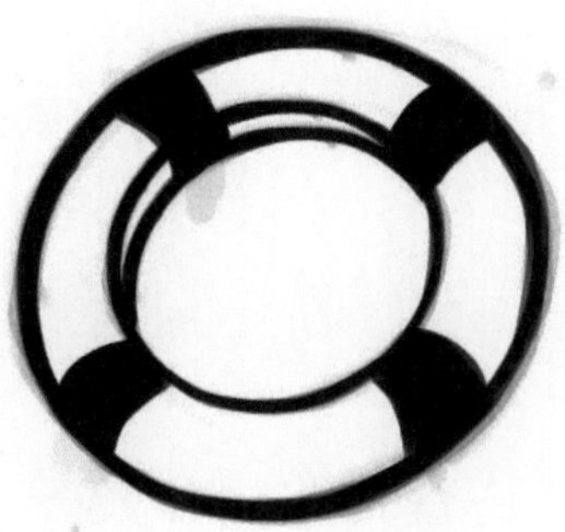

Excursus: Communication in Everyday Life and with the Physician

Contents

M. Kleinstäuber et al., *Cognitive Behavior Therapy for Persistent Somatic Symptoms and Somatic Symptom Disorder*, https://doi.org/10.1007/978-3-662-69726-9_12

12.1 Communication in Everyday Life

12.1.1 Exploration of Communication Problems in Everyday Life

Contents and Materials
- **Contents**
  - Exploration of communication problems of patients in their everyday life
  - Therapy approaches for selected interpersonal problems of patients with persistent somatic symptoms
- **Materials**
  - Worksheet 12.1: My interpersonal problems

■ Exploration of Communication Problems of Patients in Their Everyday Life

Patients suffering from persistent somatic symptoms may experience difficulties in communicating with their environment in very different interpersonal areas—such as with their family and friends, with their (spousal) partner or with colleagues and supervisors at work. In the first step it is important to explore the situations in which the patient has difficulties in communicating with their environment, in order to work out starting points for therapy in the second step. The following questions can serve as orientation:

- Can you recall situations where you talked about your symptoms and received negative feedback or observed negative reactions from others?
- Are there people in your environment with whom you tend to avoid talking about your symptoms? For what reasons?
- Do you experience difficulties or restrictions in interpersonal relationships with certain people in your environment because of your symptoms? If yes, with which persons? What are the specific difficulties or limitations? Can you talk to these people about these difficulties or limitations?
- Do you have the feeling that you have encountered more rejection in your environment since you started suffering from your symptoms? If so, can you describe specific situations in which you felt rejected?
- Do you sometimes feel misunderstood in your social environment? If so, by which persons and why do you feel rejected? How do these people react to you?
- Do you have relationships with people who are very trusting and with whom you can also talk about personally very stressful topics, such as your somatic symptoms? What are the reasons why you can trust these people so well or feel understood by them?

To record the interpersonal problems, Worksheet 12.1 (My interpersonal problems) can be used as a basis.

■ Therapy Approaches for Selected Interpersonal Problems of Patients with Persistent Somatic Symptoms

In the following, we pick out two typical problem situations from our clinical experience for each of the following three areas of interpersonal relationships—family members and friends, (spousal) partners, work colleagues and supervisors—and show by way of example how one can work on them using cognitive behavior therapy. These problem situations are multifaceted, so that we address only a limited selection of them here. Moreover, possible therapeutic approaches cannot be described in detail, but only outlined. Due to the heterogeneity of communication problems of patients with persistent somatic symptoms and related conditions, a precise indication of the number of sessions and the distribution of therapeutic contents among the sessions is only possible to a limited extent. Accordingly, the following guidelines should be applied flexibly by the therapist in terms of time and content. They should serve as a suggestion for therapists and can be further developed by them. If the following difficulties do not fit your patient, you can refer to the general paradigm for a behavioral experiment on a generally difficult interpersonal situation in ► Sect. 12.1.5.

12.1.2 Communication Problems with Family Members or Friends

Contents and Materials
- **Contents**
  - Problem A: The patient is experienced as a complaining person
  - Problem B: Support for relatives of patients with persistent somatic symptoms
- **Materials**
  - Worksheet 12.2: Characteristics of complaining behavior
  - Camera for role play recording

Problem A: The Patient Is Experienced as a Complaining Person

Patients often report that as soon as they report their somatic symptoms, those around them react annoyed or irritated. Some of these patients have received feedback from others that they are experienced as a complaining person. For those affected, this is usually a difficult and hurtful feedback to process. Therefore, this topic should be approached very gently in therapy and feelings of guilt should be avoided in the patient. In addition, working through this issue requires an already stable and mutually trusting therapy relationship. The method of video feedback helps to support the patient in "guided discovery" and to make the confrontation with one's own behavior or the recognition of complaining behavioral tendencies seem less threatening. We therefore suggest the following procedure:

Video Recording of Patient Behavior

Patients are instructed to tell the therapist about their somatic symptoms in the same way as they would talk about them with a relative or friend. In doing so, they can put themselves in a specific (and not far back in time) situation. The conversation should last a maximum of 5 min and is recorded.

Change of Perspective

Patient and therapist watch the recording together. Patients are asked to put themselves in the role of their counterpart and to imagine talking to themselves about their somatic symptoms. To avoid feelings of guilt and shame on the part of the patient, the "discovering" character of the practice should be emphasized throughout.

Helpful Statements from the Therapist

» *Your environment gives you the feedback that you seem to be complaining. Let's find out together what they mean by this and how you yourself experience your behavior. When you observe yourself, do you recognise characteristics that make your behavior and appearance seem complaining? We have a protected space for you here, where you can get to know your own behavior more closely and where you can deal with it. Let's find out together what is true or not true about the claims of those around you and let's consider together if there are opportunities for you to do things differently.*

Exploration of Features in Patient Behavior: What Makes the Behavior a Complaining Behavior?

With the help of the video recording, the following aspects of the patient's behavior should be explored:

❓
- How does the person (i.e. yourself) who is talking about their somatic symptoms in the video affect you?
- How do you feel about the role of the other person?
- Can you identify lamentability in the person's behavior? If so, can you try to describe what features of the person's behavior make them seem plaintive? Try to address different levels of behavior, such as voice, gestures and facial expressions, posture, choice of words and content.

Worksheet 12.2 (Characteristics of complaining behavior) lists various characteristics of complaining behavior at different levels of behavior. Together with patients it can be checked whether these aspects apply to their own behavior and whether further behavioral characteristics can be added from observation.

Derivation of Possibilities for Change and Further Exercises

Finally, patients are supported in deducing aspects that they could change in their behavior. The suggestions for change can be recorded on Worksheet 12.2 (Characteristics of complaining behavior). The possible changes in the patient's behavior that have been worked out can be deepened and practiced in a role play (► Sect. 12.1.4, "Problem B") or a behavioral experiment (► Sect. 12.1.5).

Problem B: Support for Relatives of Patients with Persistent Somatic Symptoms

In the case of patients with persistent somatic symptoms, especially those who have limitations in their communication skills, it is significant to involve important caregivers in the therapy. The relatives should be supported, on the one hand, to be able to cope better with the affected family member and, on the other hand, to give him functional and helpful support.

Persistent somatic symptoms often have a very diffuse effect on relatives. They are a burden for the affected person, but also have a negative impact on the entire environment of the affected person. Everyday life is restricted by the symptoms. The longer the symptoms last, the more difficult it can be for relatives to understand how much a person can suffer from persistent somatic symptoms and they can become doubtful as to whether the bodily symptoms are not after all an "imagination" or an exaggeration. It is therefore quite understandable that the need to finally find a cause of the somatic symptoms is as strong in relatives as in the affected person themselves. The idea that there is no "one" cause, but that many different factors influence the symptomatology, is initially very abstract and difficult to imagine for many. Often there is rather a "black and white conception"—that is, either the affected person is *really* ill and then *an* organic cause can be found, or the person is faking or is "crazy". With the motive of actually wanting to do something good and be supportive, they try to give comfort, which can make the relationship even more difficult and even cause rejection on the part of the affected person or the feeling of not being taken seriously. Understandably, these two opposing attitudes—wanting to support and respect the loved one on the one hand, and doubting the suffering of the loved one on the other, or feeling annoyed by the strong focus on the somatic symptoms—can put relatives in a difficult emotional situation. They feel insecure and torn in an emotional dilemma. This justifies the importance of involving relatives in the therapy sessions, for which we recommend the following procedure:

▪ Provide a Safe and Neutral Space for the Expression of Feelings and Thoughts

First of all, give the patient as well as the relative space to be able to express their feelings and thoughts in connection with the somatic symptoms. The following rules for the conversation should first be presented to the participants:

- **Allow each other to talk it out** Each participant in the conversation should be given a fixed, time-limited period in which they can speak openly about their feelings and thoughts. They should only be interrupted during this time window if there are follow-up questions that serve to improve understanding.
- **Listening attentively to each other** The participants in the conversation should listen attentively to each other without immediately commenting on what is said.
- **Refrain from comments and evaluations of what is said** In everyday life we are inclined to quickly evaluate the things our counterpart says to us through "our glasses" (i.e. our attitudes towards a certain topic). This can quickly lead to misunderstandings because the other person may be pursuing a completely different motive with their statement. For this reason, direct comments and evaluations should be avoided in a safe and neutral conversation space.
- **Express feelings directly and in the first person** When people talk about feelings in their everyday lives, it can be easy to fail to anchor them within themselves. For example, many fall into generalizing man-speak ("It's easy to feel helpless when you see someone suffering."). Alternatively, accusations occur through using the pronoun you (e.g., "You make me feel helpless every time you get that pain-distorted look."). Both forms of expressing feelings should be avoided and the first person form should be chosen (e.g., "I feel helpless when I see how bad you are.").
- **Reference to concrete situations and examples** In everyday language, people are quick to speak in generalizations and absolutes (e.g., "He looks at me every morning with that pain-distorted expression."). Typical signal words include always, every time, exclusively. It would be helpful for the conversation if the participants try to refer to concrete situations and examples.
- **Paying attention to positive things and resources** Of course, it is important that the relatives in particular are first given space to talk about their concerns and the negative aspects they associate with the affected person's somatic symptoms. However, space should also be deliberately given to aspects that work well or that represent resources (e.g. "Although we are restricted in many areas due to the somatic symptoms, we regularly manage to visit our children together").

Therapists have a moderating function and make sure that the rules of the conversation are observed. If necessary, they can log the statements of the relative and the patient on a flipchart.

▪ Involvement of Relatives in Psychoeducation

Similar to the patients themselves, it is important for the relatives to broaden their causal thinking. This can best be done if they are included in the psychoeducation. For the psychoeducation of relatives, manual contents and exercises can be picked out and adapted accordingly, depending on the individual problems:

- the exercise 'What explanations do the patients have for their symptoms' (▶ Sect. 5.1),
- the explanation of the human stress response (▶ Sect. 6.1),
- the effect of attention on the perception of our body (▶ Sect. 7.1),
- the link between thoughts and physical changes or the guided imagery "A lemon" (▶ Sect. 8.1),
- the vicious circle of avoidance behavior or boom and bust behavior (▶ Sect. 9.1) or reassurance seeking (▶ Sect. 10.1),
- a summary of the explanatory symptom and treatment model (▶ Sect. 11.1).

In the context of psychoeducation, myths that are frequently encountered on the part of relatives should be challenged:

- "No medical cause can be found, from there the symptoms are made up and not real."
- "The discomfort has been going on for so long now. I cannot imagine that ... is really suffering so much, though no cause can be found."
- "There is only *one* cause and *one* treatment for the ailment."
- "You can only be physically *or* mentally ill. Physical illness is normal and believable. However, if the doctor cannot find a cause, the person has a pathological mental problem."

Support for Relatives in Dealing with the Affected Person

Depending on the specific problem that a relative reports in dealing with the affected person, helpful behavioral patterns can be worked out after the psychoeducation that support the relatives in protecting themselves and at the same time being supportive for the affected person.

The following overview includes behavioral strategies for relatives to learn to reinforce the patient less in their sick role:

Helpful Behavioral Strategies for Relatives

- Avoidance of regular inquiries about the symptoms, which draw attention to the symptoms
- Avoidance of well-intentioned consideration and thus reinforcement of avoidance behavior
- Supporting the patient in actively shaping their life and not in experiencing the illness
- Arrangement of regular appointments in which the patient and the family member together engage in a leisure activity that (if necessary, after consultation with the therapist) is realistic and easily manageable for the patient.
- Comfort is well-intentioned, but may increase the patient's attention to the somatic symptoms
- Consciously search together for small "islands" of positive experiences in everyday life. These do not have to be expensive activities. Small pleasurable activities (e.g., lunch together, a movie night on the couch) are enough.
- As soon as the patient lapses into avoidance behavior or complaining behavior, a sign can be agreed between patient and relatives that helps patients to reflect on their behavior and prevents them from following their behavioral impulse. This can also relieve the burden on the relative, who is thereby legitimized to address sick role behavior.

12.1.3 Communication Problems with the (Marriage) Partner

Contents and Materials

- **Contents**
  - Problem A: Negative influence of somatic symptoms on sexuality
  - Problem B: Withdrawal of the patient from partnership activities
- **Materials**
  - Worksheet 12.3: Explanations for our sexual problems
  - Worksheet 12.4: Sensate focus exercises and log of experiences
  - Worksheet 12.5: The consequences of my withdrawal from activities with my partner

Problem A: Negative Influence of Persistent Somatic Symptoms on Sexuality

Somatic symptoms can influence sexuality in a partnership in many different ways. Due to somatic symptoms, for example, the desire for sexuality can be limited, as this is accompanied by pain. Persistent somatic symptoms can also be accompanied by negative changes in body image—e.g., experiencing oneself as less attractive or functional—which in turn have an inhibiting effect on the enjoyment of sexual activity. If the patient's sexuality is affected in a very complex way (especially by other general problems such as partner conflicts), more comprehensive, specialized psychological treatment of this problem is necessary and understandably cannot be covered with the help of this module (for more detail, see e.g., Hoyndorf et al., 1995). The following provides guidance on how to explore sexual problems in the context of persistent somatic symptoms. This is the first important step in approaching sexual problems, since the topic is very often avoided by therapists as well as patients.

Questions for Exploration of Sexual Difficulties Related to Persistent Somatic Symptoms

First come questions that can be used to explore sexual difficulties and possible accompanying problems (see also Hoyndorf et al., 1995; Hillman, 2012). Since most patients are unaccustomed to talking about their sexual life, it is important to obtain permission to ask questions about this very personal topic before beginning the exploration. In addition, it may be useful to first explore the following questions with the partners separately in individual conversation:

Questions About Sexual Problems and the Influence of Somatic Symptoms

- First of all, can you describe the problem to me in more detail?
- To what extent do your somatic symptoms play a role in the context of your sexual problems? (e.g., pain with certain postures; lack of sexual pleasure as a result of persistent physical discomfort during sexual activities).
- Can you describe exactly during which sexual activities the problems occur? Do they refer to all your sexual activities or only to certain ones? Do they relate to reaching climax or already to your sexual pleasure and arousal?
- When did your problems start? Was the onset related to the development of your somatic symptoms or did they already exist before?
- What do you think is the cause? Do you see the cause in the somatic symptoms or do you suspect other causes? As a partner, what do you think about possible causes?
- Is the sexual problem always constant or is it sometimes better sometimes worse?
- How often do you masturbate? How do you feel about it and do your somatic symptoms influence your experience of masturbation?
- Have you already made attempts to solve the problem? Do you have confidants with whom you have already talked about your sexual problems?
- People who suffer from similar symptoms sometimes experience changes in satisfaction with their body, e.g., they have the impression that they can no longer trust their body or no longer feel attractive. How do you feel about your body?

Questions About Attitudes Towards Sexuality in General

- Sexuality can have different meanings depending on the person. What do the terms "sexuality" or "sexual activities" encompass for you?
- What does "good sex" mean to you? If it were up to you alone, what belongs to good sex for you?
- Do you find it difficult to talk about sexuality, for example with your doctor or with me?

Questions About Sexuality in the Partnership

- When were you last sexually active?
- How satisfied are you with your sex life? Do you have any concerns about your sexual health?
- If it were up to you alone, is there anything you would want to be different in your sex life?
- How often were you sexually active before the onset of somatic symptoms, and how often since the onset of symptoms?
- Who usually takes the initiative for sex in your partnership?

Questions About Partnership and Communication Between Partners

- How can you talk to your partner about the sexual problems?
- How do you express when you have sexual desires? Is it difficult for you to express them?
- What do you do when you don't feel like having sex but your partner wants to be sexually active? And vice versa: How do you react when your partner does not want to be sexually active, but you feel like intimacy?
- What are the strengths and weaknesses of your relationship?
- Do you show affection and tenderness in everyday life? If so, how?
- Are there issues where conflicts often arise between you and your partner? How do you deal with them?
- Do these conflicts affect your sex life with your partner?
- Can you tell me three things you particularly appreciate about your partner?
- If you had three wishes for your partner in general, what would they be?

Intervention for the Treatment of Loss of Sexual Desire in Persistent Somatic Symptoms

In the following, we refer to a specific case of sexual problems in persistent somatic symptoms—the loss of sexual pleasure—and provide a paradigm for which one should plan approximately 10 sessions. If there is a suspicion of sexual trauma in the patient's history as well as post-traumatic stress disorder, this treatment module is not suitable and the focus of treatment should first be directed towards post-traumatic stress symptomatology.

Understanding Problems and the Relationship Between Persistent Somatic Symptoms and Sexual Activity

First of all, the exploration of the role of somatic symptoms as well as other influencing factors (e.g., pressure of expectations, body dissatisfaction in the patient) in the development of the sexual problem (Worksheet 12.3: Explanations for our sexual problems) is in the foreground. The frequently encountered potential assumption that insufficient love is the cause of the sexual problem should be questioned.

▪ **Uncovering Negative Feelings Related to Sexual Problems and Somatic Symptoms**

The patient and partner are instructed to perform Sensate Focus exercises (Hoyndorf et al., 1995; Masters & Johnson, 1966)—graded stroking and stimulation exercises—at home and to record thoughts and feelings experienced by both during the exercises (Worksheet 12.4: Sensate Focus exercises and log of experiences). These exercises are designed to help the couple express uncomfortable feelings related to listlessness. In the Sensate Focus exercises, the couple is appropriately instructed to consciously direct the focus of attention to the disturbing thoughts, feelings, and sensations (in the patient, also to the physical discomfort). This exploration of the body, which is not aimed at experiencing a climax, is initially a new experience for many couples. This can have a very relieving effect, as this approach counteracts pressure to perform and gives space to develop strategies for an enjoyable experience of sexuality despite somatic symptoms.

▪ **Pleasurable Sexual Experience Despite Persistent Somatic Symptoms**

The staged stroking exercises have above all a diagnostic function and provide a starting point for questioning and modifying less helpful thoughts with the partners on the one hand, and on the other hand for looking for behavioral strategies that allow sexual activity in the partnership to become a positive experience again despite somatic symptoms. Possibly the stroking exercises also give room to discover new sexual activities that the partners find pleasurable and have not yet tried. If it becomes clear during the exercises that the patient in particular has developed a negatively altered body image as a result of the persistent somatic symptoms, the exercises can be used to specifically explore and name positive aspects of one's own body.

▪ **Expression of Sexual Interest or Disinterest**

Furthermore, the stroking exercises can be used very well to practice communication about sexual interest or disinterest between partners. It is very common for misunderstandings to occur between partners because one of them expects the other to be able to "read their mind". However, often the signals of sexual interest and disinterest between partners are not clear enough. In therapy, these signals should be explored and, if necessary, made clearer and more meaningful.

▪ **Transfer to Everyday Life**

The long-term goal of these exercises is not primarily to equalize the level of sexual pleasure of both partners and to set "standards" for the frequency of sexual activity. On the contrary, any kind of pressure to perform should be avoided as much as possible. The partner who is not affected by somatic symptoms should learn to cope with a possibly persistent discrepancy in sexual interest. At the same time, the sexual contacts that take place between the partners should be made as enjoyable as possible for both partners.

▪ **Problem B: Withdrawal of the Patient from Partnership Activities**

In patients with persistent somatic symptoms who exhibit pronounced avoidance behavior, these avoidant tendencies may also extend to partnership activities (e.g., joint leisure activities, holiday trips). It is advisable to explore these restrictions in discussion with the patient and their partner. You can use the strategies described in ► Sect. 12.1.2, 'Providing a safe and neutral space for the expression of feelings and thoughts', as a guide.

In the next step—similar to ► Sect. 9.1—the short- and long-term consequences of this withdrawal behavior for the two partners individually, but also for the couple relationship, should be discussed. Use Worksheet 12.5 (The consequences of my withdrawal from activities with my partner) for guidance. Finally, similar to ► Sect. 9.2, joint activities can be planned with the couple. The therapist should support the partners in the balancing act between taking into account the patient's symptom-related performance limits and avoidance behavior. In order to create a commitment in the partners to carry out these activities, the activities should be planned precisely in terms of time.

12.1.4 Communication Problems with Supervisors and Colleagues

Contents and Materials

- **Contents**
  - Problem A: Talking to supervisors and colleagues about one's own somatic symptoms in a socially competent manner.
  - Problem B: Being able to set boundaries and say no
- **Materials**
  - Worksheet 12.6: Practice log—talking about my somatic symptoms in a socially competent way at work
  - Worksheet 12.7: Role play log—setting boundaries and saying no
  - Worksheet 12.8: Assertive, insecure, and aggressive behavior: What is typical?
  - Worksheet 12.9: My behavioral experiment—planning

- Worksheet 12.10: My behavioral experiment—log
- Camera for role play recording

Problem A: Talking to Supervisors and Colleagues About One's Own Somatic Symptoms in a Socially Competent Manner

Communication about one's symptoms at work can be a problem for the patient. Worries about negative evaluation by colleagues or the supervisor, a lack of confidants at the workplace or fear of losing one's job in case of prolonged absence due to illness can be important issues for the patient. Accordingly, various problem situations and issues may arise at the workplace that the patient needs to discuss with the supervisor or colleagues. In doing so, the patient may need to disclose to the supervisor or colleagues. A typical example would be that the patient plans an inpatient stay of several weeks in a psychosomatic clinic, followed by a staged reintegration at the workplace.

In the following, we will provide you with a paradigm to guide the therapists in supporting their patients in communicating with supervisors and colleagues about their somatic symptoms. Answers and insights to the following questions can be recorded on Worksheet 12.6 (Practice log—talking about my symptoms in a socially competent way at work).

12

? Occasion for the Interview

- For what reason do you want to have the conversation?

? Target Person(s)

- With whom should the interview take place? (e.g., supervisor, colleagues)
- Is there perhaps a trusted person at work with whom you could talk again before the planned interview, from whom you can get advice and who knows the target person?

? Desired Result of the Interview

- With what desired result would you like to leave the conversation?
- Is your desired outcome realistic? What can you expect?
- Is your desired goal anchored in you, i.e. can you influence it? (A goal that is not anchored in the patient would be, for example: "I want my supervisor to agree to my staged reintegration at work." In contrast, the patient could formulate the following as an anchored goal: "I express my desire for staged reintegration and submit a proposal for reintegration to him.")

? Planned Contents of the Interview

- What content should you include in the conversation and how should you structure it?
- Is it necessary for you to disclose anything about your symptoms during the interview?
- What exactly do you want to say about your symptoms? What do you not want to talk about?
- How do you explain your discomfort or problem to the target person?

? Behavior and Communication During the Interview

- We refer here to ◘ Table 12.1, which describes characteristics of assertive and socially competent behavior, as well as behavioral strategies for reducing litigiousness.

? Potential Difficulties in the Course of the Conversation and Strategies for Dealing with Them

- What reactions and behaviors can you expect from the target person that will make the conversation difficult?
- How can you deal with these difficulties?

My Attitude Towards My Work (Only Relevant for Problem Situations Related to the Patient's Work Performance)

When dealing with problem situations that specifically involve the performance that the patient is expected to deliver at work, it may be important to make the patient aware of and question their attitude towards their work. This can have a strong influence on the patient's behavior in the interview situation. It makes a big difference, for example, whether the patient in the example chosen above hopes for early retirement in the long term after a planned inpatient treatment or plans to return completely to their job. The following questions can provide guidance:

?

- What does your work mean to you? What do you like and dislike about your work?
- Do you feel comfortable at your workplace? What do you like about your workplace and what do you like less?
- If you had a choice, would you prefer to continue in your job and your current job, or would you prefer another job or job, or would you prefer to stop working altogether?

Table 12.1 Strategies for improving the patients' communication with their doctor

Difficulties on the patient side	Strategies for dealing with the difficulties
Little self-confident appearance	Maintain eye contact with doctor Speak loudly, moderately fast, clearly and distinctly Friendly facial expression and at the same time determined appearance Posture: Sitting upright, both feet in contact with the floor, relaxed posture Use of "I" and direct expression of feelings Choice of clothing can have an impact on the external image of the patient
My counterpart perceives me as plaintive	Neutral facial expression during symptom report Objective, neutral pronunciation; avoidance of overly "emotional" language Factual description of the symptoms with emphasis on the perception of the symptoms and their consequences Report of feelings related to the somatic symptoms is important, but should be in the first person and not dominate the conversation
Patient forgets what they wanted to say in the course of the conversation	Read through notes on the contents of the discussion intensively before the discussion or take them with you into the discussion with the doctor.
Patient quickly loses the thread and gets lost in unimportant details	Notes for the doctor's consultation should have a clear structure; important information should be separated from unimportant information Self-instruction card (e.g., with questions to guide the conversation: What symptoms do I have? How long have I had them? How often do they occur? Do they always occur or only at certain times of the day?) If patients wish to bring in medical reports from previous treatment, they should carefully consider what information from the reports is important to the doctor
Patient is easily intimidated	Exploration of individual signs of intimidation Exploration of avoidance behaviors that the patient exhibits when feeling intimidated (e.g., agreeing to everything the interviewer says; lack of eye contact; behaviors to compensate for nervousness)
Patient reacts quickly angry and irritated	Exploration of individual signs of anger in the patient: Physiological and emotional reactions, triggering thoughts, impulses to act and behavior Distinction between the less functional suppression of anger and an acceptance-oriented, mindful handling of anger (see in depth Eifert et al., 2009) Detachment from the premature evaluation of the doctor's behavior and awareness of possible motives for the doctor's behavior Self-instruction (e.g., "I feel that I am angry right now. In order to achieve my goals, it is now important that I do not follow my anger thoughts and feelings, but that I distance myself from them")

- What function does your work have for your everyday life? What would your life be like if you no longer had a job overnight?
- What impact might your attitude toward your work have on the conversation you plan to have?

Appropriate interview situations can be practiced according to the role-play paradigm with video feedback, which is presented in the following section, or within the framework of a behavioral experiment, which is described in ▶ Sect. 12.1.5.

▪ Problem B: Being Able to Set Boundaries and Say No

A specific problem that is often observed in patients with persistent somatic symptoms—especially in those who have accompanying perfectionist tendencies and high demands on themselves—is the limited ability to set boundaries and the limited ability to say "no". For therapists, this issue is a balancing act, as there are patients with persistent somatic symptoms and, in particular, strongly pronounced avoidance behavior, who at the same time exhibit the opposite tendency—i.e. frequent saying no. Before the exercise from this section is used, it should therefore be clarified whether it is actually the patient's problem of not being able to set boundaries and whether the exercise does not indirectly promote avoidance behavior.

In the following we present a structure for a role play that patients can apply to a wide variety of situations in which they would like to delimit themselves more. The log on Worksheet 12.7 (Role play log—setting boundaries and saying no) can be used for implementation.

Description of the Problem Situation

- In what specific situation would you like to practice setting boundaries or saying no?

Desired Result

- What is your goal?
- Is the goal realistic? Is it a "hidden" avoidance goal?
- Can you influence the goal yourself and is it anchored in you?

Characteristics of Confident Compared to Insecure or Aggressive Behavior

- In this specific situation, how would you identify whether the person is confident as distinct from insecure or aggressive based on the following aspects? (Worksheet 12.8: Assertive, insecure, and aggressive behavior: What is typical?; adapted from Hinsch & Pfingsten, 2015).
- How are voice, choice of words and phrasing, content, gestures, facial expressions and posture?

Allocation of Roles and Intentions of the Patient for the Role Play

- What should therapists pay attention to in their role, so that the role play has as real a character as possible?
- What 1–2 characteristics of confident behavior should you look for during role-play?

Implementation and Debriefing of the Role Play

The role play should be recorded on video and limited to 5 min. After the performance, the debriefing is crucial, which is initially done without video. The following questions can serve as orientation:

- How did you feel during the role play?
- Were you able to implement your plan?
- What did you do well? (Patients who have difficulties formulating positive things about their behavior should be supported with positive feedback if necessary).
- What else could you work on? (The therapist can also give feedback to the patient, if necessary, on how they felt in their role and how the patient affected them).

During the video debriefing, patients are asked to stop the video whenever they showed behavior in the desired direction or when he has suggestions for improvement. If patients have difficulty recognizing and verbalizing where they were able to successfully implement their intentions, the therapist should support them. If necessary, the role play can be repeated and evaluated again.

The behavior that was practiced in the role play during the therapy session can also be carried out in vivo in the next step as part of a behavioral experiment. The paradigm described in ► Sect. 12.1.5 can be used for this purpose.

12.1.5 General Paradigm for Planning Behavioral Experiments on Interpersonal and Communication Problems of the Patient

Contents and Materials

- **Contents**
  - Guide for conducting a behavioral experiment
- **Materials**
  - Worksheet 12.9: My behavioral experiment: planning
  - Worksheet 12.10: My behavioral experiment—log
  - Camera for role play recording

As an introduction, Worksheet 12.1 (My interpersonal problems) is discussed with the patient in order to clarify the patient's actual problem. In the next step, it should be clarified with patients how they imagine and hope for a solution of their interpersonal problem in the future (see point 8 on Worksheet 12.1). Furthermore, solutions for the problem should then be sought and together with the therapist it should be planned how these steps can be implemented.

Interpersonal problems can vary widely. However, what is a valuable intervention for most interpersonal problems is a behavioral experiment. Therefore, we would like to give you a general guideline below on how to plan such a behavioral experiment with your patient. You will need to adapt this scheme to your patient's individual situation.

Guide: Conducting a Behavioral Experiment

The planning of the behavioral experiment should be recorded in writing (Worksheet 12.9: My behavioral experiment—planning). Here it becomes particularly clear how important it is that the patient suggests a problem to work on that is not too complex and for which improvements can already be expected with this one-time intervention. The following questions serve as a suggestion for planning the behavioral experiment:

Drawing Up a Concrete Plan for Carrying Out the Behavioral Experiment

- What situation do you want to go to? (Example: a conversation with the wife)
- When would you like to conduct the behavioral experiment? (Example: on Saturday after the current therapy session)
- What needs to be prepared in order to be able to go to the situation? (Example: postponing a meeting with a friend until Saturday afternoon).
- What would you like to do differently in detail in the situation? (Example: The patient wants to tell his wife honestly that he will not cancel a short vacation with his best friend because of her. He wants to explain to her in a calm tone why this time out is very important for him).

The next step is to explore thoughts and expectations related to the behavioral experiment. Patient note down their expectations, fears, hopes and worries that they associate with their behavioral experiment and estimate the probability of these expectations occurring. After conducting the behavioral experiment, patients log their experience (Worksheet 12.10: My behavioral experiment—log). In the debriefing, the therapist and patient compare the results of the behavioral experiment with the expectations and discuss the significance in terms of the expectations.

12.2 Communication with the Physician

12.2.1 Switching Perspectives and Different Styles of Communicating About Somatic Symptoms

Contents and Materials

- **Contents**
  - Role play to switch perspectives: How does the patient feel in the physician's role?
  - Video feedback on the role play: How does the patient feel in the patient role?
  - Practice of the week and planning of the role play for the next session: Worksheet 12.16 (Role play "A fruitful doctor-patient conversation"—preliminary ideas)
- **Materials**
  - Worksheet 12.11: Role description 1: The "fearful-catastrophizing" doctor
  - Worksheet 12.12: Role description 2: The "trivialising" doctor
  - Worksheet 12.13: Role description 3: The "balanced" doctor
  - Worksheet 12.14: Role description 4: The patient
  - Worksheet 12.15: Log of experiences from three role plays—"The three doctor-patient conversations"
  - Worksheet 12.16: Role play "A fruitful doctor-patient conversation"—preliminary ideas
  - Camera for role play recording

At the beginning, the goals of this session are discussed with the patient in order to create transparency regarding the purpose of the following role plays:

- Patient should be given the opportunity to put themselves in the role of a physician.
- They should try out different styles of communicating about the symptoms and how to deal with them.
- They should question their expectations regarding the consultation with the physician and explore what is important to them in communicating with a physician.
- They should develop strategies with which they can communicate the contents that are important to them in the conversation with the physician.

It is important to emphasize that not all of these objectives and role plays may be relevant to a patient. Some of the role plays require the ability to switch perspective, which is more or less available or trainable in patients. So before you work through this module with your patient, assess the extent to which the exercises are appropriate for your patient. You can select individual exercises from this module according to the concerns and problems of your patient.

Role Play to Switch Perspectives: How Does the Patient Feel in the Physician's Role?

In the following, three role plays are carried out with patients in which they are to assume the role of the doctor. All three role plays should be recorded with a video camera for later debriefing. Approximately 5 min should be allowed for each role play. Each of the doctor roles places different emphasis on how somatic symptoms should be addressed and treated. While the first doctor deals with the patient's symptoms in a rather catastrophizing way and orders various further diagnostic measures for reasons of self-protection, the second doctor does not take the symptom reports so seriously and trivializes them, at the same time not providing the patient with any further coping strategies. The third doctor shows a balanced attitude. On the one hand, they try to validate patients in their burden of somatic symptoms, and on the other hand, they make suggestions as to how patients can better cope with their symptoms through changing their own behavior. Patients should consciously experiment with these different styles of dealing in the context of the role plays and observe themselves how they feel and perceive themselves in the role of the doctor. Detailed instructions for the three doctor roles can be found in Worksheets 12.11–12.13 (Role Description 1–3) and for the patient role in Worksheet 12.14 (Role Description 4).

Immediately after each role play, the therapist and patient should discuss and evaluate it. The following questions may be helpful:

- How did you feel about the role of the doctor?
- Do you have any guesses as to why the doctor behaves as described in the role instruction? What could be their motives and thoughts?
- How did you feel when you gave me feedback about my symptoms as a patient in this rather catastrophizing versus downplaying versus balancing way? What did you find difficult?
- Did this shift into the doctor's perspective help you understand why a doctor might behave in different ways toward you as a patient?
- What do the experiences you had during the role play mean to you? How can you make use of them? (The patient should be guided to realize that the primary goal is not to change the doctor's behavior. Alternatively, the patient should learn to understand and adjust to the doctor's behavior or to communicate in a way that addresses their concerns).

12

Patients log their experience of each doctor's role on Worksheet 12.15 (Log of experiences from three role plays—"The three doctor-patient conversations"). The aim of this first section of the role-play exercise is for patients to learn to put themselves in the place of the other person in the doctor-patient conversation. Understanding the thoughts and feelings of the doctor on the patient side can help to reduce negative emotions such as frustration or anger and thus relax doctor-patient communication. At the same time, this creates a basis for patients to focus on those aspects that are important to them in the conversation and to steer the conversation in a desired direction through their own behavioral changes, which are practiced in the next session.

▪ Video Feedback on the Role Play: How Does the Patient Feel in the Patient Role?

In the following, therapist and patient watch the video recording of the three role plays again. Patients are instructed to consciously put themselves in the role of the patient. Immediately after each role play, the therapist and patient should discuss and evaluate it and record the patient's thoughts (Worksheet 12.15: Log of experiences from three role plays—"The three doctor-patient conversations"). The following questions may be helpful:

- How would you fare as a patient if your doctor talked to you in the catastrophizing versus downplaying versus balancing way about your symptoms?
- Which of the three role plays made you feel most comfortable? Can you explain why?

Based on the experience of the switch of perspective into the doctor's and patient's role, patients should be supported to find a helpful attitude for themselves in dealing with their symptoms and to practice their attitude also towards their doctor, independent of the behavior of the counterpart. The patient's thoughts can again be noted on Worksheet 12.15 (Log of experiences from three role plays—"The three doctor-patient conversations"). The following questions can be helpful:

- Having learned from these three role plays as a physician and your previous experience communicating with your physicians, what can you expect from them?
- Which of the three different attitudes to dealing with physical discomfort, re-enacted in these three role-plays, could you best identify with? (The patient should of course be guided to find that the balanced posture is most helpful).
- Can you imagine adopting a "balanced" posture, such as the one depicted in the third role play, for yourself?

▪ Practice of the Week and Planning of the Role Play for the Next Session

In the following session, patients should practice in a role play to assert their attitude towards the handling of the symptoms in the conversation with their doctors and at the same time to obtain the information most important for them or to assert goals. For this purpose, it is important to explore with patients what their needs are with regard to a doctor-patient conversation. If possible, the patient should have a specific upcoming conversation with their doctor in mind. The following questions can support the exploration:

- What are you hoping for in the upcoming conversation with your doctor? What is your goal? What result or information would you like to get out of the conversation? Are your goals realistic?

- What information should you provide to your doctor for this?
- In what way should you convey your information?
- What can you do if your doctor is not responsive to your needs?
- What difficulties can arise in the conversation? How can I react to them? (e.g., the time for the conversation is very short and it is difficult to quickly describe the main points of the problem; patient is interrupted and the other person does not let them finish).

Initial ideas for planning the role play in the following session can already be noted on worksheet 12.16 (Role play "A fruitful doctor-patient conversation"—preliminary ideas). As part of the practice of the week, patients should consider in more detail their concerns and needs for an upcoming doctor's consultation.

12.2.2 Practicing a Fruitful Doctor-Patient Conversation

Contents and Materials

- **Contents**
  - Discussion of the practice of the week and planning the role play
  - Planning the doctor's interview for the role plays: Content and communication skills
  - Role play with video feedback: Effective communication of the patient's needs I and II
  - Practice of the week and planning a behavioral experiment for an upcoming doctor-patient conversation (Worksheet 12.18: Log for the next doctor-patient consultation [behavioral experiment]).
- **Materials**
  - Worksheet 12.16: Role play "A fruitful doctor-patient conversation"—preliminary ideas
  - Worksheet 12.17: Log: experiences from the role play on the doctor-patient conversation
  - Worksheet 12.18: Log for the next doctor-patient consultation (behavioral experiment)
  - Camera for role play recording

▪ Discussion of the Practice of the Week and Planning the Role Play

As an introduction to this session, Worksheet 12.16 (Role play "A fruitful doctor-patient conversation"—preliminary ideas) is reviewed with the patient. The contents of the practice of the week should be used to plan two role plays in this session. Role play 1 is to be practiced under "easy" conditions (i.e. without behaviors of the counterpart that make the conversation more difficult for the patient). There are two important goals in role play 1. First, patients should try to achieve the goal they have set for the conversation (Section A on Worksheet 12.16). Second, they should be encouraged to use 1–2 strategies in the role-play that will help them overcome their own difficulties in communicating with the doctor (Section C on Worksheet 12.16). In role-play 2, the same scene from role-play 1 is to be performed under "aggravated" conditions (Section D on Worksheet 12.16).

In the debriefing regarding the practice of the week, it is important that the therapist supports the patient to be as specific as possible, since based on Worksheet 12.16, the role plays should be planned as close to reality as possible.

▪ Planning the Doctor's Interview for the Role Plays: Content and Communication Skills

Before the therapist moves into the role play with their patients, patients should be very aware of their goals. They should know what they specifically want to say or what content they want to share with the doctor. To do this, the patient should make bullet points on Worksheet 12.17 (Log: experiences from the role play on the doctor-patient conversation) in Section C. For example, if patients are presenting to a new specialist and are asked to describe their condition, they should make notes beforehand about what points they would like to share with the doctor and think about what content might be important for the doctor treating them.

The next point that should be clarified before starting the role play is possible communication difficulties that may occur on the part of the patients and what strategies they can use to overcome them (Worksheet 12.17 in Section D). On the one hand, the therapist can refer to the therapy literature on building social competence (Hinsch & Pfingsten, 2015). On the other hand, the following table (◘ Table 12.1) gives ideas about which soft skills patients could use when facing specific problems in communicating with the doctor.

Therapist and patient should note no more than two soft skills for dealing with patient difficulties in the doctor-patient interview in Section D of Worksheet 12.7 (Log: experiences from the role play on the doctor-patient conversation) that they plan to use in the role play.

▪ Role Play with Video Feedback: Effective Communication of the Patient's Needs I

Before the role play starts, the situation should be discussed briefly and concretely. If necessary, the patient can give the therapist 2–3 typical behaviors of the doctor, which the therapist, playing the role of the doctor, tries to re-enact in the role play.

In the following, the therapist, in the role of the doctor, and the patient perform the role play with video recording. The role play should not last longer than 5 min. In their role as doctor, the therapist should take care not to introduce any difficulties for the patient. The latter should have room to concentrate on the content and implementation of the 1–2 soft skills first. The debriefing of the role play can be structured with the following questions.

?
- How did you feel during the conversation? How did you feel during the conversation?
- Were you able to convey all the important information to your doctor?
- To what extent were you able to use the strategies to improve your appearance and communication with your doctor?
- What did you experience as difficult in the course of the conversation?

In the following, the role play can be watched on video and patients should be instructed to always pause the video if they did something particularly well or if they experienced something as difficult. If patients gives little feedback, the therapist should stop the video at appropriate points and give feedback. The following rules should be observed:

- It should be started with positive feedback if possible. It is important that the patient completes the role play with a sense of achievement.
- Negative feedback should always be combined with constructive suggestions for improvement or solutions, if necessary derived by the patients themselves or with the support of the therapist.

On Worksheet 12.17 (Log: experiences from the role play on the doctor-patient conversation), the patient's positive experiences should be noted, as well as difficulties and areas for improvement in Section E.

▪ Role Play with Video Feedback: Effective Communication of the Patient's Needs II

The role play is performed again. The situation, goals, contents and soft skills that the patient wants to train should not be changed. The patient should try to specifically implement the suggestions for change that resulted from the first role play. The innovation in the second role play is that an anticipated behavior of the doctor is specifically singled out, which the patient finds difficult to deal with. Together with the patient, they consider what strategies they can use to overcome this difficulty (Worksheet 12.17: Log: experiences from the role play on the doctor-patient conversation, Section F). The following table (◘ Table 12.2) provides examples of difficult communication situations and ideas for dealing with them. This table only includes suggestions and does not claim to be complete.

It can be challenging for the therapist if the "difficult situation" that the patient indicates is an expression of the patient's less helpful expectations towards the doc-

12

◘ **Table 12.2** Barriers and difficulties for the patient when talking to the doctor and coping strategies

Barriers and difficulties	Coping strategies
My doctor cuts me off	Express in the first person what feelings this behavior triggers individually To point out to the doctor in a friendly way that you would like to speak out or that you still have important things to say Bring notes with the most important facts into the conversation
Time pressure is high	Take notes with the most important facts and contents that your patients would like to convey to their doctor during the conversation If necessary, arrange an appointment during opening hours when the practice is less busy
The doctor talks about things that are less relevant to me (e.g., about his own experiences)	Using phrases such as, "I'd like to get back to ...", "it would help me a lot if we talked specifically about my situation and what I can do ..."
The doctor doesn't clearly articulate what's wrong with me	Question the extent to which it is realistic to expect a clear diagnosis from the doctor
The doctor remains vague about how to proceed	Expressing in the first person how one feels about the lack of clarity about the way forward Formulate in a friendly way the request to make concrete proposals or a plan for further action
The doctor's main feedback is that I should "just distract myself" or "just get on with my life as before"...	Express motivation to implement changes in one's own behavior Formulate in a friendly way the request to name concrete strategies that your patients can apply in their daily life or to name sources from which the patients can obtain relevant information

tor. A typical example would be that the doctor advises against a certain diagnostic procedure with a clear justification, but the patient wants to use this procedure because of their need for certainty and clarification. The therapist is therefore required to work out and question functional and less helpful parts of the patient's ideas. Realistic expectations of the doctor should be developed, which may also include the realization that one cannot necessarily change the behavior of the other person. Depending on the situation, these strategies may be aimed at changing the behavior of the other person (e.g., asking the doctor to make recommendations for specific changes in lifestyle) or helping patients to develop acceptance towards the doctor and to protect themselves. The evaluation of the role play follows the same procedure as the first role play (Worksheet 12.17: Log: experiences from the role play on the doctor-patient conversation, Section G).

- **Practice of the Week and Planning a Behavioral Experiment for an Upcoming Doctor-Patient Consultation**

Based on the experiences from the role plays, an in vivo behavioral experiment (see guidelines in ► Sect. 12.1.5) should be planned as practice of the week. The strategies practiced in the role play should now be applied to a real, upcoming conversation between your patients and their doctor. To help plan this behavioral experiment, use Worksheet 12.18 (Log for the next doctor-patient consultation [behavioral experiment]), which has similar content to the log of experiences from the role play on the doctor-patient conversation (Worksheet 12.17: Log: experiences from the role play on the doctor-patient conversation). A new addition is that the patient's expectations of the conversation are explored and recorded. Similar to the role play, patients should think about the specific content they would like to address with their doctor and write it down. In addition, he is to implement 1–2 soft skills for communicating with the doctor. Patient is instructed to log their experiences following the real doctor's interview and to note the extent to which their expectations were confirmed. It is important to discuss the results of the behavioral experiment in the follow-up session and to plan further role plays and behavioral experiments based on the results.

12.3 Worksheets

These worksheets are also available for download online at Springer Extras (► extras.springer.com).

Worksheet 12.1	My interpersonal problems	◘ Figure 12.1
Worksheet 12.2	Characteristics of complaining behavior	◘ Figure 12.2
Worksheet 12.3	Explanations for our sexual problems	◘ Figure 12.3
Worksheet 12.4	Sensate focus exercises and a log of experiences	◘ Figure 12.4
Worksheet 12.5	The consequences of my withdrawal from activities with my partner	◘ Figure 12.5
Worksheet 12.6	Practice log—talking about my somatic symptoms in a socially competent manner at work.	◘ Figure 12.6
Worksheet 12.7	Role play log—setting boundaries and saying no	◘ Figure 12.7
Worksheet 12.8	Assertive, insecure, and aggressive behavior: What is typical?	◘ Figure 12.8
Worksheet 12.9	My behavioral experiment—planning	◘ Figure 12.9
Worksheet 12.10	My behavioral experiment—log	◘ Figure 12.10
Worksheet 12.11	Role description 1: The "fearful-catastrophizing" doctor	◘ Figure 12.11
Worksheet 12.12	Role description 2: The "trivializing" doctor	◘ Figure 12.12
Worksheet 12.13	Role description 3: The "balanced" doctor	◘ Figure 12.13
Worksheet 12.14	Role description 4: The patient	◘ Figure 12.14
Worksheet 12.15	Log of experiences from three role plays—"The three doctor-patient conversations"	◘ Figure 12.15
Worksheet 12.16	Role play "A fruitful doctor-patient conversation"—preliminary ideas	◘ Figure 12.16
Worksheet 12.17	Log: experiences from the role play on the doctor-patient conversation	◘ Figure 12.17
Worksheet 12.18	Log for the next doctor-patient consultation [behavioral experiment]	◘ Figure 12.18

Fig. 12.1 Worksheet 12.1: My interpersonal problems

Worksheet 12.1: My interpersonal problems

Use the following questions to accurately describe your interpersonal problems! If some questions don't fit your problem, just leave them unanswered.

(1) With which person(s) do I have interpersonal problems?

____

____

(2) What exactly do my problems relate to? Is there a specific topic?

____

____

(3) How much does/do the person(s) with whom I have interpersonal problems mean to me?

____

____

(4) How do the interpersonal problems with this person(s) manifest?

____

____

____

____

(5) What causes the problems from my side?

____

____

____

(6) What causes the problems on the part of the other?

____

____

____

(7) What have I done so far to deal with the problem?

____

____

____

(8) What do I wish for the future regarding this problem?

____

____

____

From Kleinstäuber, M. et al: Cognitive behavior therapy for persistent somatic symptoms and somatic symptom disorders.

Fig. 12.2 Worksheet 12.2: Characteristics of complaining behavior

Worksheet 12.2: Characteristics of complaining behavior

	Features	Do these features describe my behavior?	Which other features of my behavior can I observe?	What can I change?
Voice/ Pronunciation	– little intonation – sad voice – tentative – unclear pronunciation			
Choice of words	– resigned – demanding			
Contents	– focus on somatic symptoms – lack of perspective/thoughts of hopelessness – accusations – search for help – catastrophizing			
Emotional expression	– persistent negative mood – hopelessness – resigned mood			
Gestures/mimics /posture	– sadder, more tense facial expression – painful, tensed facial expression, serious look – little eye contact – view directed downwards – seeking help look – resigning gestures: e.g., shaking head – gestures underline the severity of suffering – sunk down posture – accompanying sounds and gestures: e.g., groaning, clenching teeth			

◘ Fig. 12.3 Worksheet 12.3: Explanations for our sexual problems

Worksheet 12.3: Explanations for our sexual problems

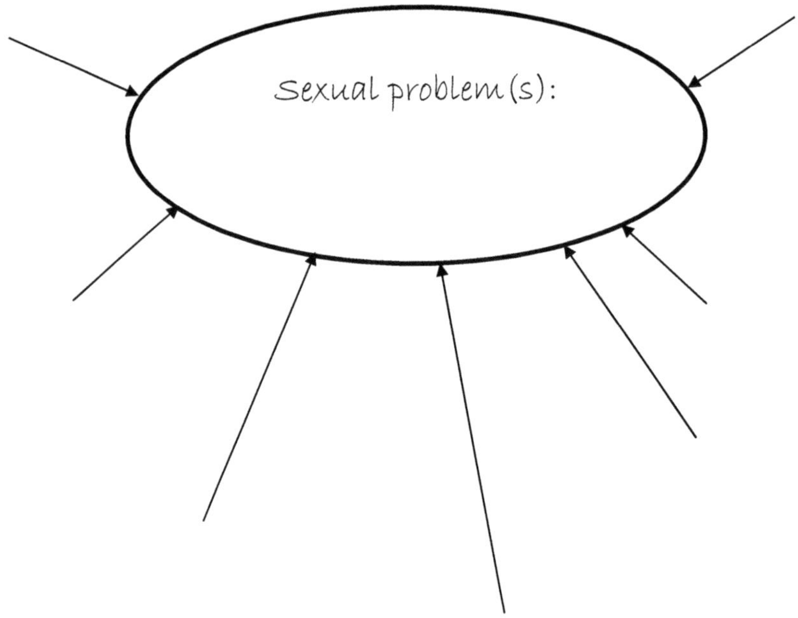

Fig. 12.4 Worksheet 12.4: Sensate Focus exercises and a log of experiences

Worksheet 12.4: Sensate Focus exercises and a log of experiences

Exercise 1:
- Caressing the body
- Breasts and genitals are not included in the exercise
- TThere should be no coitus

Exercise 2:
- Body caressing with exploratory touching of genitals
- There should be no coitus

Exercise 3 "Quiet Vagina":
- Insertion of the penis and pausing, if necessary complementary coitus movements, but without the aim of climaxing

Exercise 4:
- Coitus with exploratory and stimulating movements

The exercises focus less on the type of touch than on the exploration of subjective experiences, feelings and thoughts. The partners should find out what is good for them. The patient in particular should pay attention to where the somatic symptoms have a negative impact on the subjective experience of sexuality. For each exercise the couple should allow at least 10–15 min, and the transition from one exercise to the next depends on what the the couple experiences during the practice.

Log: experiences with the Sensate Focus exercises (Part 1)

Below you will find a few examples of thoughts that may cross your mind during the exercises. Go through the thoughts: Have you experienced one or some of these thoughts as well?

Thought applies to me	Example thoughts
	I worry about what my partner thinks of me
	These somatic symptoms are ruining everything, I can't enjoy being close to my partner anymore.
	I don't know if I can ever be attractive to my partner again?
	I don't know if I will ever be able to enjoy sexual activity with my partner again?
	I feel unattractive.
	My body doesn't work the way I want it to.
	I don't feel anything.
	I'm starting to get impatient.
	I can't relax.
	I'm afraid of disappointing my partner.
	I'm afraid of hurting my partner.
	I think I have too high standards.
	I feel responsible for making sure my partner doesn't experience somatic symptoms while we are sexually active.
	I can't stay on task.
	I'm tense.

Fig. 12.4 (continued)

Log: experiences with the Sensate Focus exercises (Part 2)

In the following, please record your experiences with the Sensate Focus exercises. Refer to both – particularly positive experiences, as well as negative experiences (or moments where your somatic symptoms negatively impacted your sexual activity).

Sexual activity	Subjective sensations	Thoughts	Emotions/feelings	In case of negative experiences: How can we deal with it?

12

Fig. 12.5 Worksheet 12.5: The consequences of my withdrawal from activities with my partner

Worksheet 12.5: The consequences of my withdrawal from activities with my partner

Enter the consequences of your withdrawal behavior in the following table! In doing so, think about positive as well as negative and short- as well as long-term consequences regarding yourself, your partner and your relationship!

	short-term consequences	**long**-term consequences
 **positive**	short-term/positive	long-term/positive
 **negative**	short-term/negative	long-term/negative

Fig. 12.6 Worksheet 12.6: Practice log—talking about my somatic symptoms in a socially competent manner at work

Worksheet 12.6: Practice log – talking about my somatic symptoms in a socially competent manner at work

Reason for the conversation

Person(s) involved in the conversation

Desired outcome of the conversation (realistic? can be influenced by the patient?)

Planned contents of the conversation

What do I want to pay attention to regarding my behavior during the conversation?

What difficulties can arise during the conversation? How can I react or deal with them?

After the interview:	
What have I done well?	What could I improve?

■ **Fig. 12.7** Worksheet 12.7: Role play log—setting boundaries and saying no

Worksheet 12.7: Role play log – setting boundaries and saying no

Description of the problem situation and allocation of roles

Desired outcome of the conversation (realistic? can be influenced by the patient?)

What does the patient want to practice in the role play

Debriefing role play	
What have I done well?	What could I improve?

My plans for the repetition of the role play

Debriefing role play (repetition)	
What have I done well?	What could I improve?

Fig. 12.8 Worksheet 12.8: Assertive, insecure, and aggressive behavior: What is typical?

Worksheet 12.8: Assertive, insecure, and aggressive behavior: What is typical?

Feature	Assertive	Insecure	Aggressive
Voice/pronunciation	▪ Moderate speaking rate ▪ Appropriate loudness ▪ clear ▪ Quiet, rather low voice pitch	▪ Rather high speaking rate ▪ Quiet ▪ Timid ▪ Unclear, "mumble" ▪ Rather high voice pitch	▪ High versus low speaking rate ▪ Yelling, screaming ▪ Hard pronunciation ▪ Partly unclear ▪ Threatening undertone ▪ Rather medium to low voice range
Choice of words	▪ Unambiguous ▪ Factual	▪ Unclear ▪ Vague	▪ Nonfactual ▪ Threatening ▪ Offending
Content	▪ Precise justification ▪ Expressing your own needs ▪ Use of the pronoun "I" ▪ Feelings are expressed directly	▪ Superfluous explanations ▪ Justifications ▪ Frequent excuses ▪ Denial of own needs ▪ Use of "man" ▪ Use of the pronoun "one" ▪ Feelings are expressed indirectly	▪ No explanation and justification ▪ Threats ▪ Insults ▪ Allegations ▪ Uncompromising ▪ Rights of others are ignored
Nonverbal behavior (gestures/facial expressions/posture)	▪ Underpining nonverbal behavior ▪ Lively and dynamic ▪ Relaxed posture ▪ Eye contact	▪ Hardly present ▪ Tensed posture ▪ Safety behavior (e.g., playing fingers with a pen) ▪ No eye contact ▪ Head directed downwards	▪ Uncontrolled ▪ Threatening ▪ Tense posture ▪ Gesticulating wildly ▪ No eye contact or "staring".

Fig. 12.9 Worksheet 12.9: My behavioral experiment—planning

Worksheet 12.9: My Behavioral Experiment – Planning

1. What will be the situation?

____

____

____

2. When will I conduct my behavioral experiment?

____

____

3. How will I have to prepare myself in order to run my behavioral experimenta and to attend the target situation?

____

____

____

____

4. What would I like to do differently in this situation?

____

____

____

____

____

____

5. What concerns, expectations, and hopes do I have?

____

____

____

____

____

____

Fig. 12.10 Worksheet 12.10: My behavioral experiment—log

Worksheet 12.10: My behavioral experiment – log

Day, time:	
Situation:	
Expectation/prediction: What exactly did you expect would happen? Probability, that expectation comes true? 0–100	
Experiment: What have you exactly done to check your expectations against reality?	
Result: What actually happened? Was your expectation correct?	
What I'm learning from this: Has my expectation changed? Probability, that expectation (in the future) comes true 0–100	
Are you satisfied with the result?	
Was it good or not so good for you, that you attended the situation?	
Next time, would you do something different?	

Fig. 12.11 Worksheet 12.11: Role description 1: The "fearful-catastrophizing" doctor

Worksheet 12.11: Role description 1: The "fearful-catastrophizing" doctor

For our role play, please put yourself in the following position: You work as a primary care physician in your own practice. This week there is another flu epidemic and your waiting room is full, you have little time for each patient. Now a patient comes to you who has been suffering from [*insert symptoms of the patient*] for 6 months. The patient was already attended an appointment with you 3 months ago, but examinations did not result in any medical explanations.
The patient is expecting help from you. You know that you have exhausted the necessary examination options and that you can't tell your patient anything new. However you are concerned because the symptoms have persisted for quite a while. You ask yourself if you could have missed something. To make sure that you do not want to do something wrong or miss something, you refer your patient to another medical specialist (e.g., neurologist, pain physician). Additionally you order some medical imaging for your patient (e.g., CT scan).

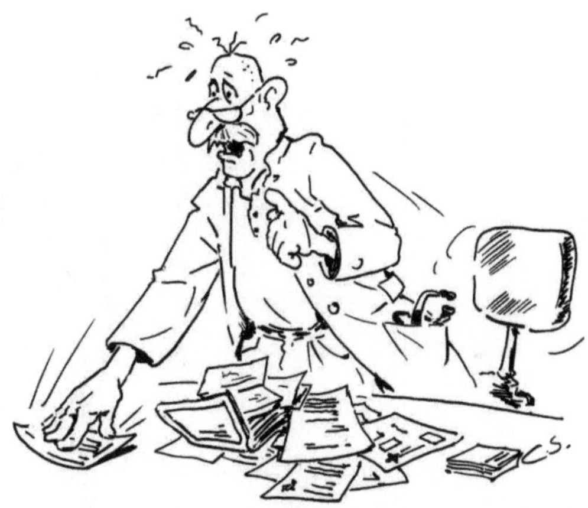

Then however you have to come to an end in the conversation with your patient, given that your waiting room is crowded with other patients. You let your patient know that it is better to be very careful and that these diagnostic means are important to eliminate possible serious causes of your patient's symptoms. You make a new appointment with your patient to discuss the results of the additional medical examinations and you offer that your patient always can give you a call when her/his/their symptoms get worse.

Fig. 12.12 Worksheet 12.12: Role description 2: The "trivializing" doctor

Worksheet 12.12: Role description 2: The "trivializing" doctor

For our role play, please put yourself in the following situation: You work as a primary care physician in your own practice. This week there is another flu epidemic and your waiting room is full, you have little time for each patient. Now a patient comes to you who has been suffering from [insert patient's symptoms] for 6 months. The patient came to see you 3 months ago, but examinations did not reveal any medical causes. The patient is expecting help from you. You know that you have exhausted the necessary examination options and that you can't tell your patient anything new. Due to the crowded waiting room, you cannot spend much time on this conversation. Under no circumstances you want to prescribe more complex examinations or therapies.

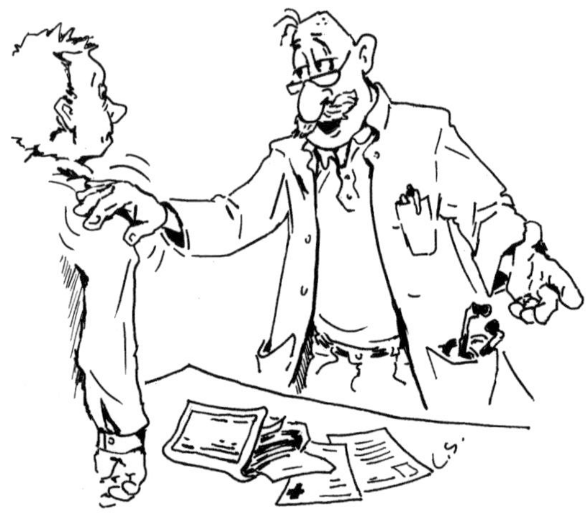

Just reassure your patient, tell him/her/them that it is not so bad, that your patient will get used to it, that your patient simply shouldn't let the symptoms get to him/her/them or take them so seriously. There is absolutely no reason to worry. Make it clear to your patient very soon that you no longer have time for him/her/them and that the next patients are already waiting.

Fig. 12.13 Worksheet 12.13: Role description 3: The "balanced" doctor

Worksheet 12.13: The "balanced" doctor

For our role play, please put yourself in the following situation: You work as a primary care physician in your own practice. Now a patient comes to you who has been suffering from [insert patient's symptoms]. Your patient came to see you 3 months ago, but examinations did not reveal any medical causes of the symptoms. Your patient is expecting help from you. You know that you have exhausted the necessary examination options and therefore do not prescribe any further unnecessary diagnostic measures.

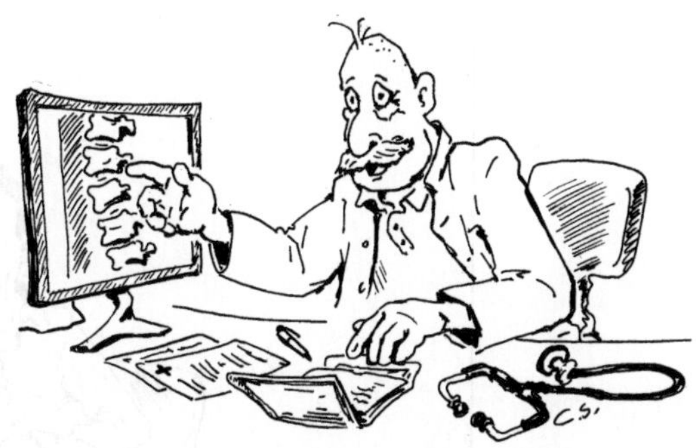

However, you take your time and talk to the patient about the issues that are bothering him/her/them. Your aim is to convey the following things: You let your patient know that you understand their concerns and take them very seriously. Although you can rule out the possibility that the somatic symptoms are due to a serious disease, it is important to make changes to the patient's lifestyle that help to prevent the symptoms from getting worse and lasting longer and longer. You will make specific suggestions on how to improve with the symptoms. The somatic symptoms should not dominate the patient's everyday life. On the contrary, it is important to continue to have a normal life despite the symptoms. It is important that the patient tries not to avoid healthy movements or adopting a relieving body posture. You discuss further measures, such as prescribing physiotherapy or taking part in rehabilitation sports at the gym. Finally, you arrange an appointment with your patient in 6 weeks to discuss with them what progress they are making in dealing with their complaints.

Fig. 12.14 Worksheet 12.14: Role description 4: The patient

Worksheet 12.14: Role description 4: The patient

For our role-play, please put yourself in the following position: You have been experiencing [*insert symptoms of the patient*] for 6 months already. Initially, you didn't give it much thought. After 3 months, the discomfort started to worry you as it became more severe. You then called your primary care physician and consulted another specialist. Both had suggested and initiated various diagnostic measures, which, however, did not result in any medical causes that could explain your symptoms. Since then, your symptoms have continued and tend to worsen rather than remit. You therefore decide to consult your primary care physician and get another doctor appointment. Briefly describe your case to your doctor and then ask your doctor some of the following questions. Don't be fobbed off with answers that are too short or general!

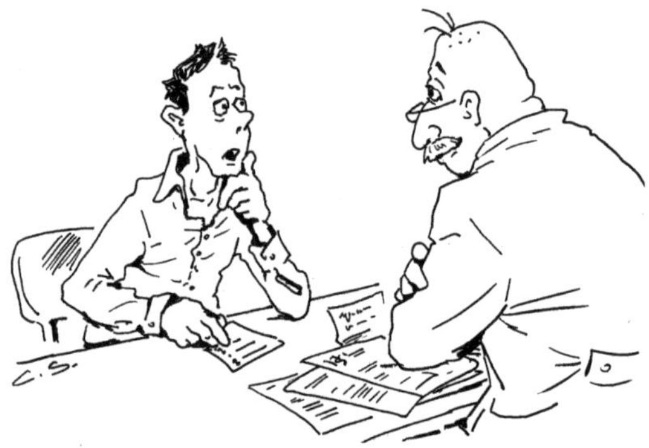

Below are some suggestions of questions you can ask your doctor:
- What can be done about the symptoms?
- Where do the symptoms come from?
- Will the symptoms ever go away?
- Is there perhaps a disease that explains the symptoms?
- Should I take it easy?
- Should I have seen the doctor earlier instead of after 3 months?

12

Fig. 12.15 Worksheet 12.15: Log of experiences from three role plays—"The three doctor-patient conversations"

Worksheet 12.15: Log of experiences from three role plays - "The Three Doctor-Patient Conversations"

(1) Physician perspective

Write down your experiences in the doctor role in the boxes below! Use the following questions for orientation:
How did you feel in the role of the doctor? Do you have any assumptions as to why the doctor behaves as described in the role instruction?
How did you feel when you had to give feedback to "your patient" about their symptoms as described in the instruction?
Did you find this difficult? What do the experiences you had during the role play mean to you? How can you make use of them?

My experience as a "fearful catastrophizing" physician:	My experience as a "trivializing" physician:	My experience as a "balanced" physician:

(2) Patient perspective (video recording)

How would you feel as a patient if your doctor talked to you about your symptoms in the manner instructed in each case? Which of the three role plays made you feel most comfortable as a patient?

My experience as a patient seeing an "anxious-catastrophizing" doctor:	My experience as a patient seeing a "trivializing" doctor:	My experience as a patient seeing a 'balanced' doctor:

(3) Summary of the experiences during the role plays

With which of the three deportments towards somatic symptoms that a re simulated in the role-plays can I best identify myself?	What can I realistically expect from a conversation with a physician?

Fig. 12.16 Worksheet 12.16: Role play "A fruitful doctor-patient conversation"—preliminary ideas

Worksheet 12.16: Role play "A fruitful doctor-patient conversation" – preliminary ideas

(A) Think about a goal for the next conversation with your doctor (e.g., specific information you want to gain from the conversation; you want to communicate your concerns more clearly to the doctor). Is your goal realistic?

(B) What would you like to say to your doctor?

(C) What could be possible weaknesses on your part in the conversation with your doctor (e.g., I let myself intimidate; I forget what I was going to say; I appear irritable or unfriendly; I appear not confident)? Do you already have ideas how to deal with your weaknesses?

D) What difficulties may arise during the consultation (e.g., the doctor does not answer my question; the doctor interrupts me; I feel under a lot of time pressure; the doctor does not address my concerns)? How can you respond to this or deal with these difficulties?

Fig. 12.17 Worksheet 12.17: Log: experiences from the role play on the doctor-patient conversation

Worksheet 12.17: Log: experiences from the role play on the doctor-patient conversation

(A)) Briefly describe the situation of the doctor's conversation: (What kind of doctor? Why do you visit the doctor? How does the room look like where you meet your doctor? Where do you sit, where does your doctor sit?)	
(B) Name a specific goal you have for the role-play doctor conversation. Check together with your therapist how realistic this goal is.	
(C) What would you like to tell your doctor? You can rank the topics that you want to talk with your doctor about by "very important" and "less important". Make sure that the order, in which you would like to discuss content with your doctor, follows a common thread.	
(D) If you fear "vulnerabilities" (e.g., I let myself intimidate; I forget what I was going to say; I appear irritable or unfriendly; I appear not confident) on your part for the conversation, choose one with which to learn want to deal with. Write down 1–2 strategies on how you could deal with this vulnerability.	
(E) What did I do well? (Feedback after role play 1)	(E) What could I improve? (Feedback after role play 1)
(F) What would cause you difficulties in the conversation (e.g., a particular behavior of your doctor, difficulties in the situation such as time pressure)? Write down each difficulty and think about 2 strategies for how you want to deal with each difficulty.	
(G) What did I do well? (Feedback after role play 2)	(G) What could I improve? (Feedback after role play 2)

Fig. 12.18 Worksheet 12.18: Log for the next doctor-patient consultation [behavioral experiment]

Worksheet 12.18: Log for the next doctor-patient consultation [behavioral experiment]

(A) Name a specific goal for the next conversation with your doctor. Check with your therapist to see how realistic this goal is.

(B) What would you like to tell your doctor? You can rank the topics that you want to talk with your doctor about by "very important" and "less important". Make sure that the order, in which you would like to discuss content with your doctor, follows a common thread.

(C) If you fear "vulnerabilities" (e.g., I let myself intimidate; I forget what I was going to say; I appear irritable or unfriendly; I appear not confident) on your part for the conversation, choose one with which to learn want to deal with. Write down 1–2 strategies on how you could deal with this vulnerability.

(E) What would cause you difficulties in conversation (e.g. a particular behavior of your doctor, difficulties in the situation, such as time pressure)? Write down each difficulty and come up with 2 strategies to deal with each difficulty.

(F) After the doctor's consultation: What did I do well?

(F) After the doctor's consultation: What could I improve?

(G) My expectations before the interview:

(G) What are my expectations regarding the conversation?

(G) Have my expectations come true?

12

References

Eifert, G. H., McKay, M., & Forsyth, J. P. (2009). *Mit Ärger und Wut umgehen. Der achtsame Weg in ein friedliches Leben*. Huber.

Hillman, J. (2012). *Sexuality and aging*. Springer.

Hinsch, R., & Pfingsten, U. (2015). *Gruppentraining sozialer Kompetenzen (GSK)*. Beltz Psychologie Verlags Union.

Hoyndorf, S., Reinhold, M., & Christmann, F. (1995). *Behandlung sexueller Störungen. Ätiologie, Diagnostik, Therapie: Sexuelle Dysfunktionen, Missbrauch, Delinquenz*. Beltz Psychologie Verlags Union.

Masters, W. H., & Johnson, V. E. (1966). *Human sexual response*. Little, Brown.

Practical Experience

Contents

A Case Study

Contents

M. Kleinstäuber et al., *Cognitive Behavior Therapy for Persistent Somatic Symptoms and Somatic Symptom Disorder*, https://doi.org/10.1007/978-3-662-69726-9_13

13.1 Symptomatology, Symptom History, and Patient's Biography

13.1.1 Symptomatology

The 25-year-old law student, who presented for psychological treatment on the advice of his primary care physician, reported various pains in his back, head, joints, limbs, and lower abdomen during the initial consultation. Occasionally, there was also a tingling sensation in the hands and feet. In addition, he has suffered from gastrointestinal symptoms such as nausea, bloating, flatulence, constipation, and diarrhea. At the present time, he is about to take important exams in his studies. Due to the symptoms he can hardly concentrate and studying is very stressful for him. The somatic symptoms have existed since his adolescence (around the age of 16). In the past years he had repeatedly consulted doctors and had been examined as an in-patient. However, no medical cause had been found to explain the pain or the gastrointestinal symptoms. In the past 3 years, the symptoms had intensified again, which increasingly restricted him in his everyday life. He could hardly relax, often reacted irritably to his environment and had problems sleeping. In connection with his complex symptoms, he had to give up many pleasant activities and hobbies. He no longer goes running and has withdrawn from university sports. He rarely plays the piano any more. Contact with his friends has also decreased significantly. He is particularly worried that the pain is sometimes so bad that he does not know how to sit, lie down or stand up. He was afraid that the symptoms would severely hinder him in carrying out his job in the future. These worries about the future are accompanied by the fact that the patient has felt increasingly depressed and hopeless and has experienced a lack of drive over the past 2 months. However, he had never experienced suicidal thoughts.

13.1.2 Symptom History

The patient states that he has been suffering from back pain for about 9 years. During the time when the pain started, there had been escalated conflicts between his parents. In addition, he was in love with a girl which remained unrequited and which had put a lot of stress on him. The pain had then subsided for about a year, but in the course of his final senior highschool year it had become even more severe than before. While the symptoms had decreased considerably at the beginning of his studies, they had intensified again in the second semester. Since then, he has suffered from the pain on a daily basis. In addition, he experiences severe headaches lasting several days almost once a month. Although he had been very active in sports at the beginning of his studies, he had given this up due to additional joint pain as well as pain in his arms and legs, which was often accompanied by feelings of numbness and tingling. Two years ago, his partner had cheated on him and they broke up. During this time he had developed persistent digestive problems for the first time. These have occurred continuously since then. He suffers from diarrhoea and nausea several times a week. Participation in university events is therefore very difficult for him. He usually looks for a seat near the exit in order to be able to reach a toilet as quickly as possible. He travels to the university by public transport, which makes things even more difficult. He could only travel on trains with toilets. Despite various medical examinations—including inpatient stays—and repeated consultations with specialists, no organic findings for his symptoms could be established. A year ago, he was diagnosed with "irritable stomach" and "fibromyalgia". These diagnoses as well as the persistent symptoms frustrated him so much and triggered such strong fears for the future in him that he had felt increasingly depressed, hopeless and lacking in drive over the last 2 months. He brooded very often about his professional future and could hardly concentrate on his studies. Activities that he had otherwise done "on the side" were difficult for him and required much more time than before. The patient has not yet sought psychiatric or psychological treatment. The patient takes painkillers (Metamizol, Diclofenac) pro re nata, which he has been prescribed by his doctor. He tries to reduce the intake of painkillers to a minimum, but this is very difficult for him. The patient is currently not diagnosed with any other conditions.

13.1.3 Patient's Biography

In the context of the family history, the patient states that his mother has also suffered from back pain for many years. The father had high blood pressure. He was not aware of any mental illnesses in his family. In connection with the biographical history, the patient reports that he is the son of a lawyer (born in 1953) and a dermatologist (born in 1956). He had a sister who is 2 years younger. The patient had experienced the atmosphere in his parental home from infancy as tense and irritable. Both parents were very achievement-oriented and often had little time for their children. The little time spent together was often marked by arguments between the parents. The patient had always experienced himself in his family as "standing behind his sister". She had been more successful than ime at school as well as in her hobbies, which was still the case today. His parents often made him feel this with comments such as "You'll never be successful, just look at your sister. Even though she's two years younger than you, she's way ahead of you." There had been a lot of pressure on the patient as a result of this behavior. Despite this competitive issue, he had always had a good relationship with his sister. She herself had experienced a problem with being favored by her parents. During adolescence there had been a phase in which the conflicts between his parents had regularly escalated and his father had even become violent towards his mother. The patient says that he would have found a divorce of the parents at that time redemptive. However, the parents had decided to continue living together. The patient reports that it had always been his dream to become a lawyer like his father. Due to his mediocre performance at school, however, his father had repeatedly made him understand that he did not believe his son to be qualified to study law. Accordingly, the senior highschool years had been extremely stressful for the patient, who had put himself under constant pressure to achieve sufficiently good results. Moving out of the parental home to begin his studies had been a liberating experience for the patient. He had been doing very well for the first few months of his studies. However, this soon changed and the pressure to perform quickly increased again.

The patient reports that so far in his life he had been in a steady relationship lasting more than 3 years. However, his partner confessed to him 2 years ago that she was cheating on him, which left him very disappointed. The couple broke up. In his youth, he had once fallen in love very unhappily, which had been a great burden on him for almost a year. Regarding his current social situation, the patient reported that he lived in a student community with a roommate. Financially he has no problems. He receives a scholarship. The contact to his parents is rather limited. He visits them from time to time and talks to them on the phone occasionally. Contact with his sister is good. The patient has a small circle of close friends. However, he had significantly reduced his social contacts and his hobbies (playing the piano, sports activities) due to his somatic and mood symptoms.

13.2 Behavior Analysis

According to the cognitive-behavioral model of somatoform disorders or persistent somatic symptoms according to Rief and Hiller (1998; ► Sect. 2.2), the patient's learning and developmental history is characterized by various risk factors for the development of persistent somatic symptoms. These include the patient's parental home, which is characterized by persistent conflicts, as well as the parents' pejorative, hardly validating behavior toward their son and their constant preference for the younger sister. In order to satisfy his parents, the patient has developed an excessively achievement-oriented behavior as well as excessive performance demands on himself. At the same time, he doubts his own ability to perform very strongly. The escalated conflicts between the parents as well as an unrequited love of the patient can be assumed as triggers for the pain symptomatology. The patient then increasingly developed avoidance behaviors and had many frustrating experiences with numerous doctor consultations that did not yield any findings for his symptoms. In connection with his graduation from school as well as the beginning of his studies, the patient's inner pressure to perform increased again. The last mentioned factors can be seen as decisive for the maintenance and chronification of the symptoms.

The following example shows a behavioral analysis of a typical problematic situation for the patient.

► Example

- **Situation:** The patient goes to bed in the evening and becomes increasingly aware of his back pain.
- **Organism Variables:**
  - Persistent pain symptoms for 9 years
  - Excessive demands on oneself
  - Low self-confidence in one's own capabilities
  - Lack of self-efficacy in coping with his symptoms
- **Reactions:**
  - Emotional: fear, helplessness, despair, anger
  - Physiological: inner tension, further aggravation of pain, nausea and diarrhea.
  - Cognitive:
    - "Again, the pain deteriorates and I'm getting sick. I just don't know what else I can do."
    - "I can't fall asleep. It's driving me crazy. I have to be fit tomorrow. If I'm not focused tomorrow, I'll miss half of that exam prep seminar again."
    - "I just don't know how this is going to go on. How will I be able to practice my profession later? I don't even know if I can finish my degree under these circumstances. Of course, that would really confirm to my father that I'm not capable of becoming a lawyer anyway."
    - "I need to take a painkiller now, maybe it'll get better. I'd better cancel the study group meeting tomorrow morning."
  - Motor-behavioral: The patient gets up and gets his painkiller prescribed by his doctor. He texts his study group to cancel the scheduled meeting. After the painkiller has taken effect and after a longer period of brooding, he falls asleep.

- Consequences
  - $\not{C}^{-}$: The effect of the painkiller causes the discomfort to subside for a short time.
  - C^{+}: The patient can calm down.
  - $\not{C}^{+}$: The cancellation of the meeting means that he has to do without feedback on his exam preparations, cannot clarify his questions about the exam material with the others and, in addition, does not hear important things that the others are discussing.
  - C^{-}: In the time until the painkiller starts to take effect, his attention to the somatic symptoms intensifies again as well as the negative brooding and his worries about the future. This further worsens his mood and triggers strong anxiety in him. In the long term, the patient's behavior leads to him being severely restricted in his exam preparations and withdrawing more and more from his social network. Based on his catastrophizing about his professional future, the inner pressure to perform increases more and more. His confidence in being able to control his symptoms again decreases more and more. ◀

13.3 Diagnosis, Therapeutic Goals and Prognosis

13.3.1 Diagnosis

According to the ICD-10, the patient meets the criteria of a somatization disorder (F45.0). According to the DSM-5, the criteria of a somatic symptom disorder, persistent, severe (300.82) are fully given. According to the criteria of ICD-10 and DSM-IV, the patient has a mild depressive episode (ICD-10: F32.0/DSM-IV: 296.21).

13.3.2 Therapeutic Goals and Prognosis

The following therapy goals result for the patient:

- Improvement in coping with the somatic symptoms and a concomitant reduction in social impairments,
- Mediation of the connection between stress or chronic strain and somatic as well as depressive symptoms,
- Learning a relaxation technique, improving relaxation and stress management skills,
- Mediating the relationship between attention and persistent somatic symptoms,
- Learning attention-refocusing techniques,
- Identification and change of less helpful thoughts and attitudes regarding persistent somatic symptoms, one's own concept of health and one's own performance expectations,
- Reduction of illness behavior (avoidance behavior, utilization of medical services and benefits, use of medical aids),
- Promote positive experiences with his body, and enjoyment skills, and fostering trust in the functioning of his body.

Although the patient has had no experience with psychological treatments so far, he shows understanding of his illness and seems to be able to engage with biopsychosocial ideas about his symptoms. The patient is also very reflective. His suffering and the resulting motivation to change are very high.

13.4 Course of Therapy and Results

13.4.1 Course of Therapy

A total of 25 therapy sessions were conducted with the patient. Due to the complexity of the patient's symptomatology, it was necessary to stretch out individual therapy modules somewhat in terms of time. At the beginning of the therapy, the focus was on communicating the connection between stress (related to his studies as well as private life), somatic symptoms and the accompanying mild depressive symptomatology. In a psychoeducational part, information on the physical stress and relaxation reaction and its control by the autonomic nervous system was conveyed. It was worked out how stress manifests itself in the patient on a physical level and which individual stressors are present in the patient's life. The patient was able to relate very well to the explanatory concept.

In addition, progressive muscle relaxation (PMR) was practiced with him. Initial problems in the implementation were discussed promptly. Due to exam preparations, the patient often did not take the time to practice the relaxation procedure independently on a daily basis. Already at this stage, his achievement-oriented thinking was picked up and challenged. Using a collection of pros and cons to his low self-care behavior, the patient became aware of how his excessive performance orientation was limiting rather than helping him. The patient was then able to set up and follow through with a set schedule for PMR. He was able to achieve good effects with this. Especially the gastrointestinal symptoms decreased significantly. For tense situations in everyday life (e.g., when he suddenly noticed an intensification of his pain), the patient sometimes used individual exercises from PMR.

In the patient's case, attention processes played an important role in the maintenance of his somatic symptoms, especially in the evening before falling asleep. The patient was therefore taught ways of directing his attention, which he could use in bed at night, but also in everyday life (e.g., journaling positive experiences, training in pleasurable experiences, mindful walk). Within the framework of specific exercises as well as practice of the week, he was to train himself to direct his attention away from the symptoms towards pleasant stimuli in his environment. The patient found the following distraction strategies particularly helpful: Listening to radio and music and reading.

In the further course of treatment, the patient was made aware of the connection between thoughts and somatic symptoms. After identifying previous problematic thought patterns, an attempt was made to modify the less helpful cognitions through disputation and behavioral experiments. In the process, the cognitions about his excessive performance demands were also taken up and the connection was made clear to him with which persistent inner body tension his self-induced pressure to perform is accompanied. Less helpful cognitions about his performance and his confidence in his own abilities were challenged. Furthermore, his dysfunctional mental clinging to the hope of someday proving to his father that he was a good lawyer was addressed and influenced with cognitive restructuring techniques. As a result, the patient was able to feel a strong sense of relief and reduce the self-produced pressure to perform with regard to the further course of his studies.

In addition, a realistic concept of health was developed with the patient. Ultimately, the aim was to reduce illness behaviors. The focus was placed primarily on the use of medical aids (such as medication as needed) and on changing contact behavior with doctors. The patient's avoidance behavior became apparent primarily with regard to social contacts, hobbies or sporting activities and the use of public transport. The patient was motivated to schedule regular meetings with fellow students and to initiate activities with his flat mates. In addition, the patient met a new girlfriend during the therapy.

With regard to physical exercise, a plan was worked out with the patient to gradually increase physical activity. The patient was able to gradually improve his physical condition. He regularly made time to play the piano at weekends and arranged for his instrument to be transported from his parents' home to his shared apartment. With the development of these positive activities and the reactivation of social contacts, the patient also experienced a significant improvement in mood and drive.

In relation to his avoidance behavior of public transport without a toilet, behavioral experiments were conducted to help the patient challenge his dysfunctional worries and associated fears.

Finally, the experiences that the patient was able to gain during the course of therapy were summarized in a multimodal explanatory symptom and treatment model. The strategies that were helpful for the patient were compiled in an "emergency plan" for future crisis situations.

13.4.2 Therapy Outcome

The patient's pain problem was still present at the end of therapy, but the intensity of the back pain in particular decreased significantly. However, the decisive factor for the patient was that he again experienced quality of life independent of his somatic symptoms, the pain no longer dominated his life so much and he experienced self-efficacy in dealing with his symptoms. He was able to develop significant self-confidence in his own abilities as a result. The gastrointestinal symptoms could be almost completely reduced by the end of the therapy with the help of the improvement in the ability to relax. The depressive symptoms remitted completely in connection with the development of positive activities and the reactivation of social contacts.

The positive course of therapy was also reflected in the test-diagnostic findings. At the beginning of the therapy, the patient had an above-average score in the "Brief Symptom Index" (BSI; Franke, 2000) on the global severity index GSI (T = 72). In the "Beck Depression Inventory" (BDI; Hautzinger et al., 1994) he had a score of 23, indicating clinically relevant depressive symptomatology. At the end of therapy, the total stress score (GSI) changed significantly with T = 62. The depression score (BDI) decreased to 6 points, indicating remission of depression. Based on a standard sample of patients with persistent somatic symptoms, the "Screening for Somatoform Disorders" SOMS-7T (Rief & Hiller, 2008; ▶ Sect. 1.3.4) showed a percentile rank (PR) of 71 for the number of symptoms at the beginning of therapy and a PR of 90 for the intensity of symptoms. The values for both indices could be decisively reduced by the end of therapy (number of symptoms: PR = 20, intensity of symptoms: PR = 47).

References

Franke, G. H. (2000). *Brief symptom inventory von L.R. Derogatis (Kurzform der SCL-90-R). Deutsche Version*. Beltz.

Hautzinger, M., Bailer, M., Worall, H., & Keller, F. (1994). *Beck-depressions-inventar (BDI)*. Huber.

Rief, W., & Hiller, W. (1998). *Somatisierungsstörung und Hypochondrie (Fortschritte der Psychotherapie Band 1)*. Hogrefe.

Rief, W., & Hiller, W. (2008). *SOMS – Das Screening für Somatoforme Störungen. Manual zum Fragebogen* (4. Aufl.). Huber.

Evaluation of the Cognitive-Behavioral Treatment Approach for Persistent Somatic Symptoms

Contents

M. Kleinstäuber et al., *Cognitive Behavior Therapy for Persistent Somatic Symptoms and Somatic Symptom Disorder*, https://doi.org/10.1007/978-3-662-69726-9_14

14.1 Patient Characteristics

Only patients who fulfilled the criteria summarized in the following overview were included in the treatment. This inclusion restriction was necessary in order to be able to guarantee the patients adequate treatment on the one hand and to be able to follow the treatment approach described in this manual. For example, for a patient with significant comorbid psychological symptoms, a 20-h therapy with a focus on persistent somatic symptoms does not seem appropriate or sufficient.

Inclusion Criteria for Manual-Oriented Treatment

- The patient currently has at least 3 somatic symptoms.
- The somatic symptoms reported by the patient are clinically relevant, i.e. cause subjective suffering, lead to use of medication or a change in lifestyle.
- There is **no** diagnosed medical cause that could explain/ sufficiently explain the somatic symptoms.
- If comorbidity is present (e.g., mild to moderate depression, anxiety disorder, cluster C personality disorder), somatic symptoms are the primary concern.
- The patient does **not** currently have any of the following mental disorders:
  - Major depressive episode
  - Acute suicidality
  - Eating disorder
  - Substance use disorder
  - Psychotic or manic symptoms
  - Organic psychosyndrome
  - Cluster A (paranoid, schizoid, schizotypal) or B (borderline, histrionic, dissocial, narcissistic) personality disorder
  - Post-traumatic stress disorder

The treatment could be offered to 76 patients so far according to the inclusion criteria. The present patient sample consists of two thirds women and one third men (64.5% women, 35.5% men). The mean age is 40 years (M = 40.16; SD = 12.50; age range: 20–66 years). With regard to educational status, at the beginning of therapy 20% a high school degree, 25% a university degree and 52% another school leaving certificate. There were still 3% in school education. While more than half of the patients (67.1%) were married or in a stable partnership, 18.4% were single and 14.4% were separated, divorced or widowed. Before seeking treatment at the outpatient clinic, the patients had been suffering from their persistent somatic symptoms for an average of 4 years (M = 3.69; SD = 4.25).

14.2 Outcomes

Before the actual start of therapy, the patients first received 5 preparatory sessions (includes diagnostic process and treatment plan), which were then followed by 20 therapy sessions. With the help of regular supervision and video feedback, it was possible to ensure that the treating therapists adhered to the described manualized procedure. Of the 76 patients admitted to treatment, n = 25 have already completed therapy. In 28 patients the therapy has not yet been completed. Sixteen patients discontinued therapy during the preparatory phase and 7 patients during the therapeutic sessions. In the following calculations, only data from patients who regularly completed therapy were included. Unfortunately, the data sets of 3 patients could not be evaluated due to an excessive number of missing values. Accordingly, the following results are based on the baseline and end of treatment assessment of a sample of n = 22 patients. The present results should be interpreted with caution against the background of the small sample size, the missing control intervention, the increased dropout rate (30%) as well as the missing follow-up assessments and should only be regarded as a first indication of the effectiveness of the treatment program, which needs to be investigated in more detail again within the framework of a high-quality study design.

14.2.1 Persistent Somatic Symptoms

The intensity of the persistent somatic symptoms was assessed with the "Screening for Somatoform Disorders" (SOMS-7 T; Rief & Hiller, 2008; ► Sect. 1.3.4) and the "Somatization" subscale of the "Brief Symptom Inventory" (BSI; Franke, 2000). The latter is an instrument for measuring general psychopathology and is an abbreviated form of the "Symptom Checklist" (SCL-90-R; Derogatis, 1983) described in ► Sect. 1.3.4. The SOMS-7 T initially demonstrated a highly significant decrease in the number of persistent somatic symptoms between pre-measurement (M = 7.80; SD = 7.54) and post-measurement (M = 3.95; SD = 5.50), $F(1.19) = 16.44$, $p = 0.001$. There was a mean effect size $d = 0.58$ (95% CI: −0.06; 1.23). On the intensity index of the SOMS-7 T, there was also a highly significant reduction in symptom intensity, $F(1.19) = 25.54$, $p < 0.001$, and a medium effect size (◘ Fig. 14.1). A statistically significant reduction in somatic symptoms between begin of therapy initiation (M = 0.77; SD = 0.61) and end of treatment (M = 0.36; SD = 0.42) was also confirmed for the BSI subscale, $F(1.21) = 19.71$, $p < 0.001$, yielding an effect size in the medium to large range: $d = 0.78$ (95% CI: 0.15; 1.42).

◘ Fig. 14.1 The change in symptom intensity score of the Screening for Somatoform Disorders (intensity index of the SOMS-7 T) between the beginning and the end of therapy

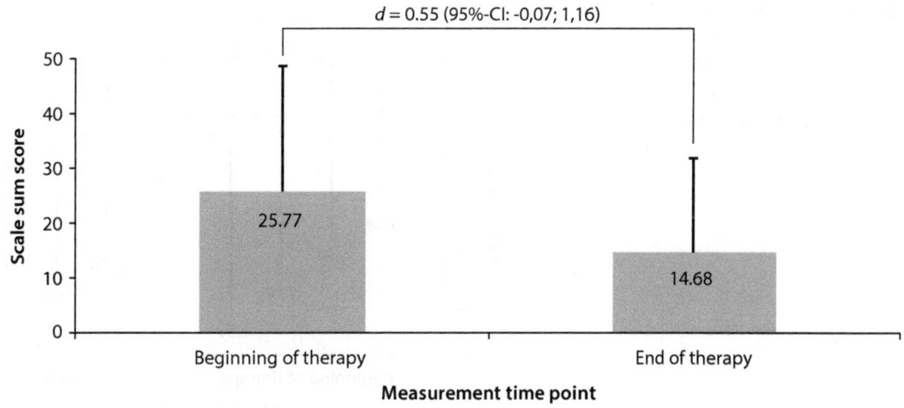

◘ Fig. 14.2 The change in total scores on the subscales of the Illness Attitude Scales (IAS) between the beginning and the end of treatment

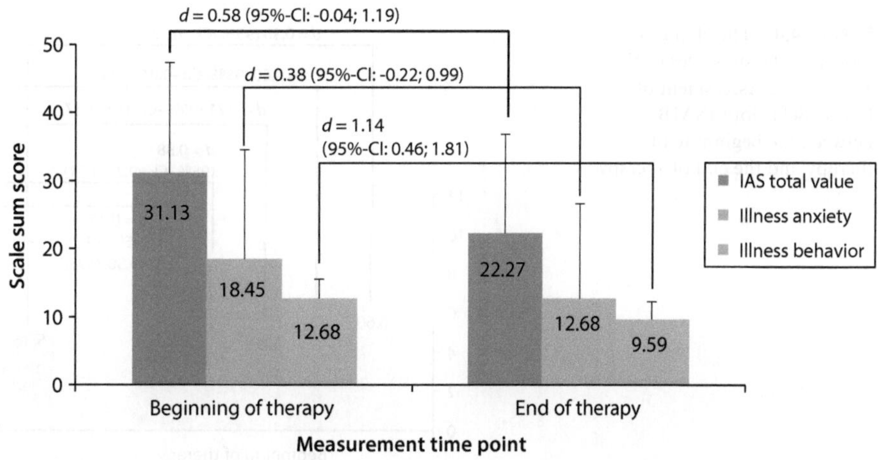

14.2.2 Somatic Symptoms-Related Outcomes

In addition to the main symptomatology—the persistent somatic symptoms—the therapy also aims primarily at changing psychopathological processes related to the somatic symptoms, such as dysfunctional cognitions and behaviors. In the context of the present therapy evaluation, the "Illness Attitude Scales" (IAS; Hiller & Rief, 2004), the "Cognitions About Body and Health Questionnaire" (FKG; Hiller et al., 1997), and the "Scale for the Assessment of Illness Behavior" (SAIB; Rief et al., 2003) were used to measure corresponding outcomes. The three instruments are described in ► Sect. 1.3.4.

▪ Illness Anxiety

Significant improvements were found with regard to the IAS subscale "illness anxiety", $F(1.21) = 6.43$, $p = 0.019$, as well as "illness behavior", $F(1.21) = 19.38$, $p < 0.001$. Total score also reduced significantly between pre- and post-measurement, $F(1.21) = 12.29$, $p = 0.002$. Effect sizes ranged from small to large values (◘ Fig. 14.2).

▪ Body-Related Dysfunctional Cognitions

Except for the subscale "Physical Weakness", $F(1.21) = 5.37$, $p = 0.031$, there are no significant improvements with the FKG. For the subscales "Catastrophizing interpretation of bodily complaints", $F(1.21) = 2.66$, $p = 0.119$, "Intolerance of physical discomfort", $F(1.21) = 2.35$, $p = 0.141$, and "Autonomic sensations", $F(1.21) = 0.07$, $p = 0.800$, no statistically significant changes were demonstrated. The effect sizes for these subscales are in the small and medium range (◘ Fig. 14.3).

▪ Illness Behavior

With the SAIB, significant improvement was also found only for one subscale—"Scanning", $F(1.20) = 12.68$, $p = 0.002$. With regard to the subscales "Diagnosis verification", $F(1.20) = 4.19$, $p = 0.055$, "Expression of symptoms", $F(1.20) = 2.11$, $p = 0.163$, "Medication", $F(1.20) = 2.67$, $p = 0.119$, and "Illness consequences", $F(1.20) = 4.27$, $p = 0.053$, there were no statistically significant changes. The effect sizes for the subscales of the SAIB ranged from small to medium (◘ Fig. 14.4).

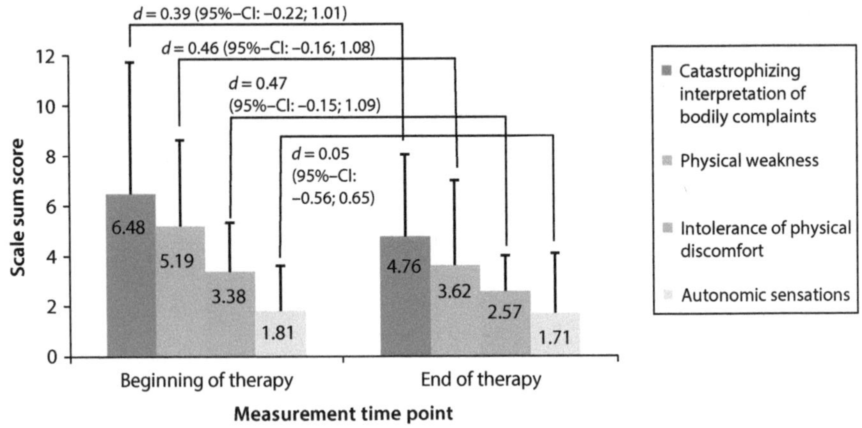

Fig. 14.3 The change in total scores on the subscales of the Cognitions About Body and Health Questionnaire (FKG) between the beginning of therapy and the end of therapy

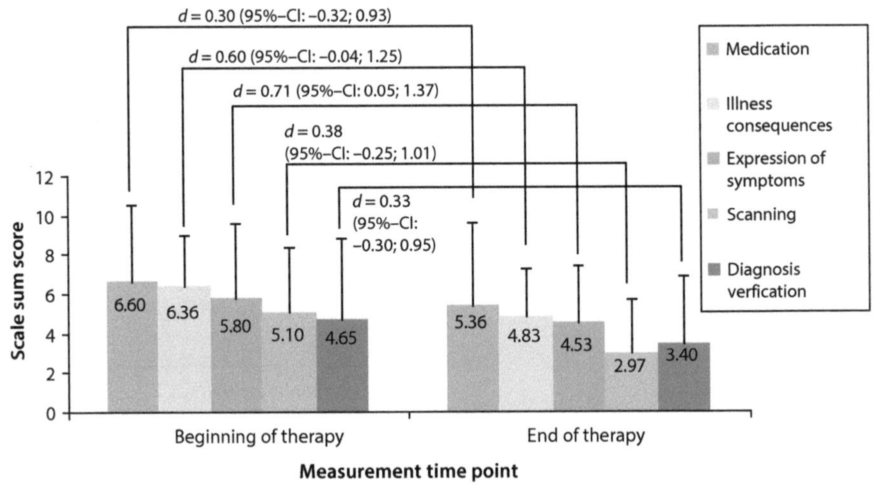

Fig. 14.4 The change in total scores on the subscales of the Scale of the Assessment of Illness Behaviour (SAIB) between the beginning of therapy and the end of therapy

14

The results of the different measurement instruments show that disorder-specific cognitive and behavioral processes could only be improved to a small extent during the course of therapy.

14.2.3 Depressive Symptoms, Anxiety, and General Psychopathology

The severity of depressives symptoms was measured using the "Beck Depression Inventory" (BDI; Hautzinger et al., 1994). This showed a highly significant decrease in depressive symptoms between pre- and post-measurement, $F(1.21) = 19.79$, $p = <0.001$, and a mean effect size of $d = 0.74$ (95% CI: 0.11; 1.37). As Fig. 14.5 illustrates, the anxiety subscale of the Brief Symptom Inventory (BSI) also showed a highly significant symptom reduction, $F(1.21) = 11.22$; $p = 0.003$. The effect size is in the high range. The BSI also allows the calculation of an overall index based on all subscales—the so-called Global Severity Index (GSI)—which permits statements about the general psychopathology (Fig. 14.5). This general index also showed a highly significant change between pre- and post-measurement, $F(1.21) = 10.49$; $p = 0.004$, with a medium effect size.

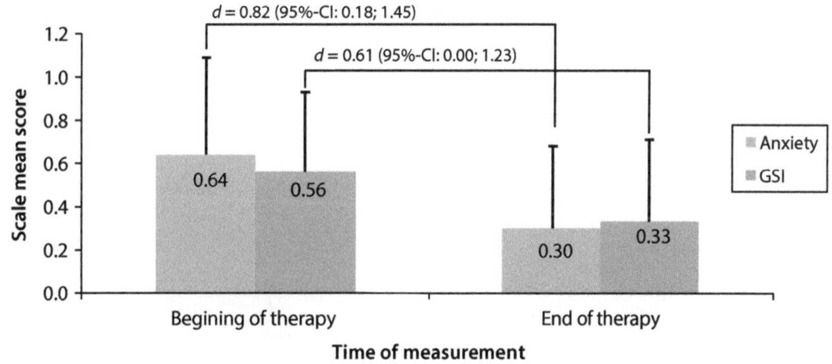

Fig. 14.5 The change of the total score on the Anxiety subscale and the Global Severity Index (GSI) of the Brief Symptom Inventory (BSI) between the beginning of therapy and the end of therapy

14.2.4 Impairment in the General Level of Functioning

As already known, patients with persistent somatic symptoms usually also experience considerable limitations in their ability to function. These were measured in the present therapy evaluation with the aid of the "Pain Disability Index" (PDI; Dillmann et al., 1994). A significant reduction in functional limitations between pre-measurement ($M = 3.50$; $SD = 1.52$) and post-measurement ($M = 1.45$; $SD = 1.21$) could be determined, $F(1.16) = 26.68$, $p < 0.001$. The effect size is in a very high range: $d = 1.49$ (95%-CI: 0.65; 2.33).

14.3 Patient Satisfaction

After completion of the therapy, the patients were asked about their personal opinion on the improvement of their condition as well as their satisfaction with the therapy. Unfortunately, the response rate to the survey was only 68%. The most important results are briefly presented below.

After completion of therapy, patients were first asked to rate their current situation at the end of treatment on a 5-point scale (0 = very bad; 4 = very good). ◘ Figure 14.6 shows that 60% of the patients rated their situation after the end of therapy as "very good" or "quite good".

Furthermore, the patients were asked after the end of treatment to what extent their "main problem", for which they had sought therapy, had improved. The assessment was made on a 5-point scale (1 = significantly improved, 5 = significantly worsened). ◘ Figure 14.7 shows that 80% of the patients stated that their main problem had improved significantly or somewhat. In addition, patients were asked whether they believed that they would be able to cope better with psychological difficulties and problems in the future as a result of therapy. ◘ Figure 14.8 shows that 80% of respondents rated this question as "very likely" or "somewhat likely".

Finally, the patients were asked how satisfied they had been overall with the therapy. Ratings were found exclusively on the two highest scales: 73% of the respondents stated that they were "completely satisfied" and 27% "very satisfied" with the therapy. Overall, however, it must be emphasized once again that the data on therapy satisfaction must be interpreted with caution due to the low response rate.

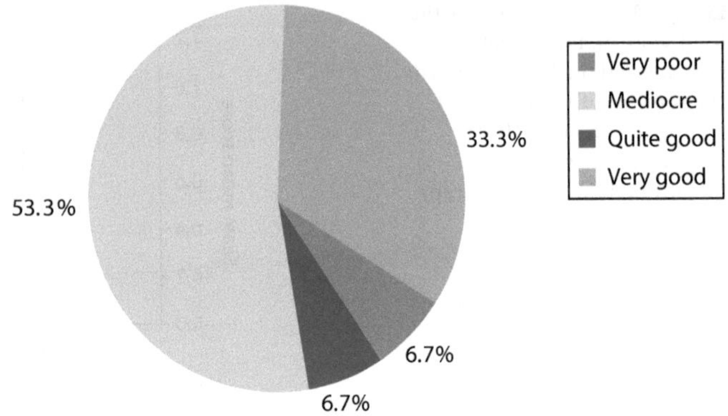

Fig. 14.6 Patients' evaluation of their health and symptom status after completing therapy

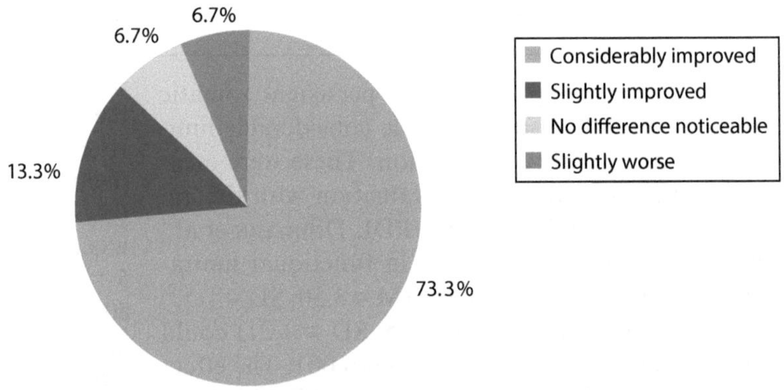

Fig. 14.7 Patients' evaluation of the improvement of their main problem after completing therapy

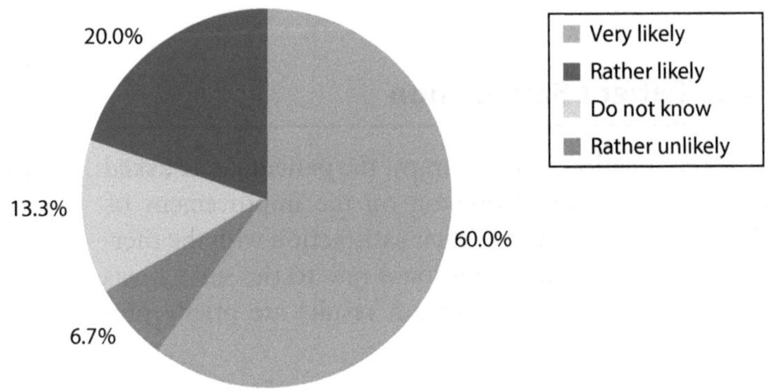

Fig. 14.8 Patients' evaluation of their change in dealing with future psychological problems after completing therapy

References

Derogatis, L. R. (1983). *The SCL-90-R manual. Scoring and adminstration procedures for SCL-90-R*. John Hopkins University School of Medicine.

Dillmann, U., Nilges, P., Saile, H., & Gerbershagen, H. U. (1994). Behinderungseinschatzung bei chronischen Schmerzpatienten. *Schmerz, 8*(2), 100–110. https://doi.org/10.1007/BF02530415

Franke, G. H. (2000). *Brief Symptom Inventory von L.R. Derogatis (Kurzform der SCL-90-R). Deutsche Version*. Beltz.

Hautzinger, M., Bailer, M., Worall, H., & Keller, F. (1994). *Beck-depressions-Inventar (BDI)*. Huber.

Hiller, W., & Rief, W. (2004). *Internationale Skalen für Hypochondrie. Deutschsprachige Adaptation des Whiteley-Index (WI) und der Illness Attitude Scales (IAS) (Manual)*. Huber.

Hiller, W., Rief, W., Elefant, S., Margraf, J., Kroymann, R., Leibbrand, R., et al. (1997). Dysfunktionale Kognitionen bei Patienten mit Somatisierungssyndrom. *Zeitschrift für Klinische Psychologie – Forschung und Praxis, 26*(3), 226–234.

Rief, W., & Hiller, W. (2008). *SOMS – Das Screening für Somatoforme Störungen. Manual zum Fragebogen* (4. Aufl.). Huber.

Rief, W., Ihle, D., & Pilger, F. (2003). A new approach to assess illness behaviour. *Journal of Psychosomatic Research, 54*(5), 405–414. https://doi.org/10.1016/S0022-3999(02)00401-4

FSC
www.fsc.org
MIX
Papier aus verantwortungsvollen Quellen
Paper from responsible sources
FSC® C105338

If you have any concerns about our products,
you can contact us on
ProductSafety@springernature.com

In case Publisher is established outside the EU,
the EU authorized representative is:
Springer Nature Customer Service Center GmbH
Europaplatz 3, 69115 Heidelberg, Germany

Printed by Libri Plureos GmbH
in Hamburg, Germany